Errors in Radiology

Luigia Romano • Antonio Pinto
Editors

Errors in Radiology

Springer

Editors
Luigia Romano
Department of Diagnostic
Radiological Imaging
"A. Cardarelli" Hospital
Naples, Italy

Antonio Pinto
Department of Diagnostic
Radiological Imaging
"A. Cardarelli" Hospital
Naples, Italy

ISBN 978-88-470-2338-3 ISBN 978-88-470-2339-0 (eBook)

DOI 10.1007/978-88-470-2339-0

Springer Milan Dordrecht Heidelberg London New York

Library of Congress Control Number: 2012936593

5 4 3 2 1 2012 2013 2014 2015

Cover design: Ikona S.r.l., Milan, Italy
Typesetting: Graphostudio, Milan, Italy

Springer-Verlag Italia S.r.l. – Via Decembrio 28 – I-20137 Milan
Springer is a part of Springer Science+Business Media (www.springer.com)

Preface

Errors in medicine have become headline news in recent years, and legal action against physicians for alleged malpractice is an increasing problem in all industrialized countries and in all specialties. Radiology has not been immune to these events. Moreover, many of its unique aspects make radiologists particularly vulnerable, due to the inherent characteristics of the discipline and its latest developments, which together call for careful assessment of the images produced by increasingly sophisticated imaging modalities.

Mistakes are unavoidable. As health-care professionals, we must admit that they can happen, but, once discovered, make sure they are not repeated. The study of errors provides the necessary foundation for radiologists to apply professional standards and exercise personal ability, as well as responsibility, to improve the quality of their own work and that of their department.

Diagnostic errors fall into recurrent patterns. Error traps need to be uncovered and highlighted in order to prevent repetition of the same mistakes.

The purpose of this book is to discuss and illustrate many of the errors occurring in radiology practice. The 28 chapters cover a large spectrum of diagnostic errors and present a wide series of cases related to diagnostic errors involving plain film, ultrasonography, computed tomography, magnetic resonance, and angiography studies. In addition, medico-legal issues related to Interventional Radiology, radiology reporting, child abuse, foreign bodies, body-packing, and contrast medium administration are addressed.

A culture of safety must be developed within radiology departments such that whenever we come across an error made by a colleague, we bring that error to his or her attention in a sensitive and constructive manner. At the same time, it is essential that radiologists and radiology departments continue to improve the process of recording and addressing errors.

The expertise, breadth of knowledge, and thoroughness conveyed by the authors of this volume provide a valuable source of information on the spectrum of potential errors in radiology. We hope that this book will allow radiologists to reduce the rate of errors in their work and to improve the quality of their departments.

April 2012

Luigia Romano
Antonio Pinto

Contents

Contributors

Ciro Acampora, Department of Diagnostic Radiological Imaging, "A. Cardarelli" Hospital, Naples, Italy

Manal Azzouz, Department of Diagnostic Radiology, Copenhagen University Hospital, Herlev, Denmark

Domenico Barbuti, Department of Radiology, "Bambin Gesù" Children's Hospital, Rome, Italy

Antonio Barile, Department of Radiology, "San Salvatore" Hospital, University of L'Aquila, L'Aquila, Italy

Emilio Bassi, Institute of Radiology, Foundation IRCCS "San Matteo" University Hospital, Pavia, Italy

Franco Bocchini, Department of Diagnostic Imaging, "Pineta Grande" Medical Center, Castelvolturno (CE), Italy

Adriana Bonifacino, Breast Unit, "Sant'Andrea" Hospital, Sapienza University of Rome, Rome, Italy

Luca Brunese, Department of Health Science, Chair of Radiology, University of Molise, Campobasso, Italy

Vitaliano Buffa, Department of Cardiovascular Radiology, "San Camillo-Forlanini" Hospital, Rome, Italy

Elisa Buzzi Rizzi, Department of Radiology, National Institute for Infectious Diseases IRCSS "L. Spallanzani", Rome, Italy

Corrado Caiazzo, Breast Screening Unit "Corso Vittorio Emanuele", ASL Napoli 1 Centro, Naples, Italy

Stefano Canestrini, Department of Radiology, "G.B. Rossi" University Hospital, Verona, Italy

Ferdinando Caranci, Department of Diagnostic Imaging and Radiotherapy, Neuroradiology Unit, "Federico II" University, Naples, Italy

Onofrio Catalano, Department of Radiology, Massachussetts General Hospital, Harvard Medical School, Boston, MA, USA

Carlo Cavaliere, Department of Diagnostic Radiological Imaging, MR Body Unit, "A. Cardarelli" Hospital, Naples, Italy

Roberta Cianci, Department of Neurosciences and Imaging, Section of Radiological Imaging, "G. d'Annunzio" University, Chieti, Italy

Teresa Cinque, Department of Diagnostic Radiological Imaging, "A. Cardarelli" Hospital, Naples, Italy

Marco Cirillo, Department of Radiology, "Bambin Gesù" Children's Hospital, Rome, Italy

Armando Conchiglia, Department of Radiology, "San Salvatore" Hospital, University of L'Aquila, L'Aquila, Italy

Laura Conti, Department of Radiology, "San Salvatore" Hospital, University of L'Aquila, L'Aquila, Italy

Antonio R. Cotroneo, Department of Neurosciences and Imaging, Section of Radiological Imaging, "G. d'Annunzio" University, Chieti, Italy

Roberta Cotti, Radiology Unit, "Regina Margherita" Children's Hospital, Turin, Italy

Massimo Cristofaro, Department of Radiology, National Institute for Infectious Diseases IRCSS "L. Spallanzani", Rome, Italy

Federico D'Orazio, Department of Radiology, "San Salvatore" Hospital, University of L'Aquila, L'Aquila, Italy

Stefania Daniele, Department of Diagnostic Radiological Imaging, "A. Cardarelli" Hospital, Naples, Italy

Carlo Nicola De Cecco, Department of Radiological, Oncological and Pathological Sciences, Sapienza University of Rome – Polo Pontino, Latina, Italy

Giuseppe De Magistris, Department of Diagnostic Radiological Imaging, Vascular and Interventional Radiology Unit, "A. Cardarelli" Hospital, Naples, Italy

Rosaria De Ritis, Department of Diagnostic Radiological Imaging, MR Body Unit, "A. Cardarelli" Hospital, Naples, Italy

Claudio Defilippi, Radiology Unit, "Regina Margherita" Children's Hospital, Turin, Italy

Giovanni Di Leo, Department of Medical and Surgical Sciences, University of Milan; Radiology Unit, "San Donato" Hospital IRCCS, San Donato Milanese (MI), Italy

Roberto Dore, Institute of Radiology, Foundation IRCCS "San Matteo" University Hospital, Pavia, Italy

Roberto Farina, Department of Diagnostic Radiological Imaging, "A. Cardarelli" Hospital, Naples, Italy

Antonella Filippone, Department of Neurosciences and Imaging, Section of Radiological Imaging, "G. d'Annunzio" University, Chieti, Italy

Anna Frezza, Surgery Unit, "Villa delle Querce" Clinic, Naples, Italy

Nicola Gagliardi, Department of Diagnostic Radiological Imaging, "A. Cardarelli" Hospital, Naples, Italy

Michele Galluzzo, Department of Emergency Radiology, "San Camillo" Hospital, Rome, Italy

Gianluigi Guarnieri, Department of Diagnostic Radiological Imaging, Neuroradiology Service, "A. Cardarelli" Hospital, Naples, Italy

Franco Guida, Department of Diagnostic Imaging, "Pineta Grande" Medical Center, Castelvolturno (CE), Italy

Isabella Iadevito, Department of Diagnostic Radiological Imaging, MR Body Unit, "A. Cardarelli" Hospital, Naples, Italy

Roberto Izzo, Department of Diagnostic Radiological Imaging, Neuroradiology Service, "A. Cardarelli" Hospital, Naples, Italy

Giuseppe Lanni, Department of Radiology, "San Salvatore" Hospital, University of L'Aquila, L'Aquila, Italy

Franco Maglione, Department of Diagnostic Radiological Imaging, Vascular and Interventional Radiology Unit, "A. Cardarelli" Hospital, Naples, Italy

Fabio Martino, Department of Radiology, ASL BARI, Mola di Bari (BA), Italy

Gianluigi Martino, Faculty of Medicine, University of Bari, Bari, Italy

Carlo Masciocchi, Department of Radiology, "San Salvatore" Hospital, University of L'Aquila, L'Aquila, Italy

Vittorio Miele, Department of Emergency Radiology, "San Camillo" Hospital, Rome, Italy

Mario Muto, Department of Diagnostic Radiological Imaging, Neuroradiology Service, "A. Cardarelli" Hospital", Naples, Italy

Carlo Muzj, Department of Diagnostic Radiological Imaging, "A. Cardarelli" Hospital, Naples, Italy

Yousef W. Nielsen, Department of Diagnostic Radiology, Copenhagen University Hospital, Herlev, Denmark

Raffaella Niola, Department of Diagnostic Radiological Imaging, Vascular and Interventional Radiology Unit, "A. Cardarelli" Hospital, Naples, Italy

Pasquale Paolantonio, Department of Radiology, "San Giovanni – Addolorata" Hospital, Rome, Italy

Nicoletta Pignatelli di Spinazzola, Department of Diagnostic Radiological Imaging, "A. Cardarelli" Hospital, Naples, Italy

Antonio Pinto, Department of Diagnostic Radiological Imaging, "A. Cardarelli" Hospital, Naples, Italy

Fabio Pinto, Department of Diagnostic Radiological Imaging, "A. Cardarelli" Hospital, Naples, Italy

Gianluca Ponticiello, Department of Diagnostic Radiological Imaging, "A. Cardarelli" Hospital, Naples, Italy

Roberto Pozzi Mucelli, Department of Radiology, "G.B. Rossi" University Hospital, Verona, Italy

Alfonso Ragozzino, Department of Radiology, "Santa Maria delle Grazie" Hospital – ASL Napoli 2 Nord, Pozzuoli (NA), Italy

Alfonso Reginelli, Department of Internal and Experimental Medicine " Magrassi-Lanzara", Section of Radiology, Second University of Naples, Naples, Italy

Luigia Romano, Department of Diagnostic Radiological Imaging, "A. Cardarelli" Hospital, Naples, Italy

Stefania Romano, Department of Diagnostic Radiological Imaging, "A. Cardarelli" Hospital, Naples, Italy

Giovanna Russo, Department of Diagnostic Radiological Imaging, "A. Cardarelli" Hospital, Naples, Italy

Francesco Sardanelli, Department of Medical and Surgical Sciences, University of Milan; Radiology Unit, "San Donato" Hospital IRCCS, San Donato Milanese (MI), Italy

Mariano Scaglione, Department of Diagnostic Imaging, "Pineta Grande" Medical Center, Castelvolturno (CE), Italy

Stefano Schininà, Department of Radiology, National Institute for Infectious Diseases IRCSS "L. Spallanzani", Rome, Italy

Maria Giuseppina Scuderi, Department of Diagnostic Radiological Imaging, "A. Cardarelli" Hospital, Naples, Italy

Giacomo Sica, Department of Diagnostic Imaging, "Pineta Grande" Medical Center, Castelvolturno (CE), Italy

Amelia Sparano, Department of Diagnostic Radiological Imaging, "A. Cardarelli" Hospital, Naples, Italy

Ciro Stavolo, Department of Diagnostic Radiological Imaging, "A. Cardarelli" Hospital, Naples, Italy

Henrich S. Thomsen, Department of Diagnostic Sciences, Faculty of Health Sciences, University of Copenhagen, Copenhagen, Denmark

Margherita Trinci, Department of Emergency Radiology, "San Camillo" Hospital, Rome, Italy

Adele Valentini, Institute of Radiology, Foundation IRCCS "San Matteo" University Hospital, Pavia, Italy

Errors in Radiology: Definition and Classification

1

Antonio Pinto, Maria Giuseppina Scuderi, and Stefania Daniele

1.1 Introduction

As indicated by the title of the landmark report of the Institute of Medicine, "To Err is Human" mistakes are part of the human condition [1]. They cannot be prevented by trying harder. At best, systematic changes are needed to prevent physician's from doing the wrong thing while making it more likely that they will do the right thing. This is accomplished by hardwiring functions into medical systems and providing information at the point of care [2].

There are four health-care-related factors contributing to medical errors that can lead to patient harm: (1) human fallibility, (2) complexity, (3) system deficiencies, and (4) a vulnerability of defensive barriers. All of these must be addressed to significantly improve patient safety [3].

Errors in medicine have become headline news in recent years, and legal action against physicians for alleged malpractice is an increasing problem in all industrialized countries and in all specialties.

Radiology is not immune to this phenomenon and presents a number of unique features linked to both the inherent characteristics of the discipline and its latest developments, which call for careful assessment [4].

Diagnostic radiology must aim for the complete detection of all abnormalities in an imaging examination and their accurate diagnosis [3].

It offers a presumptive rather than a histological or microbiological diagnosis and diverges from the normal path of other medical specialties, in that it depends entirely on visual perception and on the identification of specific characteristics on a radiograph. Mechanical, physiologic, and psychological factors contribute to an intricate diagnostic interplay that has yet to be fully

A. Pinto (✉)
Department of Diagnostic Radiological Imaging, "A. Cardarelli" Hospital, Naples, Italy

appreciated [5]. Yet, it is clear that the technician and radiologist can perform their jobs in a more efficient and focused manner if physicians have provided adequate clinical information to the radiology department [5].

Diagnostic error in radiology is an important topic, with both medico-legal and quality control implications. To improve diagnostic accuracy, it is imperative to understand the nature and source of diagnostic errors. Traditionally, the study of radiological errors was limited to errors in radiologists' reports, often out of context of the whole diagnostic episode and omitting the integral role of referring physicians. Radiological investigation begins at the point of clinical suspicion of a condition, and ends with the receipt of the radiologist's opinion by the treating team. Radiologists become personally involved only after a request has been initiated and the desired images acquired, but these two stages also generate diagnostic errors that affect the episode's outcome.

Radiological problems that have led to medical malpractice lawsuits most frequently have been due to "failure to diagnose." The three main categories of claims are misdiagnoses, complications, and miscellaneous [6, 7]. Diagnostic errors often go unrecognized or unreported and may be associated with high patient morbidity. But malpractice lawsuits have adverse effects on a physician's health because physicians who have committed a severe error can experience an abrupt change in the quality of life and an increased frequency of burnout [8].

1.2 Definition of Error

The issue of patient safety plays a prominent role in health-care. Its prominence is fueled by an expanding body of literature that shows a high incidence of error in medicine [9-11] coupled with well-publicized medical error cases that have raised public concern about the safety of modern health-care delivery. Historically, patient safety researchers investigating the impact of medical error have adopted outcome-dependent definitions and surrogate terms, while limiting their focus to patients experiencing adverse outcomes or injury as a consequence of medical care [1-3]. Perhaps this tendency stems from the guiding principle of medical practice, credited to Hippocrates, *prium no nocere* ("First, do no harm") [12]. Moreover, the manner in which patient safety has been defined promotes an outcome-dependent approach to defining medical error.

In the 1990s, the publication of the three most extensive investigations on medical error – the Harvard Medical Practice Study [9, 10], the Quality in Australian Health Study [11, 13], and the Utah and Colorado Medical Practice Study [14] – gave prominence to the term "adverse event" defined as an unintended injury to patients caused by medical management (rather than the underlying condition of the patient) that results in measurable disability, prolonged hospitalization or both [9, 10, 14]. Alternatively, an adverse event can be considered as an unintended injury or complication that results in disability, death, or prolonged hospital stay and is caused (including acts of omission and acts of commission) by health-care management rather than the patient's disease [11].

Definitions of medical error in the published literature include:

- The failure of a planned action to be completed as intended (an error of execution), or use of the wrong plan to achieve an aim (an error of planning) [15];
- An unintended act (either of omission or commission) or one that does not achieve its intended outcome [16];
- Deviations from the process of care, which may or may not cause harm to the patient [17].

But what is an error in radiology? An error is a deviation from the expected norm, regardless of whether it results in any harm. Errors may be categorized in a variety of ways and we have methods in place to facilitate their identification so that steps can be introduced to minimize their occurrence. In addition, medical errors can be further classified in terms of the outcome or harm suffered by the patient, if any, allowing assessment of the episode and the proper assignment of accountability [18].

In broad terms, factors contributing to errors are categorized as being system-related (latent errors) or person-related (active errors). The latter are human cognitive errors and are thus more likely to be preventable but also more likely to have an adverse outcome than technical errors. As applied to diagnostic radiology, three main categories of error are responsible for the majority of "missed" or misinterpreted observations on radiological examinations: technical (latent or system-related), active (errors in perception, knowledge, and/or judgment), or a combination thereof [18].

1.3 Classification of Errors in Radiology

In order for a radiologist or any other physician to be found liable for medical malpractice, four elements must be established. There must be a radiologist–patient relationship, the radiologist must have committed a negligent act (a breach of the standard of care), the negligent act must have caused injury to the plaintiff–patient (proximate cause), and the patient must have sustained an injury [19]. In general, there are four main reasons why radiologists are sued: (1) observer errors, (2) errors in interpretation, (3) failure to suggest the next appropriate procedure, and (4) failure to communicate in a timely and clinically appropriate manner [5].

1.3.1 Observer Errors

Kundel et al. [20] described the following types of observer error: scanning error, recognition error and decision-making error. The first results from failure of the radiologist to fixate on the area of the lesion.

Recognition error involves fixating on the territory of the lesion yet failing to detect the lesion, while decision-making error is the incorrect interpretation of a malignant lesion as a normal structure.

Another form of observer error that may contribute to lesions being overlooked is satisfaction of search (SOS) error [21]. An SOS error is the result of the radiologist's attention being diverted from a tumor by an eye-catching but unrelated finding. Another issue that may affect observer performance is intentional under-reading, that is, a conscious tendency to interpret equivocal radiographic shadows as negative [22]. This may occur because of collegial pressure to reduce the number of false-positive interpretations, and thereby decrease unnecessary work-ups.

Failures of abnormality detection in film reading (i.e. perceptual errors) are subject to psychophysiological factors of human visual perception [23]. They are common to visual perceptual tasks in general and are relevant to other professions (e.g. air traffic controllers, professional drivers) in which active observation is a key part of professional activity. Perceptual errors, in general, are likewise related to multiple psychophysiological factors, including level of observer alertness, observer fatigue, duration of the observation task, any distracting factors, and conspicuity of the abnormality, among many others [24]. An additional source of perceptual error results from the influence a radiology report has over another radiologist: this error occurs because the radiologist reads the first report before looking at the films [25, 26].

1.3.2 Errors in Interpretation

An error of interpretation, as its name implies, occurs at the interpretation phase of film reading and usually comprises an incorrect diagnosis given to an abnormal finding (or, rarely, to a normal finding). There are many reasons why radiologists make errors in identifying and interpreting abnormalities.

Poor ergonomics and ambient light, frequent telephone disturbances, working with an inexperienced resident, clinical history and other factors are various sources of error.

Errors of interpretation in diagnostic radiology are analogous to errors of interpretation in other branches of medicine. The closest similarity is to physical diagnosis, in which signs may be misinterpreted, an organ position is unrecognized, heart sounds are mistaken for one another, and so on. The principles of whether an error of interpretation can be considered negligence are the same in diagnostic radiology as in other branches of medicine. It is very important that errors of interpretation are judged against the standard of an average competent medical practitioner rather than against the unachievable standard of perfection.

1.3.3 Failure To Suggest the Next Appropriate Procedure

Most ordering physicians actually know the next appropriate procedure to suggest when an abnormality is found on the imaging study they originally ordered. However, if the patient becomes a plaintiff in a lawsuit against the ordering physician, the radiologist can almost be assured that the ordering physician will claim ignorance as to what to do next because no such order was specified by the radiologist. Radiologists must ensure that their recommendations or suggestions for any additional radiological procedures are appropriate and will add meaningful information to clarify, confirm, or rule out the initial impression [27, 28].

1.3.4 Failure To Communicate in a Timely and Clinically Appropriate Manner

In addition to rendering an official interpretation (a final written report), the radiologist is responsible for communicating these findings directly to the referring physician [29]. A radiologist who interprets an imaging examination and writes a report of the results controls what happens to them next. The radiologist is at that moment the only person with knowledge of those findings and how those findings might affect the patient. Documentation should include the date, time, name of the person spoken to, and what was discussed [5]. Moreover, the communication of unexpected findings directly affects the ability of radiologists to deliver quality patient care. These are findings that may seriously affect a patient's health but do not require immediate or urgent intervention. The ACR's Practice Guideline recommends communicating such findings "in a manner that reasonably insures receipt of the findings" [27]. However, an unexpected finding becomes significant when there is a failure to communicate that results in additional patient injury or death.

1.4 Conclusions

An error is a deviation from the expected norm, regardless of whether it results in any harm. It is frequently merely a symptom of a flawed underlying process that can be remedied. The consequences of radiological errors can impact the patient and his or her immediate circle, as well as members of the imaging staff directly involved in the case and those of the medical team. There are also more global consequences of error that may negatively affect the practice, the institution, the profession, the procedure, or even the imaging study.

To reduce the incidence of errors, health-care providers must identify their causes, devise solutions and measure the success of improvement efforts. Moreover, accurate measurements of the incidence of error, based on clear and consistent definitions, are essential prerequisites for effective action.

Unfortunately and understandably, what is considered a medical error is influenced by differing contexts and purposes, such as research, quality control, ethics, insurance, legislation, legal action, and statutory regulation.

References

1. Kohn LT, Corrigan JM, Donaldson MS (editors) (1999) To err is human: building a safer health-system. National Academy Press, Washington, DC
2. Reason J (1997) Managing the risks of organizational accidents. Ashgate Publishing Limited, London
3. Gluck PA (2007) Patient safety in women's health care: a framework for progress. Best Pract Res Clin Obstet Gynaecol 21:525-536
4. Fileni A, Magnavita N, Mirk P et al (2010) Radiologic malpractice litigation risk in Italy: an observational study over a 14-year period. AJR Am J Roentgenol 194:1040-1046
5. Pinto A, Brunese L (2010) Spectrum of diagnostic errors in radiology. World J Radiol 2:377-383
6. Berlin L (1986) Malpractice and radiologists, update 1986: an 11.5-year perspective. AJR Am J Roentgenol 147:1291-1298
7. Spring DB, Tennenhouse DJ (1986) Radiology malpractice lawsuits: California jury verdicts. Radiology 159:811-814
8. West CP, Huschka MM, Novotny PJ et al (2006) Association of perceived medical errors with resident distress and empathy: a prospective longitudinal study. JAMA 296:1071-1078
9. Brennan TA, Leape LL, Laird NM et al (1991) Incidence of adverse events and negligence in hospitalized patients: results of the Harvard Medical Practice Study I. N Engl J Med 324:370-376
10. Leape LL, Brennan TA, Laird N et al (1991) The nature of adverse events in hospitalized patients: results of the Harvard Medical Practice Study II. N Engl J Med 324:377-384
11. Wilson RM, Runciman WB, Gibberd RW et al (1995) The Quality in Australian Health Care Study. Med J Aust 163:458-471
12. Grober ED, Bohnen JMA (2005) Defining medical error. Can J Surg 48:39-44
13. Wilson RM, Harrison GB, Gibberd RW et al (1999) An analysis of the causes of adverse events from the Quality in Australian Health Care Study. Med J Aust 170:411-415
14. Thomas EJ, Studdert DM, Burstin HR et al (1999) Incidence and types of adverse events and negligent care in Utah and Colorado. Medical Care 38:261-271
15. Reason J (1990) Human error. Cambridge University Press, Cambridge
16. Leape L (1994) Error in medicine. JAMA 272:1851-1857
17. Reason JT (2001) Understanding adverse events: the human factor. In: Vincent C (editor). Clinical risk management: enhancing patient safety. BMJ Publishing Group, London pp 9-30
18. Siewert B, Sosna J, McNamara A et al (2008) Missed lesions at abdominal oncologic CT: lessons learned from quality assurance. RadioGraphics 28:623-638
19. Berlin L (2007) Radiologic errors and malpractice: a blurry distinction. AJR Am J Roentgenol 189:517522
20. Kundel HL, Nodine CF, Carmody D (1978) Visual scanning, pattern recognition and decision-making in pulmonary nodule detection. Invest Radiol 13:175-181
21. Samuel S, Kundel HL, Nodine CF et al (1995) Mechanism of satisfaction of search: eye position recordings in the reading of chest radiographs. Radiology 194:895-902
22. Woodring JH (1990) Pitfalls in the radiologic diagnosis of lung cancer. AJR Am J Roentgenol 154:1165-1175
23. Yerushalmy J (1969) The statistical assessment of the variability in observer perception and description of roentgenographic pulmonary shadows. Radiol Clin North Am 7:381-392

24. Pitman AG (2006) Perceptual error and the culture of open disclosure in Australian radiology. Australas Radiol 50:206-211
25. Berlin L (2000) Malpractice issues in radiology. Alliterative errors. AJR Am J Roentgenol 174:925-931
26. Pinto A, Acampora C, Pinto F et al (2011) Learning from diagnostic errors: a good way to improve education in radiology. Eur J Radiol 78:372-376
27. American College of Radiology (2005) ACR practice guideline for communication of diagnostic imaging findings. In: 2005 Practice guideline & technical standards. American College of Radiology, Reston, VA pp 5-9
28. Berlin L (2005) Errors of omission. AJR Am J Roentgenol 185:1416-1421
29. Harrigal CL, Erly WK (2007) On-call radiology: community standards and current trends. Semin Ultrasound CT MR 28:85-93

Malpractice Claims in Mammography

2

Adriana Bonifacino and Corrado Caiazzo

2.1 Introduction

Mammography is the standard of reference for the early detection of breast cancer.

Each year, radiologist reads millions of mammograms, whether as a part of a screening program (to detect an abnormality) or diagnostically (to evaluate the abnormality or a clinical problem). However, data from the Breast Cancer Detection Demonstration Project point out the limits of mammography. The false-negative rate is 8%–10% [1] and the rate of missed breast cancers is as high as 35%, according to retrospective evaluation versus blinded interpretations of mammograms [2].

Although there are differences in legal systems between Anglo-Saxon and Latin countries, in both mammography has become the most prevalent procedure involved in malpractice lawsuits filed against radiologists in the last 10 years. Indeed, among all physicians, errors in the diagnosis of breast cancer represent the most prevalent condition leading to medical malpractice lawsuits [3].

In a 14 year Italian observational study, Fileni found that the most common cause of error was failure to diagnose cancer (43.5%); the anatomic area most commonly involved by claims was the breast (60% of missed cancers in all body areas), and the number of claims filed for missed breast cancer has increased markedly. The value of the claims made to insurance companies for these cases is €93,294,509 ($132,414,303) [4].

According to the Physician Insurers Association of America, in 1995 and in 1997 radiologists were the specialists most frequently sued in malpractice lawsuits involving breast cancer [5].

C. Caiazzo (✉)
Breast Screening Unit "Corso Vittorio Emanuele", ASL Napoli 1 Centro,
Naples, Italy,

L. Romano, A. Pinto (eds.), *Errors in Radiology*, © Springer-Verlag Italia 2012

The most common lesion types reported in studies of missed breast cancers are mass or density in 19–64%, calcifications in 18–28%, mass with calcifications in 2%, and architectural distortion in 4–12% [6].

Possible causes for missed breast cancers include dense parenchyma obscuring a lesion, poor positioning or technique, perception error, incorrect interpretation of a suspect finding or subtle features of malignancy, and the slow growth of a lesion [7]. In this chapter, we discuss the most common reasons for a missed breast carcinoma, the differences in screening and diagnostic mammography, and the reasons underlying malpractice claims in mammography.

2.2 Role of the Patient

The most important reason for a missed breast cancer is *dense parenchyma.*

Unfortunately, however, a mammographic density is related to breast cancer, as women whose breasts are within the highest categories of mammographic density have a 4-to 6-fold higher risk than women whose breasts are within the lowest categories [8].

Breast parenchyma that is inherently dense compromises the radiologist's ability to detect a mass, especially a non-calcified, non-distorting lesion. The radiologist must be particularly attentive in searching for areas of architectural distortion; in some cases faint microcalcifications may be the only signs of malignancy in a dense breast.

In screening modalities it is not possible recall all patients with dense parenchyma but without a suspect sign. By contrast, in clinical modalities recall under these conditions is mandatory, as an integration study with ultrasound has a negative predictive value near 100% [9].

2.3 Role of the Technique

If radiologists read a mammogram in which the breast is in an incorrect *position*, a breast cancer may be missed.

Proper positioning and image contrast are absolutely necessary in all aspects of radiology, but especially in mammography. The technician must adhere to the positioning standards to maximize the amount of tissue included on the image.

Good *technique* requires that the technician also optimizes the image contrast, to avoid obtaining over- or underpenetrated images. This, in turn, requires proper positioning of the photocell to achieve an image with the correct optical density .

Careful attention to daily processor quality control is also integral to optimized contrast. While with the recent advent of digital mammography this point is of reduced importance, but it remains a critical consideration in most analogue-based devices. Here, we do not include a discussion of correct breast positioning or imaging technique, but we do emphasize that radiologists are responsible for the images even if it is the technician who obtains them [7].

2.4 Role of the Radiologist

2.4.1 Detection

An error may arise because, although the lesion is included in the field of view and is evident, it is not recognized by the radiologist.

This includes lesions with subtle features of malignancy that make them less visible.

The majority of missed lesions are small non-spiculated masses, areas of architectural distortion (Figs. 2.1a, b) and asymmetry, and small clusters of amorphous or faint microcalcifications (Fig. 2.2). If the radiologist "simply" does not read the lesion, it is considered a missed lesion and thus a detection error.

There are other cases of missed lesions, due to detection errors , such as the failure to diagnose multifocal and multicentric breast cancers. In fact, these types of cancer are likely to be missed in a "satisfaction of search" error, in which the radiologist, having detected a suspect lesion, then either stops reading or less carefully reads other parts of the breast image and that of the contralateral breast. However bilateral, multifocal and multicentric cancers have different outcomes and contraindications for breast-conserving therapy [10].

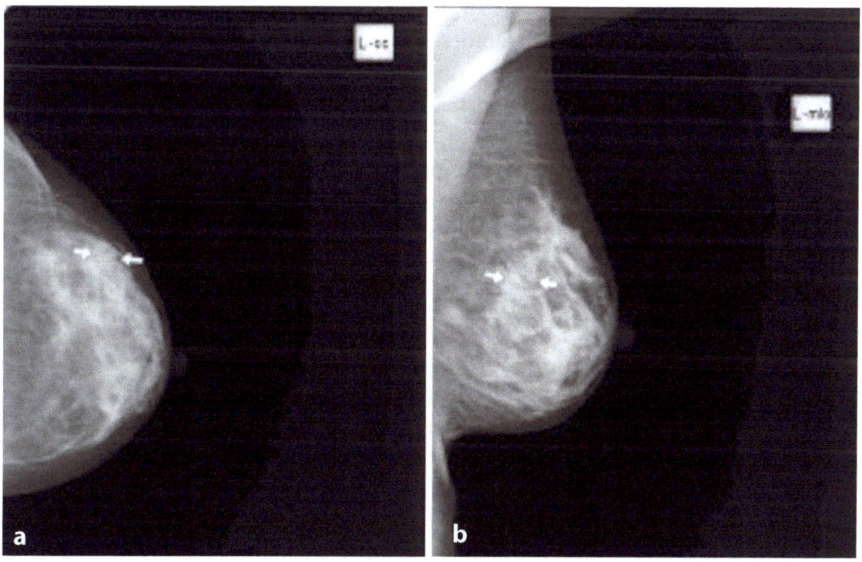

Fig. 2.1 a, b A palpable mass larger than 1 cm with hardly evident architectural distortion in the two projections (*arrows*). Final histological diagnosis: carcinoma

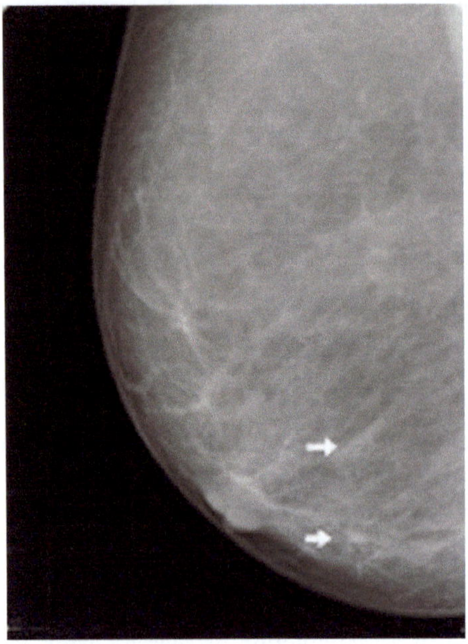

Fig. 2.2 Two clusters of faint microcalcifications (*arrows*). Final histological diagnosis of an in situ carcinoma

2.4.2 Incorrect Interpretation

The second major cause of missed breast cancers that is related to radiologist error is incorrect interpretation of a lesion. This occurs when an abnormality with suspect features is observed but is misinterpreted as being definitely or at least probably benign. Several factors may lead to misinterpretation, such as lack of experience, fatigue, or inattention on the part of the radiologist. Misinterpretation may also occur if the radiologist fails to obtain all the views needed to assess the characteristics of a lesion or if the lesion is slow growing and prior images are not used for comparison. The radiologist may erroneously judge the abnormality by its most benign features and miss important malignant clues indicating the need for biopsy. Characterization of a lesion that is identified at screening mammography should be based on diagnostic mammographic findings and not on screening findings alone [7]. It should be noted that a summary of several studies shows that 61% of non-palpable cancers are detected solely by recognition of either "subtle," "indirect," or "minimal" mammographic signs. These signs include areas of architectural distortion (54–59%), small groups of benign-appearing calcifications (34–48%), focal asymmetric densities(7–18%), and relatively well circumscribed masses (22%) [11-13], or a combination of findings (Figs. 2.3a, b) (2%) interpreted as benign [14]. While in isolation these findings have a low positive predictive value for malignancy, when considered together the risk of malignancy is higher [15]. A subtle or minimal sign of malignancy represents an important source of false-negative diagnoses, especially in screening programs, while in diagnostic

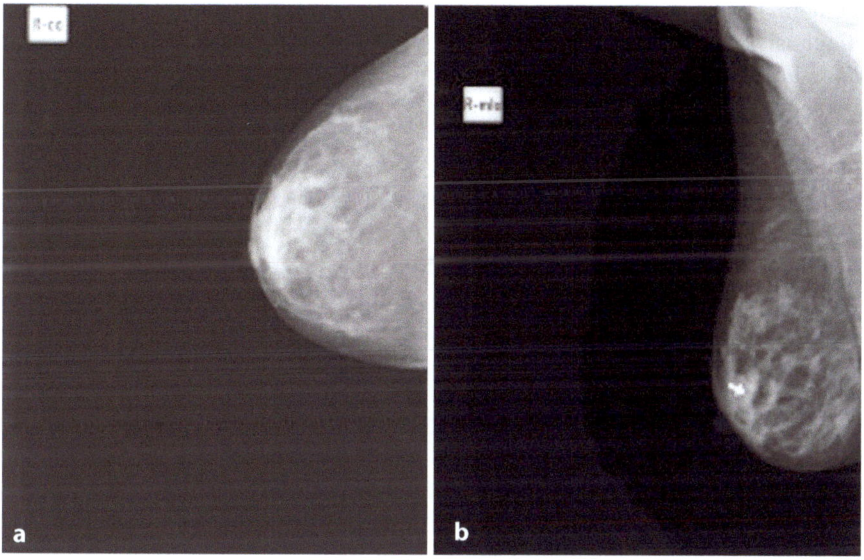

Fig. 2.3 a, b A well circumscribed mass with a recent appearance of a cluster of microcalcifications, as seen in the two projections (*arrows*). Final histological diagnosis: carcinoma

mammography the added use of ultrasound lowers this percentage [16]. On the other hand, non-specific findings occur frequently in mammographic screening programs and most of them do not represent cancer. According to Ikeda, despite non-specific findings (subtle or minimal signs) in previous screening mammograms, patient recall is not necessary, even if cancer later develops; nor does this necessarily represent error or a reduction in the standard of care [13]. Lev-Toaff observed that in slow-growing cancers malignant calcifications are frequently stable at mammography for as long as 63 months [17]. Caution should be used in evaluating stable masses (1–2 years) that suggest malignancy as they may represent slowly growing cancer, and small differences from older images are difficult to accurately evaluate.

2.4.3 Screening and Diagnostic Mammography

The factors influencing the performance of breast imagers are multiple and complex. A key determinant seems to be the training and experience of the interpreting radiologist, including years of mammographic experience, number of CME hours, and number of examinations interpreted. Specific training requirements have been established in the USA for the interpretation of mammograms while in Europe there are guidelines in screening mammography. In the USA, the Mammography Quality Standards Reauthorization Act of 1998 requires radiologists to interpret 960 mammograms per 2-year period and to accumulate 15 mammographic CME hours every 3 years. In Europe, the 2006 guidelines for satisfactory quality assurance in breast cancer screening and diagnosis require that a minimum of 5,000 screening cases be read per year and the completion of specific training in both diagnostic (symptomatic) mammography and screening mammography. If performance were only linked to the number of mammograms read, there should be huge differences between the number of malpractice claims in the USA and in Europe. But the results of an Italian study Fileni A et al. [18] are in line with those of an American survey [19], despite differences in the approach of the respective healthcare systems and in the litigation rates. Although reading a greater number of mammograms could be reasonably expected to improve performance in terms of a reduction in the number of errors and ultimately in malpractice claims, this assumption is strongly disputed in the literature. According to Beam et al., individual radiologists' current reading volume was not statistically significantly associated with accuracy in reading screening mammograms [20]. Barlowe et al. also found no evidence that greater volume or experience at interpreting mammograms is associated with better performance. The two measures of experience (years of practice and percentage of time spent on breast imaging) had different impacts on the threshold for recommending a biopsy. More years of interpreting mammography examinations was associated with a higher threshold, and more time spent in breast imaging with a lower threshold [21]. These studies have been countered by claims that accurate field screening is independent from radiologists' experience and/or performance but is instead mainly related to the number of mammograms that have been read.

Mammography facilities vary in their size, organization, services, and processes, but it is not known whether any of these differences affects the interpretive performance of diagnostic mammography. In diagnostic mammography it is particularly important to maximize sensitivity even at the expense of higher false-positive rates because the pretest probability of cancer is higher than in screening mammography. It may also be the case that radiologists in diagnostic facilities perceive a higher probability of cancer in general and are therefore more likely than other radiologists to make a positive interpretation. This is in part due to the tendency to practice defensive medicine [18], i.e., "ordering expensive tests and procedures that are not indicated medically but the absence of which may render physicians vulnerable in a malpractice lawsuit" [22]. A defensive medicine strategy is not possible in screening mammography, as a study by Jackson et al. quantitatively demonstrated that a defensive response to malpractice concerns should be associated with a lower overall accuracy of screening mammography due to the higher false-positive rate [23].

Radiologists' discomfort with clinical uncertainty is also associated with higher recall rates, lower specificity, and lower positive predictive value when interpreting diagnostic mammograms [24]. Although this leads to an increase in costs, it does not seem to have reduced the number of claims, which are relatively high in proportion to the radiologist's actual work volumes. This could indicate a greater tendency to litigate on the part of women who have chosen their specialist and paid for the service themselves [18]. Use of the BI-RADS(TM) reporting criteria rather than a positive/negative system or personal assessment increases the performance of screening and diagnostic mammography [21] and reduces the number of disputes. Radiologists' double reading in screening mammography also improves performance but whether the accuracy is the same as achieved with the introduction of CAD (computer-aided diagnosis) [25] plus a single reading is not yet known. We are not aware of reports on CAD being cited in malpractice claims. Since computers are perceived by most people to be infallible, their increasing use should reduce the number claims. On the other hand, it could also increase the number of claims if this available technology is not used.

2.5 Communication

"Errors" related to communication are probably most responsible for the dramatic increase in claims. Such errors can be divided into errors in media representation and those which are radiologist-related. The message conveyed by public and interest-group initiatives to increase the secondary prevention of breast cancer "a mammogram saved my life" is misleading as it essentially implies "saved my life because the radiologist found my breast cancer on a mammogram in which the tumor was the size of the head of a pin." The people responsible for placing such advertisements or testimonials apparently do not realize that the unstated implication is that "the radiologist who missed my breast cancer on the mammogram cost me my life." Many women wrongly believe that the act of getting a mammogram reduces their chances of developing breast cancer. Yet, it is difficult to encourage women to get a mammogram even if in about 14% of cases the tumor will not be visible. Now, despite repeated warnings by radiologists over the years that mammography does not depict all cancers and does not save all lives, the damage (women's belief that screening mammography is guaranteed to save their lives) has been done and perfection is expected. Moreover, not only the public but also medical colleagues have not received meaningful education from the radiologist community regarding the true fallibility of mammography [26].

In medical education, both in Europe and the USA, there are no communication courses. This deficiency is even greater for a specialty such as radiology, in which patient contact, and thus patient knowledge, is seldom portrayed in the media. The absence of a patient interview or an improper interview can be considered an error and it is certainly partly responsible for damage claims.

Radiologists, and physicians in general, should be taught communication skills. It is only by making full use of these skills and implementing reasonable corrective measures that the answer to the question of Kopans et al., "Will mammography survive malpractice?" be "yes" [27].

2.6 Conclusions

The discussion in this chapter, while providing an accurate analysis of the literature on malpractice in mammography, nevertheless requires three points as conclusions:

1. Mammography screening is the only structured system of possible reference. The data cited in the literature exclusively refer to this system. Therefore, whether a senologic program within an established Breast Unit could modify the percentage of mammographic interpretation errors remains unclear;
2. A Breast Unit promotes a new type of education for radiologists in terms of communication skills, thereby improving the relationship with the patient. Certainly, more effective communication leads to better results in image evaluation;
3. In the coming years, mammography screening will no doubt develop in terms of anamnesis, medical examination, echography, and selection of risk categories. This evolution will lead to the integration of mammography screening, as a structured system, and a personalized senologic program within Breast Units, thereby overcoming the present difficulties related to breast density, detection limits, and the knowledge deficit regarding the peculiarities of every single patient's clinical history.

References

1. Baker LH (1982) Breast Cancer Detection Demonstration Project: five-year summary report. Cancer J Clin 32:194-225
2. Harvey JA, Fajardo LL, Innis CA (1993) Preview mammograms on patients with impalpable breast carcinomas: retrospective vs blind interpretation. Am J Roentgenol 161:1167-1172
3. Pinto A, Brunese L (2010) Spectrum of diagnostic errors in radiology. World J Radiol 2:377-383
4. Fileni P (2010) Radiologic malpractice litigation risk in Italy: an observational study over a 14-year period. AJR 194:1040-1046
5. Berlin L (2001) Dot size, lead time, fallibility, and impact on survival: continuing controversies in mammography. Am J Roentgenol 176:1123-1130
6. Bird RE, Wallace TW, Yankaskas BC (1992) Analysis of cancers missed at screening mammography. Radiology 184:613-617
7. Aneesa S (2003) Missed breast carcinoma: pitfalls and pearls. RadioGraphics 23:881-895
8. McCormack VA, dos Santos Silva I (2006) Breast density and parenchymal patterns as markers of breast cancer risk: a meta-analysis. Cancer Epidemiol Biomarkers Prev 15:1159-1169
9. Skaane P (1999) Ultrasonography as adjunct to mammography in the evaluation of breast tumors. Acta Radiol Suppl 420:1-47
10. Heron DE, Komarnicky LT, Hyslop T et al (2000) Bilateral breast carcinoma: risk factors and outcomes for patients with synchronous and metachronous disease. Cancer 88:2739-2750
11. Sickles EA (1986) Mammographic features of 300 consecutive nonpalpable breast cancers. Am J Roentgenol 146:661-663
12. van Dijck JA, Verbeek AL, Hendriks JH, Holland R (1993) The current detectability of breast cancer in a mammographic screening program: a review of the previous mammograms of interval and screen-detected cancers. Cancer 72:1933-1938

13. Ikeda DM, Birdwell RL, O'Shaughnessy KF et al (2003) Analysis of 172 subtle findings on prior normal mammograms in women with breast cancer detected at follow-up screening mammography. Radiology 226:494-503
14. Wolverton DE, Sickles EA (1996) Clinical outcome of doubtful mammographic findings. Am J Roentgenol 167:1041-1045
15. Ikeda DM, Andersson I, Wattsgard C et al (1992) Interval carcinomas in the Malmo Mammographic Screening Trial: radiologic appearance and prognostic considerations. Am J Roentgenol 159:287-294
16. Stavros AT, Thickman D, Rapp CL et al (1995) Solid breast nodules: use of sonography to distinguish between benign and malignant lesions. Radiology 196:123-134
17. Lev-Toaff AS, Feig SA, Saitas VL et al (1994) Stability of malignant breast microcalcifications. Radiology 198:153-156
18. Fileni A, Magnavita N, Pescarini L (2009) Analysis of malpractice claims in mammography: a complex issue. Radiol Med 114:636-644
19. Farria DM, Schmidt ME, Monsees BS et al (2005) Professional and economic factors affecting access to mammography: a crisis today, or tomorrow? Cancer. 104:491-498
20. Beam CA, Conant EF, Sickles EA (2003) Association of volume and volume-independent factors with accuracy in screening mammogram interpretation. J Natl Cancer Inst 95:282-290
21. Barlow WE, Chi C, Carney PA et al (2004) Accuracy of screening mammography interpretation by characteristics of radiologists. J Natl Cancer Inst 96:1840-1850
22. Litvin SG (2005) An overview of medical malpractice litigation and the perceived crisis. Clin Orthop Relat Res 433:8-14
23. Sara L. Jackson (2009) Variability of interpretive accuracy among diagnostic mammography facilities. J Natl Cancer Inst 101:814-827
24. Carney PA, Yi JP, Abraham LA et al (2007) Reactions to uncertainty and the accuracy of diagnostic mammography. J Gen Intern Med 22:234-241
25. Gruppo di studio GISMa-SIRM, Chersevani R, Ciatto S, Del Favero C et al (2010) "CADEAT": considerations on the use of CAD (computer-aided diagnosis) in mammography. Radiol Med 115:563-70
26. Leonard Berlin (2004) Mammography screening can survive malpractice if radiologists take center stage and assume the role of educator. Radiology 233:641-644
27. Kopans DB (2004) Mammography screening is saving thousands of lives, but will it survive medical malpractice? (editorial). Radiology 230:20-24

Errors in the Diagnosis of Lung Neoplasms 3

Luigia Romano, Antonio Pinto, and Carlo Muzj

3.1 Introduction

Imaging diagnosis of lung cancer frequently occurs in the context of screening. In other cases, nodules may be detected on a routine CT scan or chest radiograph in asymptomatic patients. These tumors, which tend to be smaller at diagnosis, are referred to as central or peripheral as they have not spread beyond their local confines. While the features of the lesions' borders can be suggestive of malignancy, they are not diagnostic. However, the presence of spiculation is thought to indicate a higher likelihood of malignancy [1] whereas clearly defined edges [2] may indicate an inflammatory process. Cavitation, frequently an indication of long-standing or advanced lung cancer, is most commonly seen in squamous cell lung cancer [3].

The diagnosis of a subtle lung cancer at chest radiography remains a formidable challenge. Several investigators [4-8] have described the substantial pitfalls of interpretation created by overlapping structures and by the small size and low conspicuity typical of many lesions. Notwithstanding the difficulty in making the diagnosis, missed lung cancer is the second-leading cause of malpractice claims against radiologists [9].

Chest images contain a range of perceptual ambiguities that contribute to a significant error rate in diagnosis [10]. Indeed, is not unusual to retrospectively discover significant radiological abnormalities in patients who are later diagnosed with lung cancer [8]. The term *missed cancer* can refer to a lesion that was detected but misinterpreted by the radiologist [6]. The failure to detect a lung cancer, under any conditions, would be considered as negligence.

L. Romano (✉)
Department of Diagnostic Radiological Imaging, "A. Cardarelli" Hospital, Naples, Italy

3.2 Misdiagnosis of Lung Cancer on Chest Radiograph

The chest radiograph is a two-dimensional projection of a complex array of three-dimensional structures. Each of these structures, i.e., the pulmonary vessels, bones, and parts of the mediastinum, may project over the lung and thereby partly or totally obscure pulmonary lesions at chest radiography. Some lung nodules are small or inconspicuous because of ill-defined margination or low opacity. Consequently, a radiologist may fail to detect the lesion or may discount it as a benign structure.

Most overlooked lung neoplasms on chest radiographs are solitary pulmonary nodules. Missed cancer usually has a substantial upper lobe predilection [4, 11]. This predominance probably reflects the tendency of bronchogenic carcinoma to involve the upper lobes more frequently than other regions [4]. The perihilar regions are less common sites of overlooked lung cancer. Radiologist-missed lung cancers on chest radiographs have been reported to share the following characteristics: (a) most missed nodular cancers are visually subtle, but they are not always very small (median diameter, 16–20 mm); (b) missed cancers are located predominantly in the upper lobes; (c) superposing structures and distracting lesions are frequently present; and (d) image quality is commonly poor [4, 5, 9, 11]. The findings in the radiologist-missed cancer series that served as the basis for those conclusions were similar to those reported in previous studies [5, 7], although image quality was generally high.

The role of the lateral chest radiograph in the detection of lung cancer has been discussed for over 30 years [12, 13]. In the series by Shah et al. [7], only the lateral chest radiograph revealed the lung neoplasm retrospectively in two patients (5%) and the cancer was better seen on the lateral radiograph than on the frontal projection in one other patient (2%) in the same series. These results are comparable to those of other series, in which the detection rate for lung cancer on the lateral radiograph vs. the frontal chest radiograph was 2–4% [14, 15].

Lung cancer nodules are frequently missed on chest radiographs by radiologists in clinical practice, with reported error rates of 20–90% [14, 16] (Fig. 3.1). Even in observer performance studies, in which the participating radiologists are aware that many lung cancers are included, up to 40% of previously missed cancers remain undetected [17]. In one classic study [14] of lung cancer detected during the Mayo Lung Screening Project, 45 (90%) of 50 peripheral and 12 (75%) of 16 central lung lesions were visible in retrospect on films obtained 4 months prior to the radiograph on which the diagnosis was established (Fig. 3.2a, b). In several clinical series of missed lung cancer, in which the numbers of patients ranged from 27 to 40, the median diameter of such lesions was fairly large (> 1.5 cm) [4-7]. Missed tumors were attributed to multiple factors, including failure of perceptual analysis by the radiologist, lack of comparison with previous radiographs, inadequate awareness of clinical information, and deficiencies in film quality [6, 7].

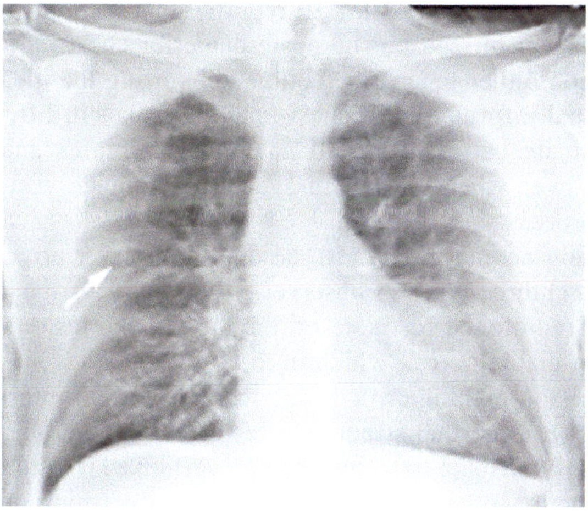

Fig. 3.1 Missed cancer of the middle pulmonary right field: a subtle low-density small nodule (*white arrow*) is partially hidden by the superposing ribs

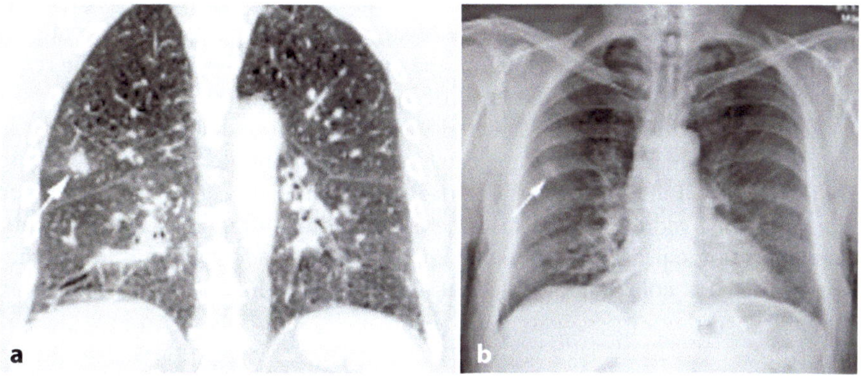

Fig. 3.2 a Coronal reformatting CT image shows an irregular rounded nodule with a poorly defined border, localized at the right upper pulmonary lobe (*white arrow*). Biopsy revealed a poorly differentiated cancer. **b** A lung nodule was visible (*white arrow*) retrospectively on the X-ray film obtained 4 months previously

3.3 Source of Errors in Chest Film Interpretation

There are many sources of error in the radiographic diagnosis of lung cancer: image quality, lesion detection, lesion recognition, and communication of the radiological findings to the referring physician [18]. Lesion size is an important factor influencing detectability on chest radiographs; according to some reports, only 50% of 1-cm lesions are detected [19]. Lesion shape may also influence detectability, as sharply marginated lesions are found more easily than spiculated or poorly defined cancers.

In addition, technical features play an important role in the failure to diagnose lung cancer [19]. On chest radiography, film contrast, density, and kVP all influence lesion detection [9]. Manning et al. [20] reported that the majority of errors related to lung cancer missed on the posteroanterior chest radiograph were failures of decision rather than of detection, supporting the idea that the complexity of the visual information in chest imaging makes it difficult for observers to discriminate between normal anatomic structures and nodular pathological features, even when such features have been made visually obvious by the imaging process.

A missed diagnosis of a lung neoplasm can also be due to observer error. In the study of Kundel et al. [21] three types of observer error were described: scanning error (failure of the radiologist to fixate on the area of the lesion), recognition error, and decision-making error, which in the authors' series was the most common [21]. A decision-making error is due to the incorrect interpretation of a malignant lesion as a normal structure after detection. Another form of observer error that may contribute to lesions being overlooked (including lung cancer) is the satisfaction of search (SOS) error [10], in which an abnormality is missed because another abnormality has been detected and further image interpretation subsequently discontinued. Sources of error in interpretation include the patient's clinical history, the presence or absence of previous studies, the index of suspicion, the presence of an abnormality, the reading room environment, and the level of interpreter vigilance.

In case of evidence of a suspected lung neoplasm on chest plain film, it is important that the radiologist suggests the next appropriate imaging procedure (Fig. 3.3a, b). Indeed, the failure to do so is another cause of malpractice claims against radiologists. These recommendations or suggestions for additional radiologic procedures must be appropriate and add meaningful information to clarify, confirm, or rule out the initial impression. The American

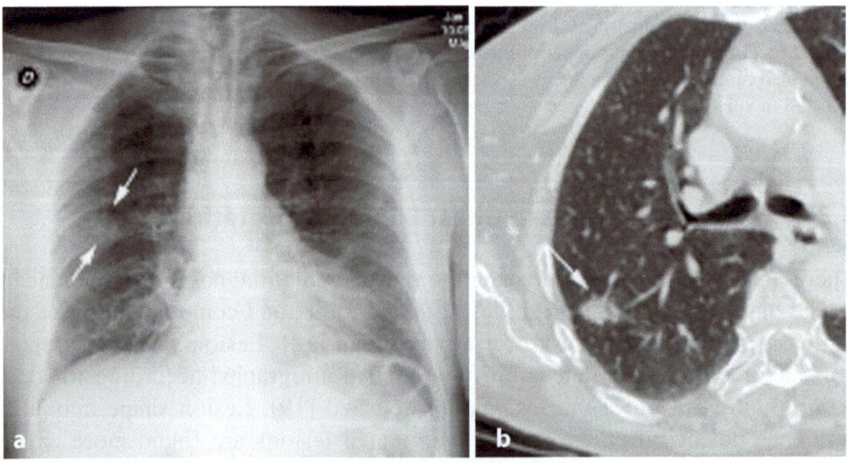

Fig. 3.3 a A chest X-ray film shows a poorly marginated opacity (*white arrow*) of the right lung in an asymptomatic smoker. **b** The axial CT image shows the irregular infiltrating edge of the nodule (*white arrow*) with distortion of the adjacent small vessels

College of Radiology "Practice Guideline for Communication of Diagnostic Imaging Findings" [22] states that "follow-up or additional diagnostic studies to clarify or confirm the impression should be suggested when appropriate."

3.4 Errors in the Diagnosis of Lung Cancer on Chest Computed Tomography

The number of lung cancers missed at CT, as cited in the literature, has been limited probably because it is difficult to identify the missed cases among the many routine CT examinations performed in most medical centers [23, 24]. Gurney [23] reported that nine lung cancers missed at CT were identified from a monthly tumor registry that was maintained for about 10 years; five of these tumors were peripheral lung cancers < 3 mm in diameter, which was considered as the threshold size for detectability. White et al. [24] reported 14 lung cancers overlooked at CT from about 37,500 chest CT scans at more than three institutions; the most common characteristic among these cases was an endobronchial location.

A more recent study of seven lung cancers missed at low-dose CT was reported on by Kakinuma et al. [25], based on 5,418 lung cancer CT screening studies performed over a period of more than 3 years. In the study by Li et al. [26], 83 primary lung cancers were found during an annual low-dose CT screening program and confirmed histopathologically at either surgery or biopsy. Of these lung cancers, 32 were missed on 39 CT scans: on 23 scans owing to detection errors and on 16 scans owing to interpretation errors (Fig. 3.4a-d). In their interpretation error cases, 88% of the missed cancers, or the features of these tumors, mimicked benign lesions and/or were associated with underlying lung disease. Missed cancers with linear, triangular, and irregular patterns, similar to the patterns of benign lesions, were common findings, and the underlying lung diseases were due to other abnormalities, such as residual tuberculosis (including pleural thickening) or residual or new inflammatory lesions, emphysema, or lung fibrosis [26].

Due to improvements in CT imaging technology, the detection of small pulmonary nodules has improved. The ability to detect small nodules is of paramount importance in finding early-stage lung cancer. However, nodules < 1 cm in diameter often pose a dilemma, for both clinicians and patients, as they may be difficult to biopsy and can easily be confused with normal anatomic structures within the lung.

3.5 Conclusions

Lung cancer is the most frequently occurring cancer in the world; in the USA it is the second most commonly diagnosed cancer. Accurate imaging-based staging can have a significant impact on appropriate treatment and surgical

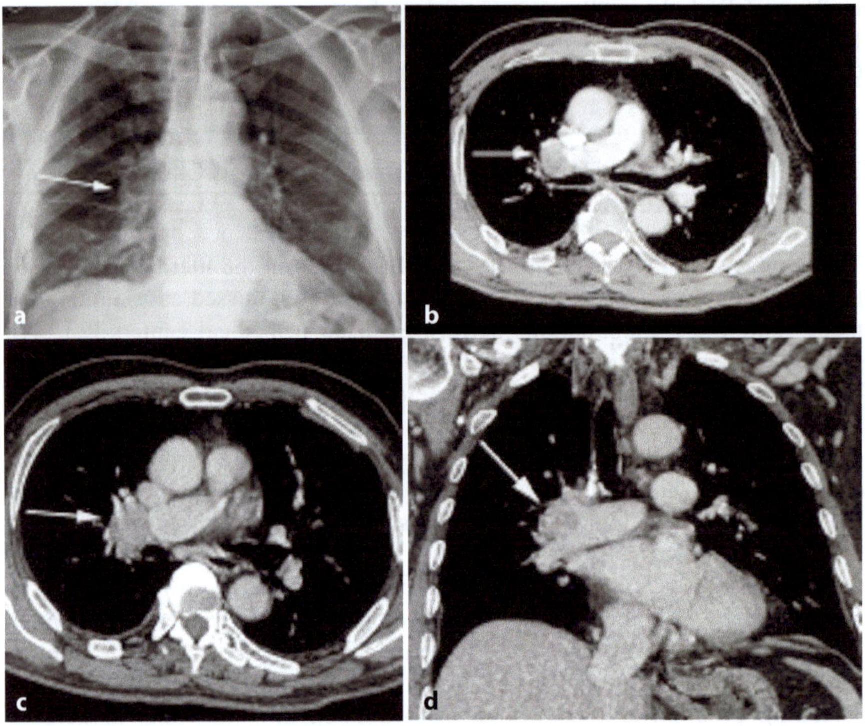

Fig. 3.4 a Admission radiograph from a young male with chest pain, hemoptysis, and breathlessness: the right pulmonary artery is enlarged. **b** Axial CT scan obtained during the arterial phase shows a typical filling defect of the right pulmonary artery (*white arrow*) due to a thromboembolism. **c, d** After 2 weeks of anticoagulant therapy, the axial CT scan obtained during the portal phase demonstrates contrast enhancement of the embolus (*white arrow*): the filling defect of the right pulmonary artery is due to hilar cancer

options. The failure to detect, identify, or describe an abnormality that on a plain chest radiograph is subsequently shown to be lung cancer has potentially very serious consequences in medical malpractice litigation.

Multiple strategies have been recommended to reduce the rate of missed lung cancer. These include scrupulous comparison of the current radiographic study with the results of previous examinations, avoidance of distracting findings leading to SOS errors, and the double reading of images. Each of these approaches has drawbacks related to workflow and the limitations of human perception. Computer-aided detection (CAD) systems are increasingly being introduced as a "second reader" to assist in the evaluation of images of complex anatomic structure, and they can mark many visually subtle lung cancers that may be missed by radiologists. Although false-positive detections are numerous and potentially distracting, the majority of them are clearly due to superposing anatomic structures. Accordingly, the reduction of false-positives should be a priority in the development of CAD programs.

References

1. Kuriyama K, Tateishi R, Doi O et al (1987) CT-pathologic correlation in small peripheral lung cancers. AJR Am J Roentgenol 149:1139-1143
2. Theros EG (1977) Varying manifestations of peripheral pulmonary neoplasms: a radiologic-pathologic correlative study. AJR Am J Roentgenol 128:893-914
3. Chaudhuri MR (1973) Primary pulmonary cavitating carcinomas. Thorax 28:354-366
4. Austin JH, Romney BM, Goldsmith LS (1992) Missed bronchogenic carcinoma: radiographic findings in 27 patients with potentially resectable lesion evident in retrospect. Radiology 182:115-122
5. Quekel LG, Kessels AG, Goei et al (1999) Miss rate of lung cancer on the chest radiograph in clinical practice. Chest 115:720-724
6. Monnier-Cholley L, Arrive L, Porcel A et al (2001) Characteristics of missed lung cancer on chest radiographs: a French experience. Eur Radiol 11:597-605
7. Shah PK, Austin JH, White CS et al (2003) Missed non-small cell lung cancer: radiographic findings of potentially resectable lesions evident only in retrospect. Radiology 226:235- 241
8. Turkington PM, Kennan N, Greenstone MA (2002) Misinterpretation of the chest x ray as a factor in the delayed diagnosis of lung cancer. Postgrad Med J 78:158-160
9. White CS, Salis AI, Meyer CA (1999) Missed lung cancer on chest radiography and computed tomography: imaging and medicolegal issues. J Thorac Imaging 14:63-68
10. Samuel S, Kundel HI, Nodine CF et al (1995) Mechanism of satisfaction of search: eye position recordings in the reading of chest radiographs. Radiology194:895-902
11. Forrest JV, Friedman PJ (1981) Radiologic errors in patients with lung cancer. West J Med 134:485-490
12. Tala E (1967) Carcinoma of the lung: a retrospective study with special reference to pre-diagnosis period and roentgenographic signs. Acta Radiol Diagn (Stockh) 26:1-127
13. Forrest JV, Sagel SS (1979) The lateral radiograph for early diagnosis of lung cancer. Radiology 131:309-310
14. Muhm JR, Miller WE, Fontana RS et al (1983) Lung cancer detected during a screening program using four-month chest radiographs. Radiology 148:609-615
15. Stitik FP, Tockman MS (1978) Radiographic screening in the early detection of lung cancer. Radiol Clin North Am 16:347-366
16. Heelan RT, Flehinger BJ, Melamed MR et al (1984) Non-small-cell lung cancer: results of the New York screening program. Radiology 151:289-293
17. Monnier-Cholley L, Carrat F, Cholley BP et al (2004) Detection of lung cancer on radiographs: receiver operating characteristic analysis of radiologists', pulmonologists', and anesthesiologists' performance. Radiology 233:799-805
18. Potchen EJ, Bisesi MA (1990) When is it malpractice to miss lung cancer on chest radiographs? Radiology 175:29-32
19. Brogdon BG, Kelsey CA, Moseley RD (1983) Factors affecting perception of pulmonary lesions. Radiol Clin North Am 21:633-654
20. Manning DJ, Ethell SC, Donovan T (2004) Detection or decision errors? Missed lung cancer from the posteroanterior chest radiograph. Br J Radiol 77:231-235
21. Kundel HL, Nodine CF, Carmody D (1978) Visual scanning, pattern recognition and decision making in pulmonary nodule detection. Invest Radiol 13:175-181
22. American College of Radiology (2005) ACR practice guideline for communication of diagnostic imaging findings. In: 2005 Practice guideline & technical standards. American College of Radiology; Reston, VA, pp 5-9
23. Gurney JW (1996) Missed lung cancer at CT: imaging findings in nine patients. Radiology 199:117-122
24. White CS, Romney BM, Mason AC et al (1996) Primary carcinoma of the lung overlooked at CT: analysis of findings in 14 patients. Radiology 199:109-115
25. Kakinuma R, Ohmatsu H, Kaneko M et al (1999) Detection failures in spiral CT screening for lung cancer: analysis of CT findings. Radiology 212:61-66

26. Li F, Sone S, Abe H et al (2002) Lung cancers missed at low-dose helical CT screening in a general population: comparison of clinical, histopathologic, and imaging findings. Radiology 225:673-683

Errors in Polytrauma

4

Franco Guida, Giorgio Bocchini, Giacomo Sica, Anna Frezza, and Mariano Scaglione

4.1 Introduction

In the managing of traumatized patients, and even more so in dealing with normal dynamic diagnostics, an error can increase the rate of mortality and morbidity. While procedural or clinical-diagnostic errors are more frequent in medical facilities that are not dedicated to trauma, they can involve patients in highly specialized trauma centers as well. The occurrence of these errors, in a wider sense, can be explained by the different dynamics in relation to the seriousness of the trauma (minor or major). Most diagnostic errors (downgrading of an injury) in radiology occur using traditional imaging studies, i.e., plain films and ultrasound, because of their intrinsic low resolution and/or limited field of view. On the other hand, the use of MDCT in trauma patients requires the adoption of tailored protocols and skill to highlight subtle or even minimal signs of injuries, especially in the subclinical status [1].

Death after trauma statistically assumes a trimodal distribution; an immediate peak due to the seriousness of any injury before any medical intervention (at the scene); a second peak due to injuries of rapidly evolving character, such as hemorrhage (first cause of early death), which is only partially preventable; and a third peak, at a distance of weeks, months, or even years after the traumatic event, that is determined by systemic complications, e.g., sepsis and multisystem organ failure, or by later complications of unrecognized injuries in which downgrading was mainly diagnostic (e.g., pseudoaneurysms or post traumatic arteriovenous fistula) [2].

M. Scaglione (✉)
Department of Diagnostic Imaging, "Pineta Grande" Medical Center, Castelvolturno (CE), Italy

4.2 Errors in Traditional Imaging

Diagnostic errors made with traditional imaging (X-ray and ultrasound) are statistically more common, accounting for 75% of all misdiagnoses [3]. In various studies, echographic diagnosis has been shown to have a sensitivity and specificity that are high enough for the identification of some types of injuries and in particular for those which are easily explored [4]. However, the sensitivity and specificity of ultrasound are highly inadequate for other types of traumatic injuries, especially those involving some parenchymatous organs, the hollow bowels, and the retroperitoneum. These limitations are largely due to differences in operator ability but also to physical limits posed, for example, by overweight patients or those with meteorism.

Traditional radiography for an initial and widespread approach to study skeletal segments of the torso, appendicular skeleton, and the chest is limited by its low intrinsic resolution. The failed or late diagnosis of skeletal injuries, especially those of the appendicular skeleton and the articulations, statistically account for the majority of claims in radiography malpractice suits [3]. For example, posterior glenohumeral dislocations are very rare, with an incidence of 1–4% of all dislocations of the same shoulder [5, 6]. However, failure to recognize this injury can determine a permanent disability and lead to a malpractice claim [7, 8]. The anatomic complexity of the wrist, with its many small bone elements, frequently results in a misdiagnosis, particularly in patients with semilunar dislocations of the carpal and scaphoid bones, both of which can be the cause of disability as well as neurological complications. Indeed, one multicenter study showed the misdiagnosis of 25% of these patients [9, 10]. It should be kept in mind that a fracture of the scaphoid bone accompanies 60–70% of all carpal injuries and is the most common form of wrist fracture [11-16].

Injuries of the vertebral column are involved in 10% of all misdiagnoses occurring in the initial phase. Such injuries are much more common at the cranio-cervical junction (40–50%) and at the cervical-dorsal transition. However, the identification of an injury in one segment of the spine should raise suspicion of similar injuries in the other segments, especially since the timely identification of a spinal injury is absolutely fundamental in dealing with the traumatized patient. Standard radiographic evaluation of the cervical spine provides at least three projections: antero-posterior, cross-table lateral, and open mouth odontoid views, sometimes integrated with oblique projections [17]. Yet, standard radiographic projections were shown to be inadequate in the identification of 50% of the fractures detected [18, 19]. In 2009, the American College of Radiologists (ACR) recommended multidetector computed tomography (MDCT) with multiplanar reconstruction (MPR) as the method of choice in suspected spinal trauma, replacing traditional imaging studies for patients who show a suspicious clinical framework according to the criteria of NEXUS or the Canadian Cervical Spine Rules [20]. Similar conclusions have been reached by the Eastern Association for the Surgery of

Trauma (EAST) [21, 22]. A meta-analysis of ten studies showed that the sensitivity and specificity of MDCT in the identification of traumatic cervical spinal injury are 90–100% and 98–100% compared to 38.9–93% and 95–100% using traditional methods [23]. For injuries of the dorso-lumbar spine, the sensitivity of MDCT is > 97%, compared to 33% with traditional imaging; the specificity of both modalities is > 97% [24, 25]. Under-staging of a lumbar spine fracture is more likely in overweight patients or when there are coexisting intra-abdominal injuries, especially in the presence of ecchymosis of the abdominal wall, which can increase diagnostic errors by as much as 45%. The frequency of unrecognized spinal injuries seems to be higher when injuries of the hollow viscera are also present, followed by those of the mesentery, solid organs, and large vessels [26]. Transverse process fractures, in which only 60% are identifiable with traditional radiology, are associated with similar fractures elsewhere in the spine in approximately 10% of cases [27]. Compared to fractures of the appendicular skeleton, unrecognized visceral thoraco-abdominal injuries are less common: 10–15% for the liver and the spleen and 15–20% for the large and small bowel.

In thoracic trauma, pneumothorax (PNX) is underestimated (when visible in retrospective studies) in 50% of patients examined by chest X-ray. With the increased diffusion of contrast-enhanced MDCT in the evaluation of trauma it has been determined that > 72% of all PNX remain hidden with traditional imaging [28]. Many trauma centers erroneously consider the width of the mediastinum at chest radiography to be predictive of thoracic vascular injuries; however, many studies have shown the presence of aortic lesions in patients with a normal mediastinum [29, 30].

Another common cause of errors in traditional radiology involves costal fracture, which usually can be recognized only several days after the trauma. Injuries to the sternum are also frequently underestimated; however, as these fractures bring intense pain more appropriate diagnostic exams are usually performed to identify the cause (e.g., MDCT) [31, 32].

Among polytraumatized children with known skeletal and solid visceral organ injuries, ureteropelvic junction injuries are missed in approximately 50% of cases on initial evaluation with radiography and ultrasound [33]. In addition, in more than 80% of polytraumatized female patients with a previously unknown first-trimester pregnancy, the initial evaluation did not identify the pregnancy, thus exposing the embryo to a dose of radiation that could induce malformations or death [34]. However, under circumstances of polytrauma, in which a rapid diagnosis is needed, this cannot be considered as an absolute management error.

This brief summary shows that traditional radiology is often inadequate in the correct staging of skeletal and visceral trauma. Thus this modality cannot be considered as comprehensive and its use is best restricted to the staging of minor traumas or to guide further decision-making by the radiologist and clinician. Contrast-enhanced MDCT is the most effective method in terms of sensitivity and specificity. Nonetheless, in every radiological investigation, both radiation exposure and cost-benefit issues must be taken into account. The radiologist is obligated, in every case, to assume the role of imaging manager, guiding the complex and multidisciplinary management of patients with minor and major trauma, because he or she is the only person with a full understanding of the available imaging techniques and their most effective use.

4.3 Errors in MDCT

The appropriate use of advanced diagnostic imaging, which in the trauma patient almost exclusively consists of contrast-enhanced MDCT, may objectively and noticeably reduce the percentage of errors associated with the use of traditional methods. This is due to the high sensitivity and accuracy intrinsic to this method provided that several fundamental conditions in the management of the injured patient and in the execution of the examination are respected. In blunt trauma, clinical evidence is at best equivocal in 20–50% of the cases, regardless of patient collaboration [35]. Autopsy examination of polytrauma patients has shown that the primary cause of death is severe hemorrhage and severe post-traumatic broncho-pulmonary injuries [36].

The important information obtained from correctly performed contrast-enhanced MDCT studies accounts for the "gold standard" rating of this technique in the assessment of major trauma. Moreover, with the introduction of new equipment allowing rapid "whole-body" scanning, the patients who can benefit from MDCT are no longer only those who are hemodynamically stable but now also includes semi-instable and borderline patients. However contrast-enhanced MDCT as with other methods, is not devoid of errors, with the most common sources of errors related to the lack of experience on the part of the radiologist and, above all, to incorrect patient management [37]. The latter implies a failure to follow the established protocol for whole-body CT in trauma patients [1], including minimum slice thickness, which is necessary for the MPR and maximum-intensity projections (MIP).

A strict collaboration with the trauma team is necessary even before the MDCT examination in order to avoid various types of common errors. The patient should be undressed, with a correct venous access of at least 18G positioned as proximally as possible and, if not collaborating, adequately sedated, thus saving time. His or her upper limbs should be either raised above the head or semi-flexed at the sides of the body to reduce artifacts and dose exposure. Since one of the main causes of death in decelerated trauma is massive mono- or bilateral PNX, it is important that the radiologist searches it in the scout view at the start of the contrast-enhanced MDCT study. Another frequent condition that may determine errors in interpretation and, especially, under-staging is the inadequate flow of intravenously injected contrast material. Thus, adequate catheter access and a flow rate of intravenous contrast of 3,5ml/s or higher should be established, as these conditions will facilitate the search for and correct identification of vascular injuries. In polytrauma patients, the identification and characterization of such injuries is of primary importance and it demands more than just determining the site of vascular contrast extravasation (blush); rather, the nature of the extravastion must be characterized, which is possible with the most recent MDCT equipment. A correct multi-phase study will distinguish all sites of active arterial bleeding in the early contrast-enhanced phase from the slower venous bleeding characteristic of the portal and late phases, enabling the detection and characterization of pseudo-aneurysms and arterio-venous fistulas, which would otherwise remain underestimated [38, 39] (Fig. 4.1).

Among the many sources of CT-related errors, some occur more frequently at the multicenter level. A missed identification or incorrect characterization of active bleeding may have inauspicious consequences whereas their correct recognition determines whether the patient is best managed conservatively, with an endovascular approach, or by traditional surgery. On the other hand, a false positive will cause unnecessary hospitalization or treatment [37].

In a contrast-enhanced MDCT study, the correct phase must be analyzed to obtain the maximal amount of diagnostic information. Use of the pre-contrast phase allows the detection of even the smallest clots, which point to the nature of the underlying injuries as well as to vascular intramural hematoma, which may be difficult to see in the contrast-enhanced phase (Fig. 4.2). The pre-contrast-phase is a also useful to diagnose entero-mesenteric injury. Patients with this type of injury should receive a thorough abdominal examination using the pulmonary parenchyma window, to avoid underestimating the presence of very small collections of intraperitoneal or retroperitoneal free air [38]. Late-phase studies are performed at the discretion of the radiologist, who must be present in the CT room during the examination. This phase (excretion phase) provides information on the dynamics of extravasation and, importantly, on traumatic pathologies involving the urinary system, most of which are treatable conservatively or by interventional surgery [39] (Fig. 4.3).

In the cranial-cervical region, two frequent errors in procedure may result in a serious increase in morbidity and mortality: under-staging of the supra-aortic trunks and underlying vascular damage due to the intra parenchymal hematomas of the brain. The first type can be avoided by extending the study of the arterial chest-abdominal phase to the neck, as the frequency of traumatic injuries in this vascular district is high enough (1–5%), and with obviously serious consequences in terms of morbidity and mortality, to warrant assessment [40, 41] (Fig. 4.4). In the second, an intra-parenchymal hematoma in a polytraumatized patient is often indicative of either an arteriovenous malformation or the spontaneous bleeding of an intracranial aneurysm. The latter may be the cause of the hematoma and probably of the trauma itself. Such cases are best evaluated by integrating the pre-contrast study of the skull with a cerebral angio-CT or angio-MRI.

Injuries of the diaphragm are not very common but represent 5% of under-

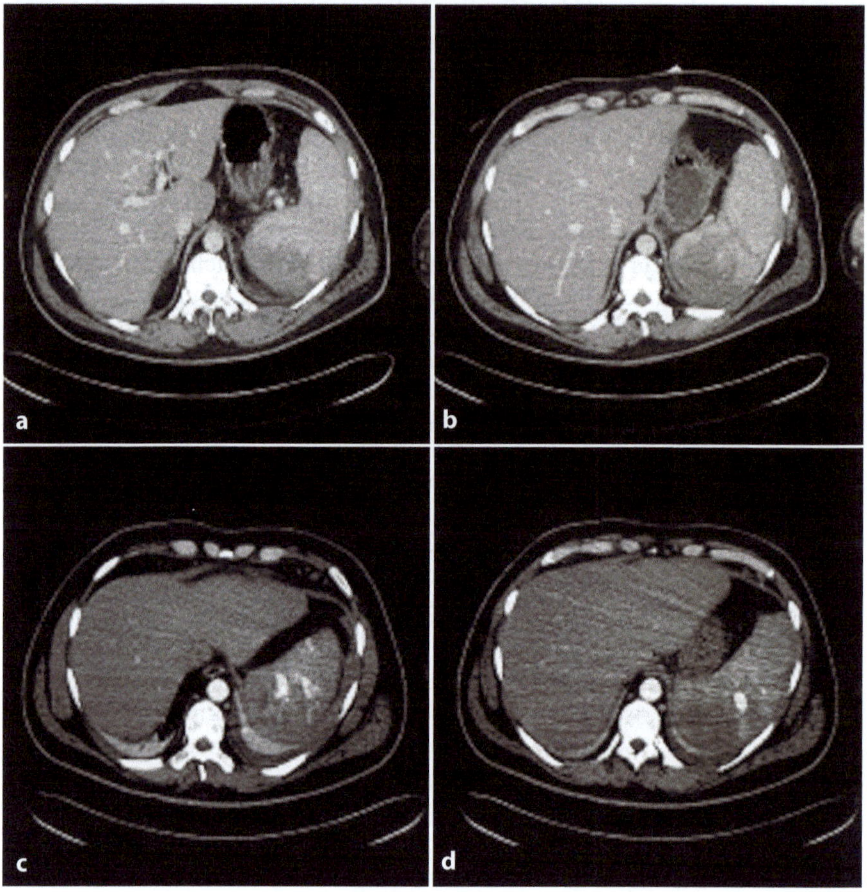

Fig 4.1 High-grade splenic injury. The extent of the parenchymal damage may not be the most significant factor in terms of patient management. A correct CT splenic/solid organ injury evaluation requires a high-flow (4–6 ml/s) injection of intravenous contrast-medium through an 18-16 gauge antedecubital vein. **a, b** A low-flow injection of contrast material does not show significant vascular injury in the context of an injured parenchyma on a portal-venous phase acquisition. **c, d** High-flow contrast material injection shows multiple contained vascular injuries (pseudoaneurysms) in the context of splenic injury. The presence of vascular injuries changes the splenic injury grade, and the patient's management and outcome

estimated injuries, half of which are not identified in the first 24 h [42]. Diagnosis of the injured diaphragm is particularly difficult [43], resulting in a late diagnosis. If the injury is clinically suggestive, it is generally visible on a traditional examination as herniation of the abdominal viscera; but this is a rare occurrence in the most serious cases. Various studies have shown that even with CT examination the sensitivity for fractures of the diaphragm is relatively low (50–73%) [43, 44].

In abdominal traumas, an important cause of error is respiration artifacts

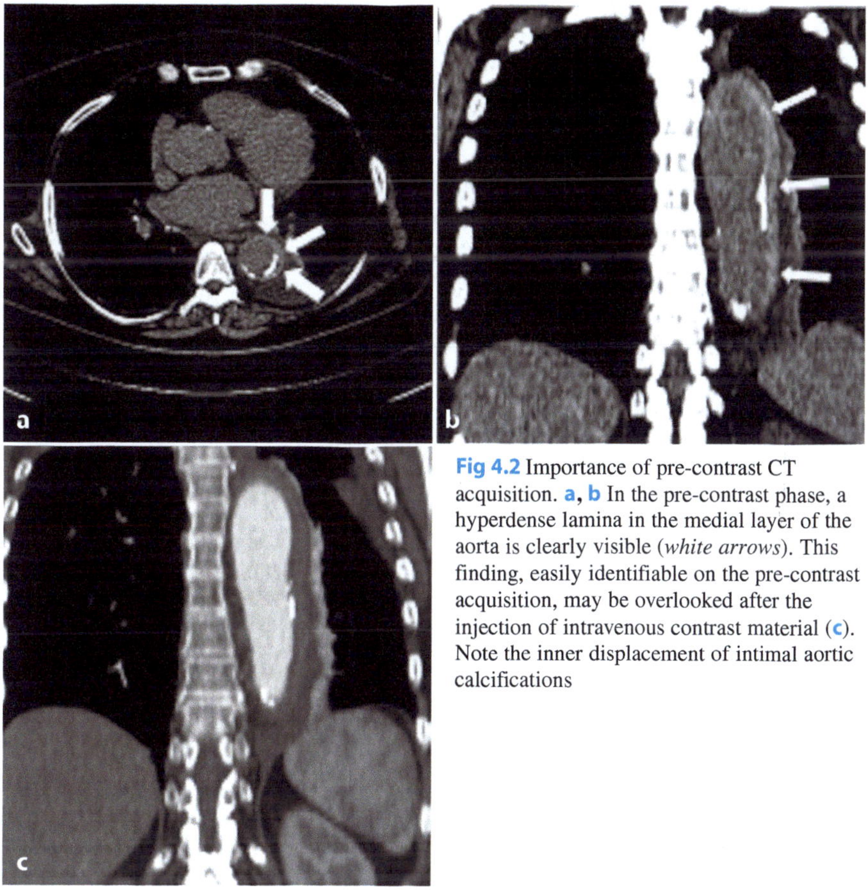

Fig 4.2 Importance of pre-contrast CT acquisition. **a, b** In the pre-contrast phase, a hyperdense lamina in the medial layer of the aorta is clearly visible (*white arrows*). This finding, easily identifiable on the pre-contrast acquisition, may be overlooked after the injection of intravenous contrast material (**c**). Note the inner displacement of intimal aortic calcifications

on the images. These are usually easily recognized, appearing as an indistinct margin of the examined vessels and associated with bands of hyperdensity at the level of the adjacent parenchymatous organs and hollow viscera, whereas modern ultra-rapid MDCT has notably reduced this source of artifact. Young radiologists must familiarize themselves with the anatomy of the retroperitoneal area and the intricate relationships between the retroperitoneum and peritoneal cavity. In fact, in the diaphragmatic pillars, adrenal glands, and liver, the only sign of small lacerations may be a retroperitoneal hematogenous collection along the hepato-duodenal ligament, exposed hepatic area, etc. Periportal tracking (hypodense liquid film along the main portal tract or its intrahepatic branches) is another non-specific sign of hepatic laceration that is often incorrectly interpreted or underestimated.

Periportal tracking can also be found in cases of high central venous

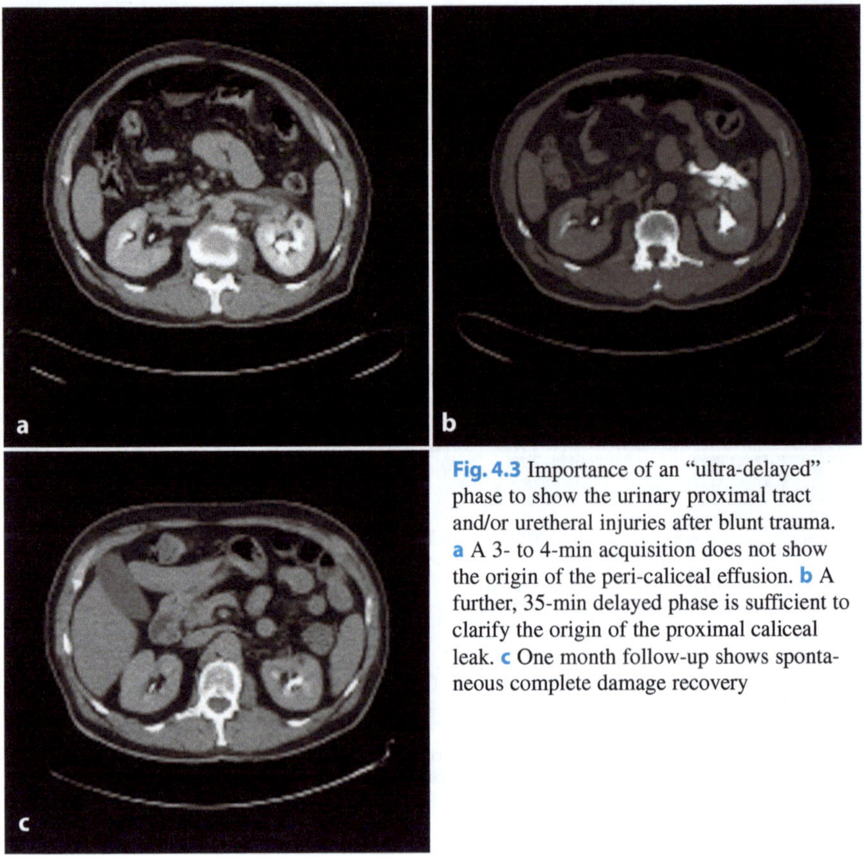

Fig. 4.3 Importance of an "ultra-delayed" phase to show the urinary proximal tract and/or uretheral injuries after blunt trauma. **a** A 3- to 4-min acquisition does not show the origin of the peri-caliceal effusion. **b** A further, 35-min delayed phase is sufficient to clarify the origin of the proximal caliceal leak. **c** One month follow-up shows spontaneous complete damage recovery

pressure, as in the presence of pericardial tamponade or PNX [37]. At the spleen, a lobulation or a cleft, typically located in the upper pole, can be easily misinterpreted as a splenic laceration. However, the two can be distinguished by bearing in mind that lobulations and clefts demonstrate regular and well-defined edges unlike those of lacerations. Respiratory artifacts may also simulate a subcapsular parenchymal hematoma. The differential diagnosis is based on the fact that a true hematoma distorts the underlying parenchyma while the respiratory artifact tends to produce a shadow on the extracapsular side.

Lastly, relatively frequently underestimated abdominal lesions are "entero-mesenteric" injuries. Oral contrast should be carefully considered and selectively used because it may simulate or hide even serious mesenteric and/or intestinal injuries [38]. Entero-mesenteric injuries are rarely detected on a first contrast-enhanced MDCT examination due to its inherent, evolutionary nature;

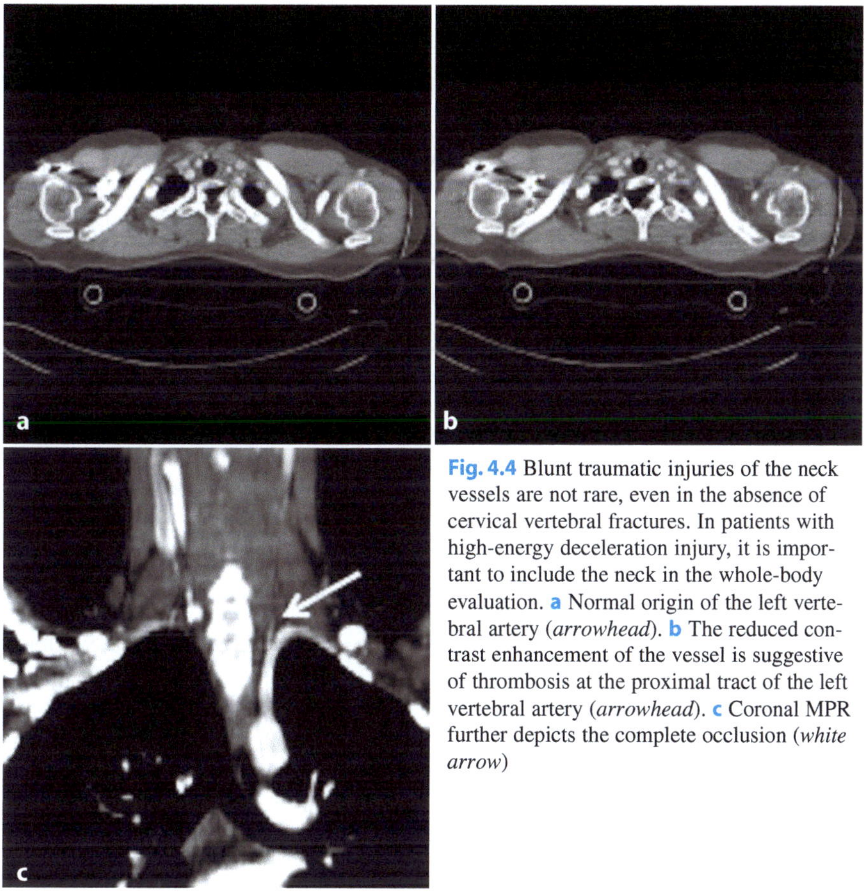

Fig. 4.4 Blunt traumatic injuries of the neck vessels are not rare, even in the absence of cervical vertebral fractures. In patients with high-energy deceleration injury, it is important to include the neck in the whole-body evaluation. **a** Normal origin of the left vertebral artery (*arrowhead*). **b** The reduced contrast enhancement of the vessel is suggestive of thrombosis at the proximal tract of the left vertebral artery (*arrowhead*). **c** Coronal MPR further depicts the complete occlusion (*white arrow*)

therefore, close clinical and diagnostic follow-up is required to obtain the correct diagnosis. Polytraumatized patients are often catheterized, which may conceal even large bladder lacerations. If these are suspected, then during the first or subsequent contrast-enhanced MDCT examination the catheter should be used to fill the bladder with iodinated contrast, which allows identification of even the smallest traumatic fractures, as these are otherwise underestimated.

Trauma is a systematic, evolving illness that requires tightly coordinated clinical and instrumental monitoring. The reduction of errors in polytrauma patients is the responsibility of the trauma team. The radiologist plays an essential role in the initial critical examination. The key elements to a successful diagnosis are fundamental knowledge, experience, and the correct application of imaging protocols.

References

1. Ptak T, Rhea T J, Novelline A R (2001) Experience of a continuous, single pass whole body multidetector CT protocol for trauma. Emergency Radiology 8:250-256
2. Potenza B, Hoyt D, Coimbra R et al (2004) Trauma research and education foundation. The epidemiology of serious and fatal injury in San Diego County over an 11-year period. J Trauma 56:68-75
3. Brooks A, Holroyd B, Riley B (2004) Missed injury in major trauma patients. Injury 35:407-410
4. Farahmand N, Sirlin CB, Brown MA et al (2005) Hypotensive patients with blunt abdominal trauma: performance of screening US. Radiology 235:436-443
5. Samilson RL, Prieto V (1983) Posterior dislocation of the shoulder in athletes. Clin Sports Med 2:369-378
6. Hawkins RJ, Neer CS, Pianta RM et al (1987) Locked posterior dislocation of the shoulder. J Bone Joint Surg Am 69:9-18
7. Neviaser TJ (1980) Old unreduced dislocations of the shoulder. Orthop Clin North Am 11:287-294
8. Schultz TJ, Jacobs B, Patterson RL (1969) Unrecognized dislocations of the shoulder. J Trauma 9:1009-1023
9. Herzberg G, Comtet JJ, Linscheid RL et al (1993) Perilunate dislocations and fracture dislocations: a multicenter study. J Hand Surg Am 18:768-779
10. Perron AD, Brady WJ, Keats TE et al (2001) Orthopedic pitfalls in the ED: lunate and perilunate injuries. Am J Emerg Med 19:157-162
11. Ring D, Jupiter JB, Herndon JH (2000) Acute fractures of the scaphoid. J Am Acad Orthop Surg 8:225-231
12. Ritchie JV, Munter DW (1999) Emergency department evaluation and treatment of wrist injuries. Emerg Med Clin North Am 17:823-842
13. Berger RA (1997) The ligaments of the wrist: a current overview of anatomy with consideration of their potential functions. Hand Clin 13:63-82
14. Nguyen DT, McCue FC, Urch SE (1998) Evaluation of the injured wrist on the field and in the office. Clin Sports Med 17:421-432
15. Zemel MP, Stark HH (1986) Fractures and dislocations of the carpal bones. Clin Sports Med 5:709-723
16. Wackerle JF(1987) A prospective study identifying the sensitivity of radiographic findings and the efficacy of clinical findings in carpal navicular fractures. Ann Emerg Med 16:733-737
17. Mower WR, Oh JY, Zucker MI et al (2001) Occult and secondary injuries missed by plain radiography of the cervical spine in blunt trauma patients. Emerg Radiol 8:200-206
18. Woodring JH, Lee C (1993) The role and limitations of computed tomographic scanning in the evaluation of cervical trauma. J Trauma 34:32-39
19. Davis JW, Phreaner DL, Hoyt DB et al (1993) The etiology of missed cervical spine injuries. J Trauma 34:342-346
20. Daffner RH, Wippold FJ II, Bennett DL et al (2009) ACR appropriateness criteria suspected spine trauma. http://www.guideline.gov/content.aspx
21. Como JJ, Diaz JJ Jr, Dunham CM et al (2009) Practice management guidelines for identification of cervical spine injuries following trauma–update from the Eastern Association for the Surgery of Trauma Practice Management Guidelines Committee. http://www.east.org/tpg/
22. Diaz JJ Jr, Cullinane DC, Altman DT et al (2006) Practice management guidelines for the screening of thoracolumbar spine fracture. http://www.east.org/tpg/tlspine
23. Cain G, Shepherdson J, Elliott V et al (2010) Imaging suspected cervical spine injury: plain radiography or computed tomography? Systematic review. Radiography 16:68-77
24. Roos JE, Hilfiker P, Platz A et al (2004) MDCT in emergency radiology: is a standardized chest or abdominal protocol sufficient for evaluation of thoracic and lumbar spine trauma? Am J Roentgenol 183:959-968

25. Wintermark M, Mouhsine E, Theumann N et al (2003) Thoracolumbar spine fractures in patients who have sustained severe trauma: depiction with multi-detector row CT. Radiology 227:681-689
26. Beaunoyer M, St-Vil D, Lallier M et al (2001) Abdominal injuries associated with thoracolumbar fractures after motor vehicle collision. J Pediatr Surg 36:760-762
27. Krueger MA, Green DA, Hoyt D et al (1996) Overlooked spine injuries associated with lumbar transverse process fractures. Clin Orthop 327:191-195
28. Ball CG, Kirkpatrick AW, Fox DL et al (2006) Are occult pneumothoraces truly occult or simply missed? J Trauma 60:294-298
29. Exadaktylos AK, Sclabas G, Schmid SW et al (2001) Do we really need routine computed tomographic scanning in the primary evaluation of blunt chest trauma in patients with "normal" chest radiograph? J Trauma 51:1173-1176
30. Wong YC, Ng CJ, Wang LJ et al (2004) Left mediastinal width and mediastinal width ratio are better radiographic criteria than general mediastinal width for predicting blunt aortic injury. J Trauma 57:88-94
31. Ziegler DW, Agarwal NN (1994) The morbidity and mortality of rib fractures. J Trauma 37:975-979
32. Palvanen M, Kannus P, Niemi S et al (2004) Hospital-treated minimal-trauma rib fractures in elderly Finns: long-term trends and projections for the future. Osteoporos Int 15:649-653
33. Onuora VC, Patil MG, al-Jasser AN (1993) Missed urologicalinjuries in children with polytrauma. Injury 24:619-621
34. Bochicchio GV, Napolitano LM, Haan J et al (2001) Incidental pregnancy in trauma patients. J Am Coll Surg 192:566-569
35. Schurink GW, Bode PJ, van Luijt PA et al (1997) The value of physical examination in the diagnosis of patients with blunt abdominal trauma: a retrospective study. Injury 28:261-265
36. Barendregt WB, de Boer HH, Kubat K (1993) Quality control in fatally injured patients: the value of the necropsy. Eur J Surg 159:9-13
37. West OC, Anderson J, Lee SJ et al (2002) Patterns of diagnostic error in trauma abdominal CT. Emergency Radiology 9:195-200
38. Guida F, Bocchin G, Chef G M et al (2010) Traumi intestinali e dei meso. Radiol med 115:S161-S165
39. Sica G, Bocchini G, Guida F et al (2010) Multidetector computed tomography in the diagnosis and management of renal trauma. Radiol med 115:936-49
40. van Wessem KJ, Meijer JM, Leenen LP et al (2011) Blunt traumatic carotid artery dissection still a pitfall? The rationale for aggressive screening. Eur J Trauma Emerg Surg 37:147-154
41. Miller PR, Fabian TC, Croe MA et al (2002) Prospective screening for blunt cerebrovascular injuries. Ann Surg 236:386-395
42. Voeller GR, Reisser JR, Fabian TC et al (1990) Blunt diaphragm injuries. A five-year experience. Am Surg 56:28-31
43. Reber PU, Schmied B, Seiler CA et al (1998) Missed diaphragmatic injuries and their long-term sequelae. J Trauma 44:183-188
44. Demos TC, Solomon C, Posniak HV et al (1989) Computed tomography in traumatic defects of the diaphragm. Clin Imaging 13:62-67

Missed Fractures in the Emergency Department

5

Vittorio Miele, Michele Galluzzo, and Margherita Trinci

5.1 Introduction

Diagnostic errors are important in all branches of medicine as they are an indication of inadequate patient care. Medically, the significance of a diagnostic error in an Emergency Department (ED) varies from minimal to potentially life threatening. In other patients a delay in diagnosis may negatively influence the long-term results, increase operative risks, and cause additional pain and suffering. However, all errors have implications for patient care. Moreover, patients are often distressed that an error has been made, which may complicate their relationship with the doctor or the hospital [1]. In the ED, clinically important diagnostic errors are relatively common among polytrauma patients, in whom orthopedic injuries predominate but also constitute 75% of missed diagnoses [2]. Spinal injuries account for approximately 10% of all initially missed diagnoses. These are especially common at the craniocervical junction (40-50% of all initially missed spinal injuries) and at the cervico-thoracic junction.

5.2 Criteria to Assess the Risk of Cervical Spinal Fractures

In response to efforts to make healthcare time-efficient, clinical criteria have been developed to identify the risk of cervical spine fractures in patients presenting to the ED. These clinical indicators include altered mentation, posterior midline cervical spine tenderness, focal neurologic deficit, neck pain on range of motion, and painful injury that may distract the patient from cervical spine pain. Among the studies supporting the use of screening tools to

V. Miele (✉)
Department of Emergency Radiology, "San Camillo" Hospital,
Rome, Italy

decrease the use of cervical spine radiography and/or spinal immobilization in patients presenting without any of these symptoms, the NEXUS and Canadian C-Spine Rule studies [3, 4] are the largest and they have validated these clinical criteria, Specifically, both concluded that, clinically, the cervical spine can be cleared without the use of cervical spine radiography.

5.3 Imaging and Screening of Cervical Spine Injuries

Standard radiographic evaluation of the cervical spine typically consists of cross-table lateral, anteroposterior, and open-mouth odontoid views, supplemented at some centers by oblique imaging [5]. Several reports concluded that standard plain radiography is unreliable in detecting bony cervical spine injury and may miss > 50% of all cervical spine fractures [6, 7]. The role of imaging in patients with suspected traumatic spinal injury has progressed significantly with the advent of increasingly sophisticated imaging hardware and techniques. The latest American College of Radiologists (ACR) appropriateness criteria for suspected spinal trauma in 2009 [8] recommends axial multidetector computed tomography (MDCT) with sagittal and coronal multiplanar reformations (MPR) as the primary imaging modality of choice over radiography for patients in whom imaging is indicated based upon established clinical criteria (NEXUS or Canadian Cervical Spine Rules) [3, 4] (Fig. 5.1). It is well established that MDCT is more sensitive than radiography. A meta-analysis of ten studies found that the sensitivity of MDCT in the detection of cervical

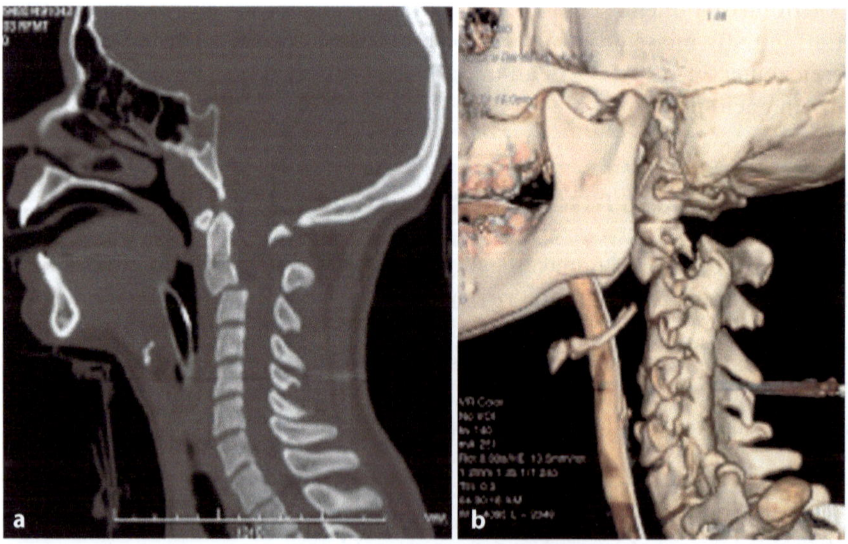

Fig. 5.1 **a** MDCT, sagittal reformation. Cervical fracture at the C2/C3 level with dislocation seen on the lateral plane. **b** Same patient. MDCT; 3D volume-rendering reconstruction

spinal injury ranged from 90% to 100% compared to 38.9% to 93% for radiography, while specificity ranged from 98% to 100% and 95% to 100%, respectively [9].

Clinical screening for cervical spine injuries earlier in the process of assessing patients for potential injuries could magnify the time benefits of early diagnosis and treatment, especially in avoiding the need for prolonged immobilization. This requires training clinicians in the appropriate method of physical examination and implementing this approach in areas of emergency medical services. In addition, the amount of time spent by patients in the ED could be reduced if at triage nurses used the examination to remove backboards and collars from patients [10].

5.4 Thoraco-lumbar Fractures

Fractures of the thoraco-lumbar spine may be difficult to diagnose radiographically. Added to the inherent diagnostic difficulty is the fact that missed diagnosis contributes to an incidence of neurologic deficits of 10.5% compared to 1.4% when these injuries are diagnosed at presentation [11]. In one study, 12.7% of lumbar spine fractures were missed radiographically in polytrauma patients. The same study further revealed a miss rate for lumbar fractures of 23.2% when diagnosis relied solely on standard transaxial abdomino-pelvic CT images [12], thus underscoring the importance of high-resolution images and MPR.

Chest radiography for the evaluation of the thoracic spine is fraught with difficulty and 50% of studies are non-diagnostic. Furthermore, there is significant overlap between the radiographic findings of thoracic spine injury and those of traumatic aortic injury [13]. Dedicated overpenetrated coned down AP and breathing lateral thoracic spine radiographs are superior to standard chest films [14].

Thoraco-lumbar fractures are missed more often among patients who have recognized intra-abdominal injury, especially those with abdominal wall ecchymosis, and contribute to diagnostic error by up to 45%. The frequency of missed spine injuries seems to be highest among patients with concordant injuries to the hollow viscus [15] (Fig. 5.2). Transverse process fractures, of which only 60% are identifiable with conventional radiography, may be associated with fractures of the vertebral body in approximately 10% of patients [16] (Fig. 5.3).

5.5 Orthopedic Injuries

Missed fractures and the inappropriate management of orthopedic injuries account for a significant proportion of malpractice claims made against emergency care providers. This finding takes on added relevance because orthopedic

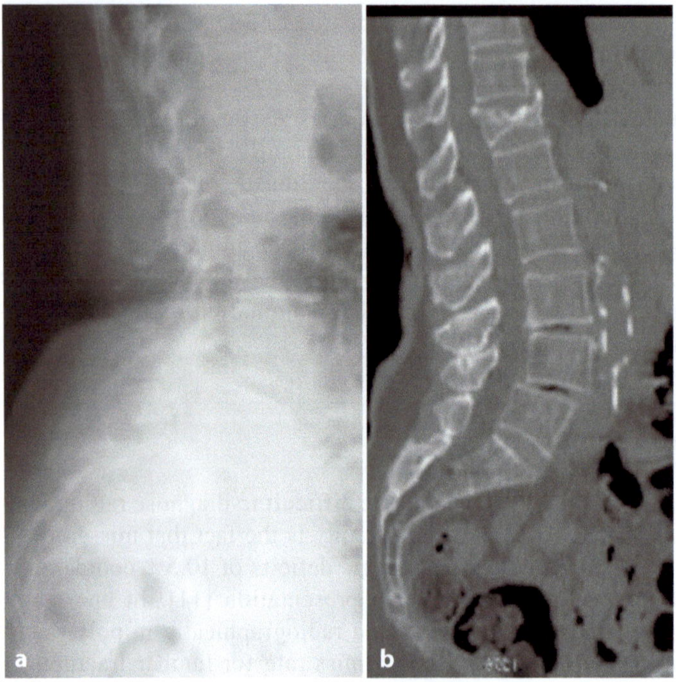

Fig. 5.2 a Post-traumatic lower back pain. Lateral plain film. b MDCT; sagittal reformation. Diagnosis: D12 body fracture. The fracture was missed on plain film

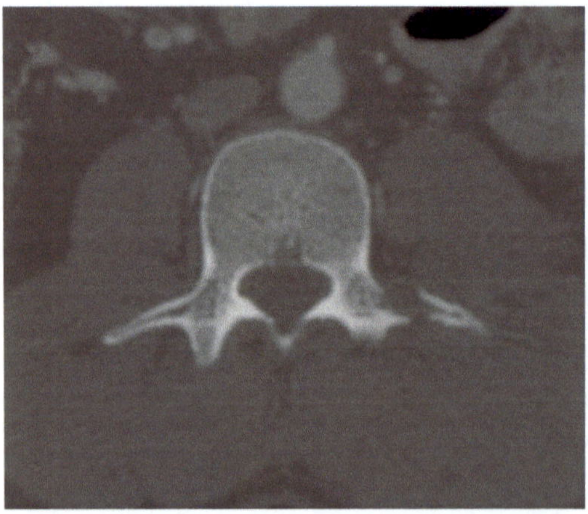

Fig. 5.3 MDCT, axial view. Images shows left transverse process fracture of the L3 lumbar vertebra

injuries are seen frequently in the ED. Missed orthopedic injuries are most common in the peri-articular regions, shoulder girdle (Figs. 5.4, 5.5), and feet. The glenohumoral joint of the shoulder is the most commonly dislocated joint in the body. Compared with anterior shoulder dislocation, posterior shoulder

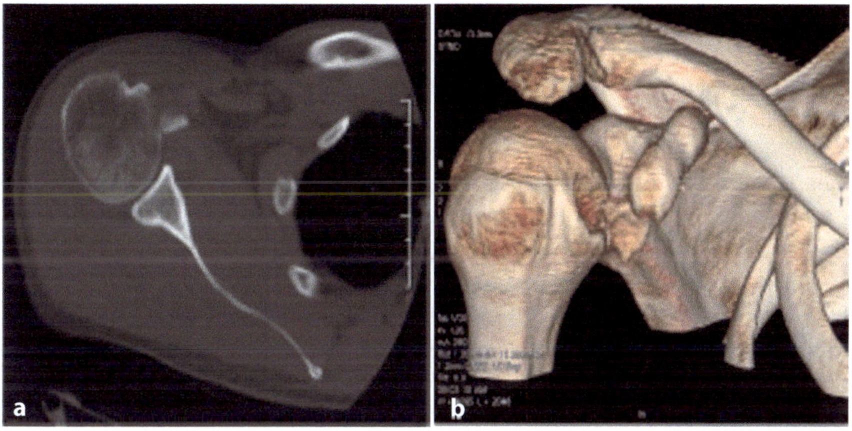

Fig. 5.4 **a** MDCT, axial plane. Diagnosis: humeral head fracture. **b** MDCT examination of the same patient; 3D volume-rendering reconstruction

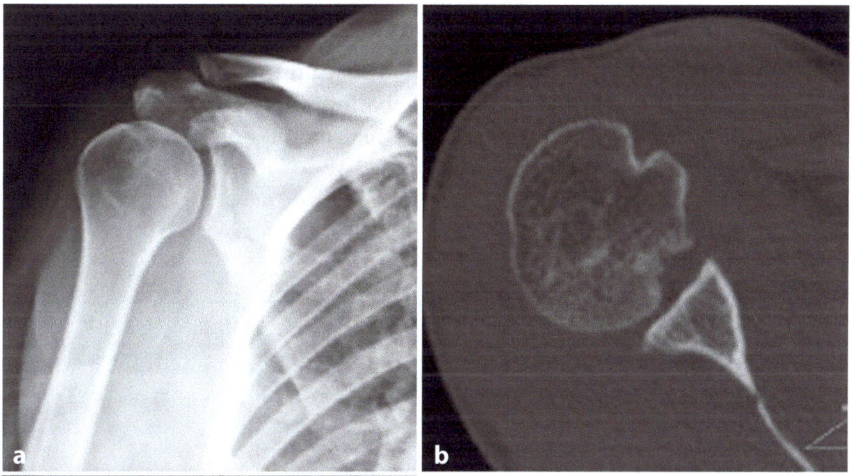

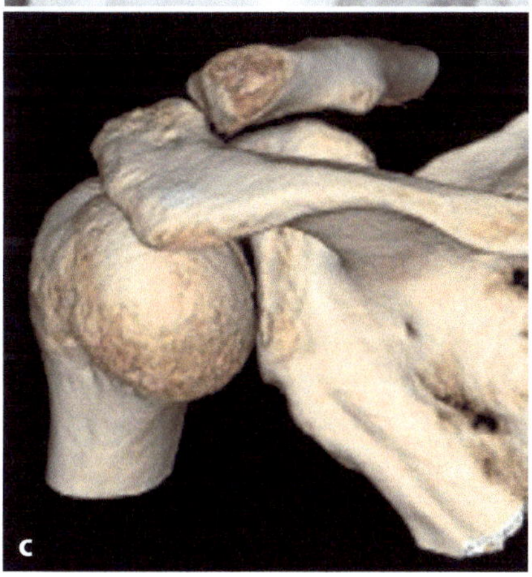

Fig. 5.5 **a** Plain film, frontal view. Normal shoulder girdle. **b** MDCT examination of the same patient; axial images. Diagnosis: reverse Bankart fracture. **c** MDCT; 3D volume-rendering reconstruction

dislocation is an infrequent event, with a reported incidence of 1–4% of all shoulder dislocations [17, 18] (Fig. 5.6). The major clinical significance of posterior dislocation is the frequency of errors in its diagnosis and thus the significant delays in treatment, which can result in permanent disability [19, 20].

The wrist is a complex structure with multiple bones and joints that allow a nearly infinite combination of positions and motions (Fig. 5.7). The effects of trauma on the wrist can be both subtle and complex. The morbidity of wrist injury is related, in part, to the frequently missed diagnosis in the ED of lunate or perilunate dislocation [21, 22]. One multicenter study reported a missed diagnosis in 25% of patients with perilunate dislocations and fracture-dislocations [21]. Unfortunately, missed injuries to the wrist are associated with a high incidence of long-term pain, dysfunction, and disability [22].

Of all the wrist injuries encountered in the ED, fracture of the scaphoid is among those most frequently missed [23, 24]. The scaphoid bone is the most commonly injured of the carpal bones, accounting for 50–80% of carpal injuries and occurring predominantly in young healthy individuals [25, 26]. Scaphoid fractures are the most problematic to diagnose in a clinical setting because they can take up to 6 weeks to become conclusive on plain X-ray films. Not surprisingly then, it is estimated that up to 40% of scaphoid fractures are missed at first presentation [27]. Failure to diagnose and immobilize scaphoid injuries can lead to osteoarthritis, mal-union, non-union. and avascular necrosis; indeed, non-union occurs in 5–12% of the cases [28, 29]. Even

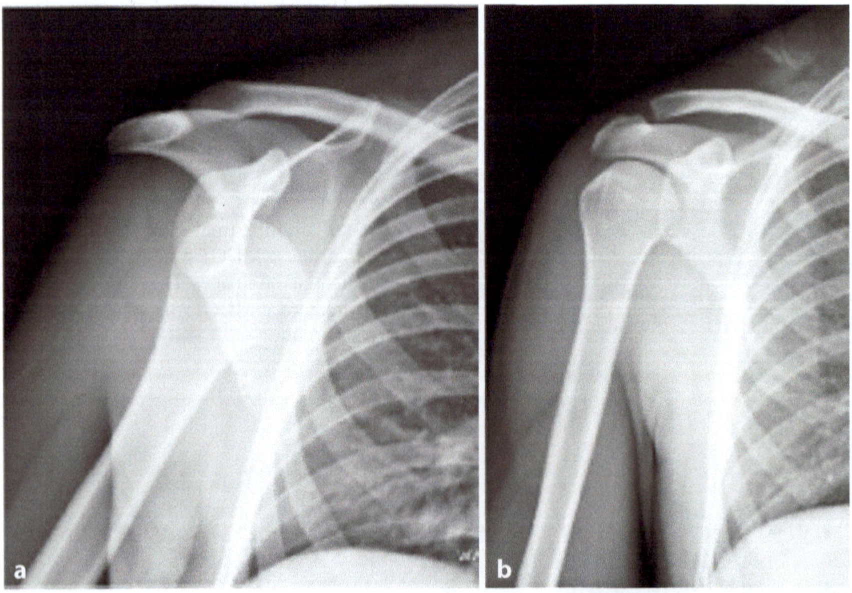

Fig. 5.6 a Plain film, frontal view. Anterior shoulder dislocation. **b** Plain film, frontal view after orthopedic treatment

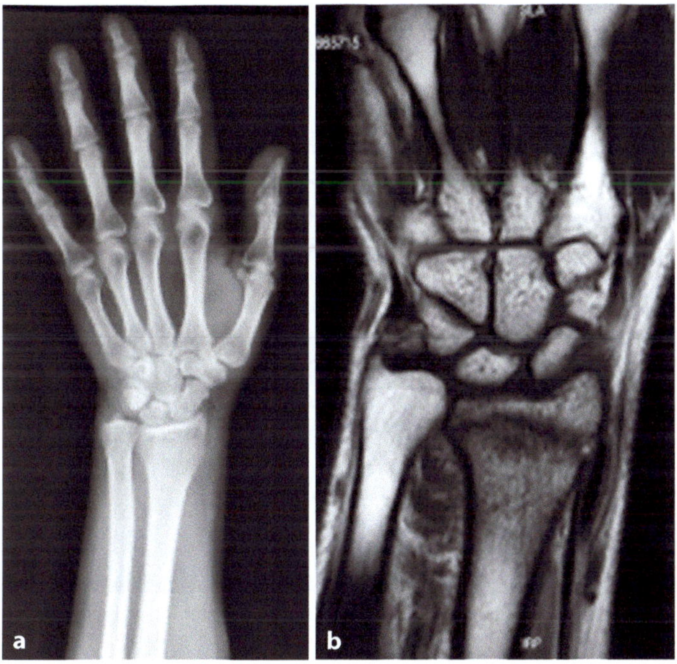

Fig 5.7 a Plain film, frontal view of a suspected fracture of the distal tract of the radius. **b** Magnetic resonance (MR), coronal T1-weighted image clearly shows the fracture

asymptomatic non-union has been shown, both clinically and radiologically, to lead to progressive deterioration [30]. Initial radiographic sensitivity is 64% and decreases on further imaging to only 30% [31]. Immobilization for a clinical scaphoid injury usually consists of a scaphoid cast for at least 6 weeks, until healing is confirmed based on imaging in conjunction with repeated clinical examination. In such cases, the available imaging options are a modified carpal view, bone scintigraphy, magnetic resonance imaging (MRI), and CT [32] (Fig. 5.8).

Elbow and forearm fractures represent 8–10% of all adult fractures [33]. Early diagnosis and treatment typically result in functional improvement and a reduction in patient morbidity whereas late diagnosis often leads to long-term patient morbidity. The potential sequelae of missed fractures are malunion, pain, instability, recurrent elbow dislocation, and/or limited motion [34]. Patients with an elbow fracture usually complain of pain and loss of function. However, small non-displaced fractures may result in mild pain and minimal loss of motion. In patients with suspected osseous injuries, the first-line imaging modality is plain-film radiography. The minimum requirements to fully visualize the injured site are two perpendicular imaging views. Imaging in two planes may not conclusively demonstrate non-displaced fractures [35].

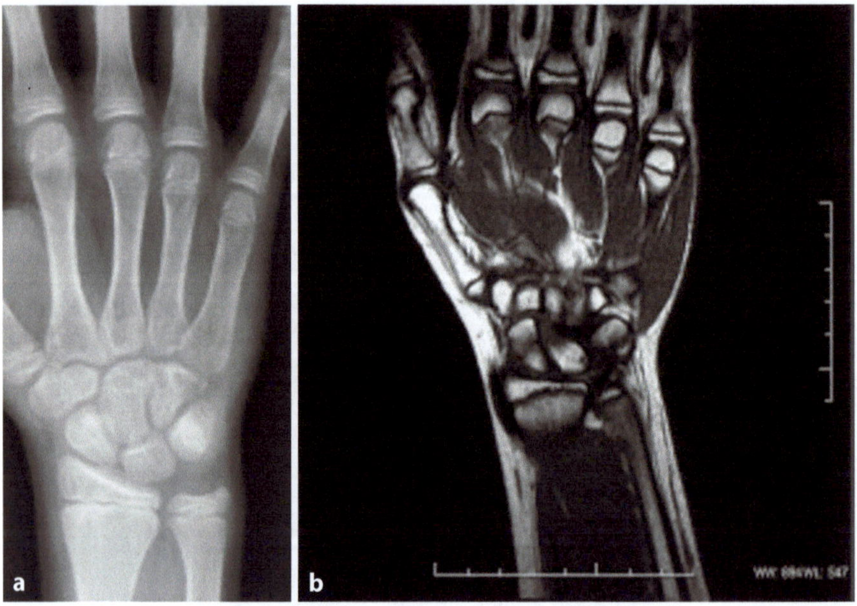

Fig. 5.8 **a** Plain film, frontal view. Normal scaphoid bone. **b** MR coronal T1-weighted image shows a scaphoid carpal bone fracture missed at first presentation

Ankle distortions are quite common and usually associated with ligamentous injury. During initial evaluation in the ED, 39% of ankle and midfoot fractures are potentially missed because of inadequate clinical and radiological evaluations in a limited time [36, 37] (Fig. 5.9). Some 50% of missed fractures due to ankle distortions involve the talus bone. Both the overlapping of bony structures in conventional radiographs and inadequate physician experience can lead to the missed diagnosis of these fractures.

The calcaneus is the largest and most commonly fractured tarsal bone, accounting for approximately 60% of all foot fractures [38]. These fractures represent 2% of all fractures treated [38]. Among patients sustaining this injury, 8090% are men in their prime working years, with the majority being industrial workers [39]. Calcaneal fractures are often associated with significant morbidity involving prolonged pain and disability (Fig. 5.10). If initially missed or treated inappropriately, these injuries may produce an even worse outcome. It should also be borne in mind that there may be associated soft-tissue complications if these injuries are not recognized and treated properly in the acute setting. In addition to anteriorposterior and lateral views of the foot, an axial view should be obtained if there is suspicion of calcaneal injury. Fractures of the calcaneus are usually best visualized on lateral view, which allows assessment of the posterior facet position and the loss of calcaneal height (Bohler's angle) in addition to providing a general impression of overall comminution.

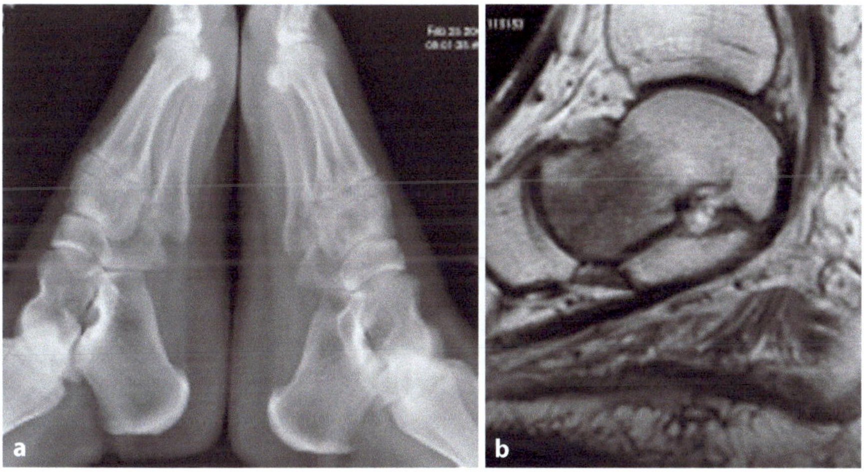

Fig. 5.9 **a** Plain film, frontal view. Normal talus. **b** Spin-echo coronal T1-weighted image shows hypointense bone marrow edema with subtle fracture line of the talus

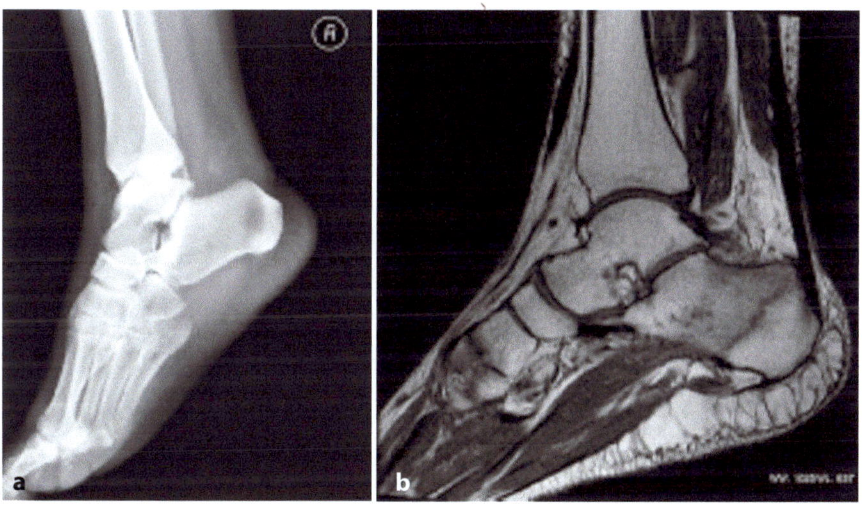

Fig. 5.10 MR sagittal T1-weighted image shows a calcaneal fracture (**a**) that was missed on plain film (**b**)

5.6 Common Errors in the Emergency Department

The main cause of diagnostic error in the ED is the failure to correctly interpret radiographs: the majority of the diagnoses missed on radiography are fractures. Some of the radiological abnormalities are subtle; of these, radiologists miss abnormalities in 3.4% of the cases [1]. However, the majority are obvi-

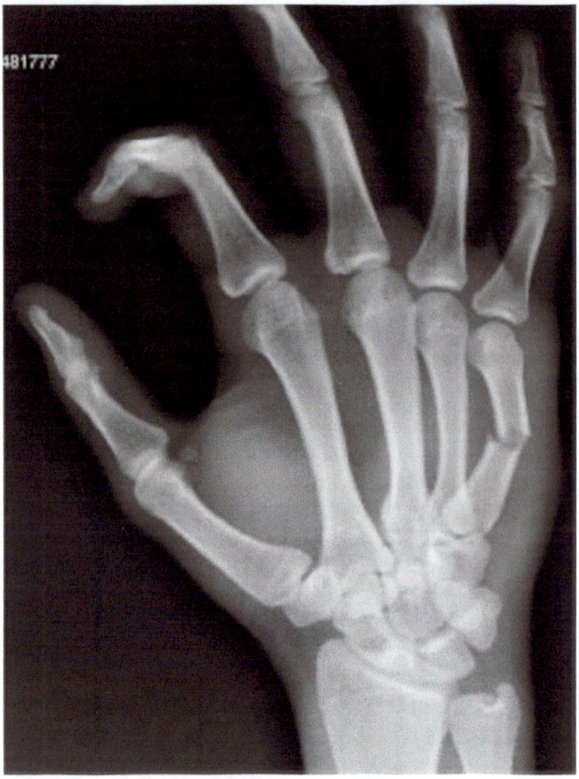

Fig. 5.11 Plain film: fifth metacarpal fracture. A fracture of the medial phalange of the fifth finger was also demonstrated

ous, which suggests inadequate training and/or poor technique in radiological interpretation. Some of the fractures are observed but misinterpreted as normal variants or old injuries. It can be assumed that many abnormalities have been misinterpreted but not recorded.

In the ED, correct identification of an injury requires that the patient is properly examined, which in turn implies that not only must physicians take greater care in specifying the exact radiographic views they wish to obtain (for example, for finger injuries, asking for finger radiographs rather than hand radiographs) but, when possible, they must also state exactly the injury they wish to exclude. In both cases, this will ensure that radiographers perform the correct views (Fig. 5.11). A good clinical examination should also lead to a reduction in the number of fractures and dislocations missed because of failure to radiograph. The decision regarding the need for radiography may be based on guidelines or on a doctor's experience but obviously depends on the findings, history, and physical examination. Injuries missed because of failure to radiograph are typically because the injury was poorly localized or because of the presence of other injuries distracting attention from the injured part.

References

1. Guly HR (2001) Diagnostic errors in an accident and emergency department. Emerg Med J 18:263-269
2. Brooks A, Holroyd B, Riley B (2004) Missed injury in major trauma patients. Injury 35:407-410
3. Hoffman JR, Schriger DL, Mower W et al (200) Validity of a set of clinical criteria to rule out injury to the cervical spine in patients with blunt trauma. N Engl J Med 343:94-99
4. Stiell IG, Wells GA, Vandemheen KL et al (2001) The Canadian C-Spine rule for radiography in alert and stable trauma patients. JAMA 286:1841-1848
5. Mower WR, Oh JY, Zucker MI et al (2001) Occult and secondary injuries missed by plain radiography of the cervical spine in blunt trauma patients. Emerg Radiol 8:200-206
6. Woodring JH, Lee C (1993) The role and limitations of computed tomographic scanning in the evaluation of cervical trauma. J Trauma 34:32-39
7. Davis JW, Phreaner DL, Hoyt DB et al (1993) The etiology of missed cervical spine injuries. J Trauma 34:342-346
8. Daffner RH, Wippold FJ II, Bennett DL et al (2009) ACR appropriateness criteria suspected spine trauma. http://www.guideline.gov/content.aspx
9. Cain G, Shepherdson J, Elliott V et al (2010) Imaging suspected cervical spine injury: plain radiography or computed tomography? Systematic review. Radiography 16:68-77
10. Moscati RM, Lerner EB, Pugh JL (2007) Application of clinical criteria for ordering radiographs to detect cervical spine fractures. Am J Emerg Med 25:326-330
11. Reid DC, Henderson R, Saboe L et al (1987) Etiology and clinical course of missed spine fractures. J Trauma 27:980-986
12. Rhee PM, Bridgman A, Acosta JA et al (2002) Lumbar fractures in adult blunt trauma:axial and single-slice helical abdominal and pelvic computed tomographic scans versus portable plain films. J Trauma 53:663-667
13. Dennis LN, Rogers LF (1989) Superiormediastinal widening from spine fractures mimicking aortic rupture on chest radiographs. AJR 152:27-30
14. Bernstein M (2010) Easily missed thoracolumbar spine fracture. Eur J Radiol 74:6-15
15. Beaunoyer M, St-Vil D, Lallier M et al (2001) Abdominal injuries associated with thoraco-lumbar fractures after motor vehicle collision. J Pediatr Surg 36:760-762
16. Krueger MA, Green DA, Hoyt D et al (1996) Overlooked spine injuries associated with lumbar transverse process fractures. Clin Orthop 327:191-195
17. Samilson RL, Prieto V (1983) Posterior dislocation of the shoulder in athletes. Clin Sports Med 2:369-378
18. Hawkins RJ, Neer CS, Pianta RM et al (1987) Locked posterior dislocation of the shoulder. J Bone Joint Surg Am 69:9-18
19. Neviaser TJ (1980) Old unreduced dislocations of the shoulder. Orthop Clin North Am 11:287-294
20. Schultz TJ, Jacobs B, Patterson RL (1969) Unrecognized dislocations of the shoulder. J Trauma 9:1009-1023
21. Herzberg G, Comtet JJ, Linscheid RL et al (1993) Perilunate dislocations and fracture dislocations: a multicenter study. J Hand Surg Am 18:768-779
22. Perron AD, Brady WJ, Keats TE et al (2001) Orthopedic pitfalls in the ED: lunate and perilunate injuries. Am J Emerg Med 19:157-162
23. Ring D, Jupiter JB, Herndon JH (2000) Acute fractures of the scaphoid. J Am Acad Orthop Surg 8:225-231
24. Ritchie JV, Munter DW (1999) Emergency department evaluation and treatment of wrist injuries. Emerg Med Clin North Am 17:823-842
25. Larsen CF, Brodum V, Skov O (1992) Epidemiology of scaphoid fractures in Odense, Denmark. Acta Orthop Scand 63:216-220
26. Mehta M, Brautigan MW (1990) Fracture of carpal navicular. Efficacy of clinical findings and improved diagnosis of six view radiography. Ann Emerg Med 19:225-231

27. Waizengger M, Barton NJ, David TR et al (1994) Clinical signs in scaphoid fractures. J Hand Surg Br 19:743-746
28. Leslie IJ, Dickson RA (1981) The fractured carpal scaphoid. Natural history and factors influencing outcome. J Bone Joint Surg Br 63:225-230
29. Dias JJ, Brenkel IJ, Finlay DB (1989) Patterns of non union in fractures in the waist of scaphoid. J Bone Joint Surg Br 71:307-310
30. Lindstrom G, Nystrom A (1993) Natural history of scaphoid non-union, with special reference to 'asymptomatic' cases. J Hand Surg Br 18:403-406
31. Tiel-van Buul MM, van Beek EJ, Borm JJ et al (1993) The value of radiographs and bone scintigraphy in suspected scaphoid fracture. A statistical analysis. J Hand Surg Br 18:403-406
32. Nguyen Q, Chaudhry S, Sloan E et al (2008) The clinical scaphoid fracture: early computed tomography as a practical approach. Ann R Coll Surg Engl 90:488-491
33. Amis AA, Miller JH (1995) The mechanisms of elbow fractures: an investigation using impact tests in vitro. Injury 26:163-168
34. Celli A, Nicoli E (2004) Fractures of the radial head associated with dislocation of the elbow. Chir Organi Mov 89:7-19
35. Greenspan A, Norman A, Rosen H (1984) Radial head-capitellum view in elbow trauma: clinical application and radiographic-anatomic correlation. AJR Am J Roentgenol 143:355-359
36. Benger JR, Lyburn ID (2003) What is the effect of reporting all emergency department radiographs? Emerg Med J 20:40-43
37. Judd DB, Kim DH (2002) Foot fractures frequently misdiagnosed as ankle sprains. Am Fam Physician 66:785-794
38. Lowery RB, Claxon JH (1996) Fractures of the calcaneus: Part 1: anatomy, injury, mechanism, and classification. Foot Ankle Nit 17:230-235
39. Barei DP, Bellabarba C, Sangeorzan et al (2002) Fractures of the calcaneus. Orthop Clin North Am 33:263-285

Missed Fractures in Children 6

Fabio Martino, Domenico Barbuti, Gianluigi Martino, and Marco Cirillo

6.1 Brief Overview of the Healthy and Injured Growing Skeleton

Fractures in children are a common occurrence. Most are overt and easily detected, others are subtle and often overlooked. Missed orthopedic injuries, such as fractures and dislocations, are a common event in accident and emergency practice, particularly in children and young adults. Such injuries can have serious consequences since delays in treatment can result in long-term disability. They are also one of the most common causes of medical-legal issues and comprise the largest source of malpractice claims in the emergency department (ED) [1]. Missed fractures occur for various reasons, among the most important of which in EDs is a junior radiologist's (or junior physician's) lack of expertise in child skeletal injuries.

Trauma-related injuries in children differ from those seen in adults, and a full understanding of pediatric injuries requires insight into the unique anatomical and biomechanical features of the growing skeleton, which involve the bone, periosteum, and particularly the epiphyseal plate, which is totally absent in adults. In children, the bone matrix has a lower density because the mesh in the spongy web is wider and the compact bone has a greater porosity, resulting in less elasticity but greater plasticity. This feature makes the bone more pliable, allowing it to considerably bend before it breaks. The periosteal sheath is much thicker (relative thickness) than in adults and less easily torn, but also more easily stripped from the bone. This feature can assure some stability to a fracture, because it limits both the extent of the break and the width of its displacement. The growth plate is present only in

F. Martino (✉)
Radiology Unit, ASL BARI,
Mola di Bari (BA), Italy

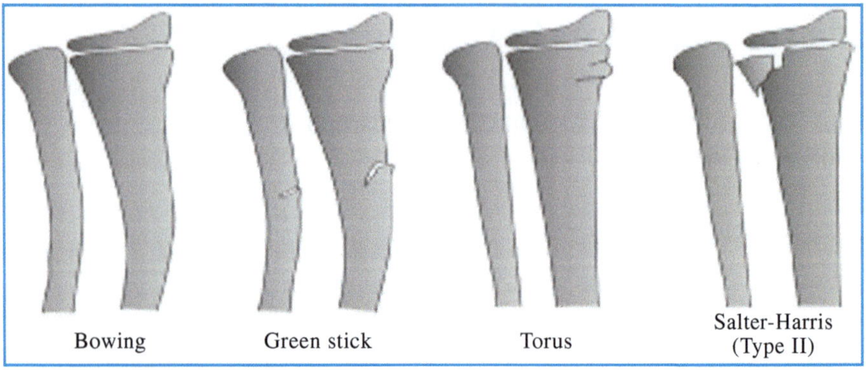

Fig. 6.1 Incomplete fractures

childhood and totally absent in the mature skeleton. The epiphyseal plate represents the weakest area of the growing skeleton and is thus more prone to damage than the nearby bones, ligaments, and tendons. However, it also acts as a shock absorber for the musculoskeletal structures, preserving them from harm and focusing the force of the trauma on itself. In fact, before the full growth spurt, an epiphyseal and/or apophyseal displacement is more likely than a ligamentous injury.

The anatomical attributes of the immature skeleton explain why incomplete fractures are found exclusively in the pediatric population. These fractures comprise plastic deformation, "greenstick" fracture, "torus" fracture, and epiphyseal-metaphyseal or apophyseal fractures, with or without detachment, in an older child (Fig. 6.1).

Plastic deformation, also termed bowing fracture, refers to the ability of immature bone to bend but remaining intact. This stable diaphyseal curvature is produced by radiographically undetectable micro-fractures occurring on the concave side of the involved bone. Bowing fractures most commonly involve the forearm, specifically, the radius and ulna; other frequent locations are the clavicle and fibula [2].

A *greenstick fracture* occurs when a bending bone breaks on its convex side in response to a distracting force, like the bending of a fresh tree branch, but it stays intact on the opposite side. This injury usually involves the diaphysis, most frequently of the forearm bones.

In a *torus fracture* (the term torus is derived from the Latin and in classical architecture refers to the convex molding placed at the base of the column), also known as a buckle fracture, a compression fracture occurs in a long bone, usually near the metaphysis. Although a torus fracture may be seen in any long bone, the distal radius is its most common site. Characteristically, the compression side of a bending bone may buckle upon itself without disrupting the other side, producing a bump. This is a stable incomplete fracture that heals rapidly.

The *epiphyseal-metaphyseal fracture* affects the growth plate, which is the softer part of a child's bones. This injury, also termed a Salter-Harris fracture, is one of the most common injuries sustained by the immature musculoskeletal system of the older child. During the period of skeletal growth, the physis is involved in 15-30% of fractures, more or less extensively [3]; 75% of these cases are seen in children over the age of 10 [4] and the wrist is the most frequent site (50%), followed by the ankle (30%), and the knee and shoulder.

There are five different main types of physeal injuries, depending on the pattern and the possible association with epiphyseal-metaphyseal fracture. As noted above, the most common fracture is the Salter-Harris type II (75% of cases), followed by types I, III, IV and V. Each may have a different prognosis.

Not only do traumatic injuries of the immature musculoskeletal system differ from those of the adult, but the prevalence of one vs. the other changes with age, because of the continuous anatomical, biomechanical and lifestyle alterations that characterize the developmental period. For example, fractures of the clavicle and femoral diaphysis are frequent in early childhood, and those of the distal end of the radius in adolescence. The same considerations apply to joint trauma. The relative weakness of the epiphyseal plate explains why the growth plate rather than the bones and ligaments are more frequently damaged, and why Salter-Harris injuries are more frequent than joint dislocation before the epiphyseal line has been completely obliterated.

Finally, as in adults, a trauma-related injury in a growing child may be linked to a non-accidental cause; particularly important in the pediatric setting is the likelihood of the battered child. Non-accidental trauma has a higher incidence in children younger than 4 years, with 80% of the fractures in abused children occurring before 18 months of age [5], often with a pattern of associated injuries that is very characteristic of child abuse.

6.2 Missed Fractures in Children

6.2.1 Which Fractures and How Many?

Fractures in infants and children are different than those seen in adults. Many are very subtle and difficult to detect with certainty. Particular consideration should be given to "incomplete fractures," i.e., hairline fractures (toddler's fracture) and subtle avulsion fractures. Moreover, assessing bone integrity after the trauma can, in some cases, be difficult. Indeed, normal variations in bone contour and epiphyseal plate configuration are endless and at first may suggest an underlying pathology. Certain fractures can be easily missed in children [6], especially those of the hand phalanges (26.4%) followed by the metatarses (9.5%), distal radius (7.7%), tibia (7.3%), and phalanges of the foot (5.5%). Other common elusive injuries on radiographs are non-displaced greenstick fractures of the wrist and fractures of the scaphoid, zygoma, skull, and radial head [7].

Missed fractures can lead to significant morbidity in all age groups, but particularly in children and young adults. Failure to diagnose a fracture can result in a lack of correct or timely treatment, potentially leading to incorrect healing and further problems within the injured area. Radiology is one of the specialties most vulnerable to claims of medical negligence; thus, it is essential that radiologists be familiar with these relatively common entities and, at the same time, aware of the limitations of radiographic investigations in diagnosing fractures.

6.2.2 The Most Frequent Causes

Missed orthopedic injuries, such as fractures and dislocations, comprise the largest source of malpractice claims in the ED. In fact, fractures account for 71% of the delayed diagnoses in pediatric trauma [8]. Since in the ED a prompt consultation with a radiologist is not universally available during daylight hours, and rarely during "off" hours, X-ray image interpretations may often be provided by emergency physicians [9]. The discrepancy rate in interpreting radiographs between an emergency physician and a radiologist ranges between 3 and 11%, and the majority of malpractice claims involving misread radiographs involve images taken during off hours. Furthermore, 63% of all malpractice events stem from incidents that took place between the hours of 6 pm and 1 am (weekends) and between midnight and 7 am (weekdays). For these reasons, the involvement of radiologists in the routine interpretation of conventional radiographs in trauma settings is encouraged in order to improve the detection of subtle fractures.

The most common reason for errors is misreading radiographs (approximately 80%), such as perceptual errors [10] and satisfaction of search (SOS) errors [11]. Other factors may also affect the accuracy of diagnosing fractures, such as failure to perform radiography [12], and insufficient clinical information [13]. Another cause, probably not as frequent, of missed fracture is the simple lack of mention of a detected injury in a radiographic report [14].

Missed diagnoses arising from radiologists' "slips and lapses" or from other previously mentioned causes may occur with respect to fracture in both adults and children and will not be treated in detail in this chapter. Hence, apart from them, the most frequent causes of failure to recognize a fracture in a pediatric patient are discussed in the following.

6.2.3 Misdiagnosis Due to Cognitive Error

A missed diagnosis may be due to a cognitive error; that is, by a lack of knowledge and expertise in pediatric radiology, even if the imaging method used is adequate and the technique has been correctly executed. In such cases, the injury is seen but is not recognized as such by the radiologist (Fig. 6.2). The

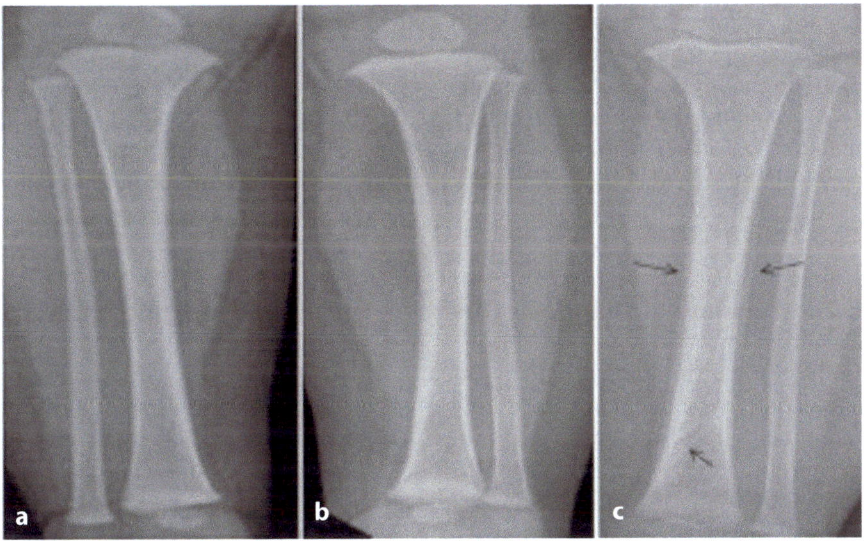

Fig. 6.2 A 1-year-old boy with an initially missed toddler's fracture of the left tibia. AP comparative radiograph of the right (**a**) and left (**b**) legs showed no obvious fracture. An X-ray control 3 weeks later (**c**) revealed an oblique hairline fracture (*single arrow*) of the tibial midshaft, which appears to be surrounded by a periosteal apposition outline (*opposing arrows*)

misreading of an X-ray demonstrating a typical fracture of growing bone indicates a radiologist's lack of adequate experience and expertise in pediatric pathology [15].

As for the incomplete fractures referred to above, a toddler's fracture or chondral injury may be missed if the radiologist is not sufficiently experienced. For example, epiphysiolysis of an unossified humeral or radial head in a very young child (which should generate suspicions of child abuse) can easily be missed because it is not visible on plain radiographs. In these case, X-ray evidence of hemarthrosis (with pain and functional limitations) should raise strong suspicion of a chondral fracture. In doubtful circumstances, an ultrasound (US) may be useful to make the final diagnosis.

6.2.4 Errors Arising from Poor Execution of an Appropriate Imaging Method

Correct technique is the first step to achieve a correct diagnosis. Accordingly, we emphasize that a technician's negligent behavior induces only a latent error (incorrect diagnosis waiting to happen); however, insufficient supervision of the radiologist will cause the latent error to evolve into active fault. Indeed, a poor technique produces films of little or no diagnostic value, while a poor imaging reading is the real threat to patient health and safety. Performing a single radiographic view of an injured bone is always a source of error, especially in the presence of an incomplete fracture. An adequate X-ray evaluation of a traumatized bone should always comprise two planes and, if possible, include two adjacent joints. The X-ray beam should, preferably, be oriented perpendicular to the injured bone segment, particularly at the level of the growth plate. Motion artifacts are unacceptable and should be prevented.

6.2.5 Failure of Diagnosis Due to an Unsuitable Imaging Method

In the clinical suspicion of a bony fracture, X-ray is always the preferred exam and another type of exam should not be considered until appropriate plain-film radiography has been performed [16, 17]. However, a fracture may be missed because it is radiologically invisible or equivocal. In fact, some non-displaced and subtle fractures may be radiographically occult, particularly physeal fractures occurring in an older child. Not infrequently, in a Salter-Harris type I fracture, initial plain radiographs may not show a fracture line, as is also the case with images of a type V injury [3]. Thus, in the presence of negative plain radiographs and high clinical suspicion of occult fracture, failure of diagnosis may occur if the radiologist does not resort to additional, more appropriate examinations. Magnetic resonance imaging (MRI) has high sensitivity and specificity in detecting radiologically occult fractures and remains the reference standard for the early diagnosis of these fractures. The ability of MRI to detect bony fractures that were not seen on radiographs is based on the visualization (obtained on T1-weighted images) of a hypointense fracture line surrounded by adjacent edema with low signal intensity. Fluid-sensitive MRI sequences facilitate the detection of marrow edema with high signal intensity at the site of fracture.

6.3 Pediatric Fractures: How To Not Miss Them

6.3.1 How To Study Skeletal Injuries in the Child

Radiologists have an important role in the diagnosis of pediatric traumatic injury, which is the first cause of emergency admittance worldwide. Injuries caused by skeletal trauma during childhood occur more frequently than in adulthood, although in most cases the extent of anatomical damage is mild. During childhood and adolescence, osteo-articular injury is common, accounting for the majority of the demand for medical care in the ED of a pediatric hospital (> 15-20% of all visits). Plain radiographs remain an important diagnostic tool in the evaluation of extremity trauma [18]. Routine use of comparison films of the contralateral asymptomatic side is not appropriate, although it may be useful in the evaluation of suspected physeal injuries or when a nor-

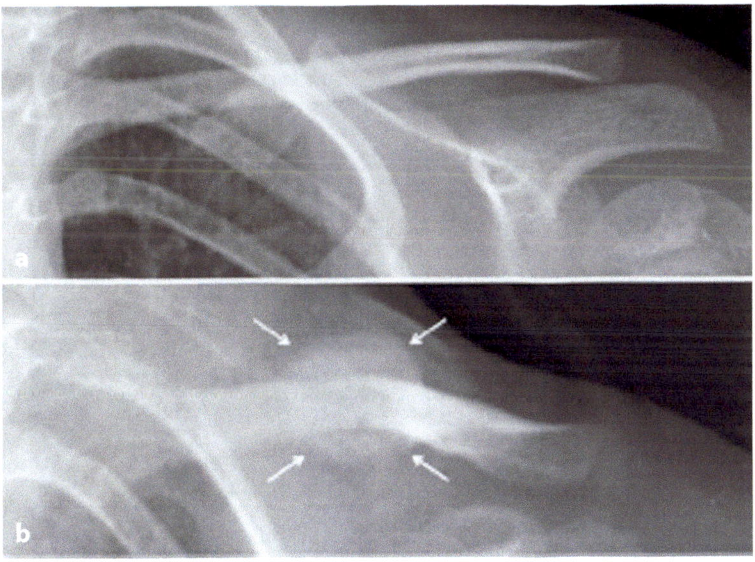

Fig. 6.3 The clavicle is the only bone routinely examined with a single correctly performed AP view. a AP radiography of an injured clavicle negative for fracture in a 4-year-old boy. b The X-ray control after 4 weeks showed a callus bump (*arrows*) surrounding the clavicle midshaft, revealing the missed fracture

mal variant is considered. Clearly, there is no consensus agreement as to whether one should obtain comparative views in all subtle cases, but in our experience this practice has proven to be very worthwhile. In fact, in some cases comparative views are invaluable to solve interpretative ambiguities, thus paving the way to the definitive diagnosis [2].

Indeed, in our experience, comparative views are indicated in case of diagnostic doubt for subtle Salter-Harris fracture after conventional radiographs. Digital imaging helps to reduce the number of repeat radiographs. An image archiving and communication system reduces the overall rate of misdiagnosis. Although conventional radiography is the mainstay of fracture diagnosis, there are multiple conditions in which a fracture can be overlooked by the radiologist. US, CT, and MRI are complementary, and repeated radiographic examination (Fig. 6.3), CT, or MRI may be indicated depending on the clinical scenario.

In the management of patients with suspected skeletal injuries, MRI plays an increasingly important role when diagnostic uncertainty persists after plain-film evaluation [19] and the correct diagnosis is mandatory for adequate treatment. MRI is useful to discover subtle physeal injuries [17, 20], particularly to diagnose non-displaced Salter-Harris type I fracture and Salter-Harris type V radiographically occult fracture, either of which can lead to growth disturbance if not treated properly. An US examination of an extremity (soft tissue, bone surfaces, and adjacent joints) in children with a history of trauma during growth can be helpful for diagnosing either radiographically occult or missed

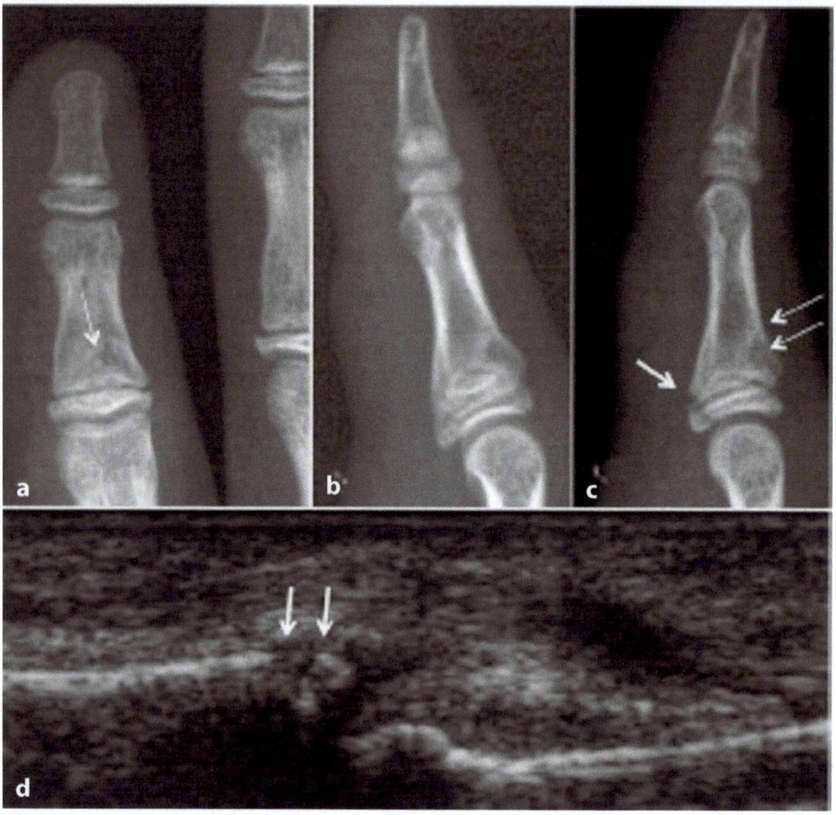

Fig. 6.4 Jammed finger from hyperextension due to a ball-handling injury in a 12-year-old boy. **a** AP X-ray of the injured index finger equivocal for buckle fracture (*single thin arrow*). **b** The suspected damage was not confirmed on the lateral view because it was incorrectly performed. In fact, the finger was obliquely oriented with respect to the X-ray beam. **c** Ultrasound showed an unsuspected small fragment of bone avulsed from the palmar aspect of the base of the middle phalanx (*double thick arrow*), joint effusion, and volar plate distortion. **d** Additional lateral radiography, correctly performed, confirmed the chip fracture (*single thick arrow*) and an angled buckle fracture also (*double thin arrows*)

fractures [21-23]. US is highly appropriate for use prior to the appearance of the secondary ossification center. The most common site of fractures that are radiographically occult and detectable by US is the elbow, followed by the knee, ischium, distal fibula, proximal femur, and humeral shaft [24].

The US diagnosis is based on a clear visualization of cortical bone discontinuity, as a direct sign of fracture, while indirect signs include step-off deformities, tiny avulsed bone fragments, and the double-line appearance of cortical margins. In our opinion, sonographic examination of an area of discomfort is warranted in case of painful soft-tissue swelling in a patient with a history of trauma and without radiographic abnormality (Fig. 6.4).

6.3.2 Skeletal Fractures in the Child: How To Not Miss Them

Literally, every fracture can be overlooked. One of the key points to avoid missing childhood fractures is knowing where they occur and what they look like. In fact, the etiology of radiological error is multifactorial and the main reason for studying diagnostic failure is to try to prevent it. Radiological diagnosis depends entirely on visual perception and on the identification of specific characteristics on radiological images. Mechanical, physiological, and psychological factors contribute in an intricate interplay. The technician and radiologist can do their jobs in a more efficient and focused manner if they receive adequate clinical information from the treating physician(s). Helpful points ("the good six") to avoid missing childhood fractures are:

1. Get appropriate, correctly performed radiographic views (Fig. 6.5);
2. Don't forget to check the bones and the surrounding soft tissues (Fig. 6.6);
3. After conventional radiographs, use ultrasound to evaluate any doubtful cases affecting an extremity (Fig. 6.7);
4. Resort to MRI in case of diagnostic doubt regarding physeal damage or spinal injuries (Fig. 6.8);

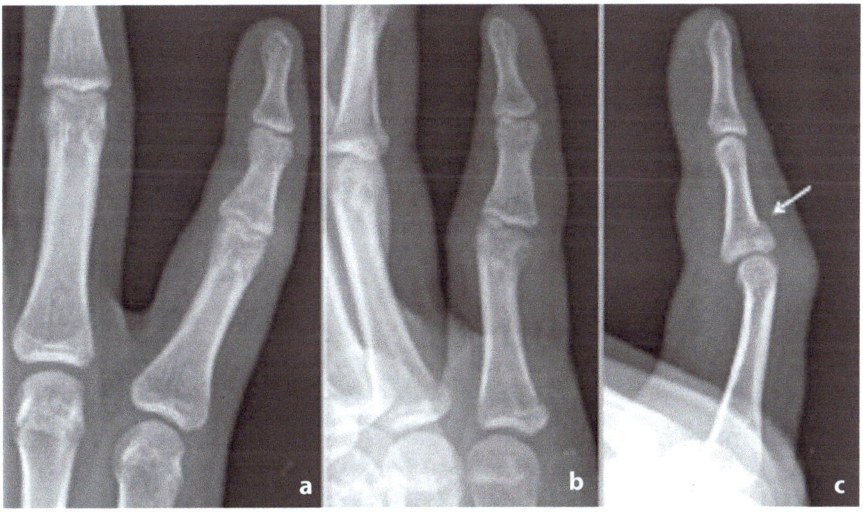

Fig. 6.5 X-ray of the right hand of a 13-year-old girl: 5th-finger fracture. Initial imaging examination (a, b) showed negative radiographic findings for bony lesions. The technically incorrect execution of the radiographic assessment produced the false-negative result. In fact, in addition to the preliminary AP radiograph (a) of the injured finger, the inexperienced technologist performed an oblique projection (b) rather than the standard lateral view, which was finally performed as an additional projection (c) and revealed the missed fracture (*arrow*) on the dorsal aspect of the middle phalanx. It must be kept in mind that chip fractures are frequently detectable only on a true lateral view

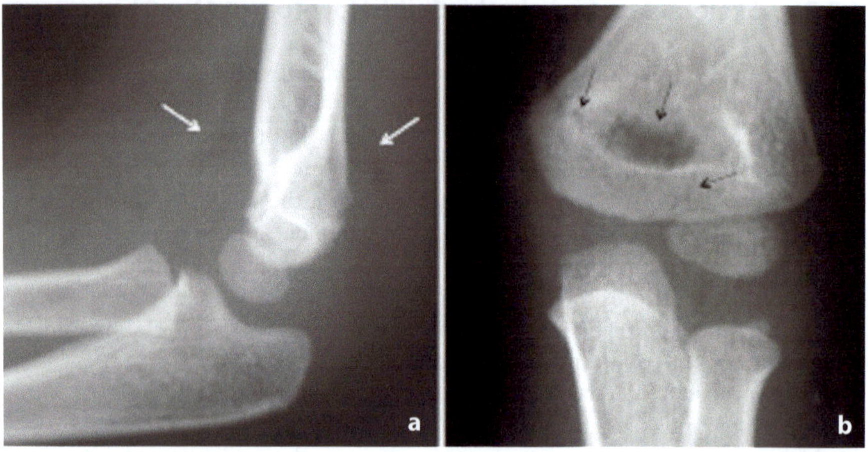

Fig. 6.6 Initial AP X-ray of an injured elbow, ruled negative for fracture. The lateral view (**a**) of the same elbow documents the presence of the fat-pad sign (*white arrows*), indicating an elbow-joint effusion, which should produce a high index of suspicion for a missed fracture. An additional AP view with moderate cephalad angulation of the X-ray beam (**b**) depicts a subtle supracondylar fracture line (*black arrows*)

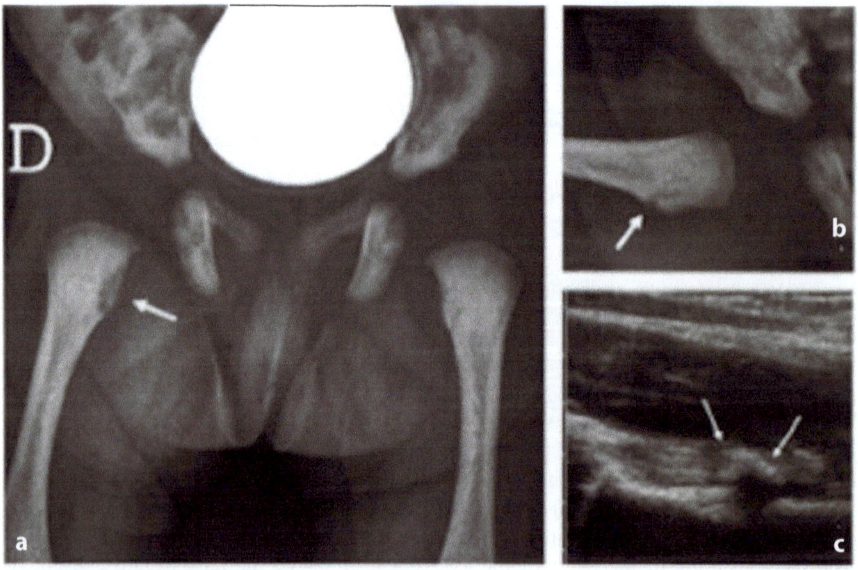

Fig. 6.7 a, b Radiographs showing an incomplete avulsion of the lesser trochanter of the right femur (*arrows*) in a newborn, which occurred during delivery. The lesion was unseen by the radiologist on the baby's initial radiographs, in AP (**a**) and oblique (**b**) views of the right hip. Later, due to persistent pain and functional impairment, an ultrasound exam (**c**) revealed the missed fracture (*double thin arrows*)

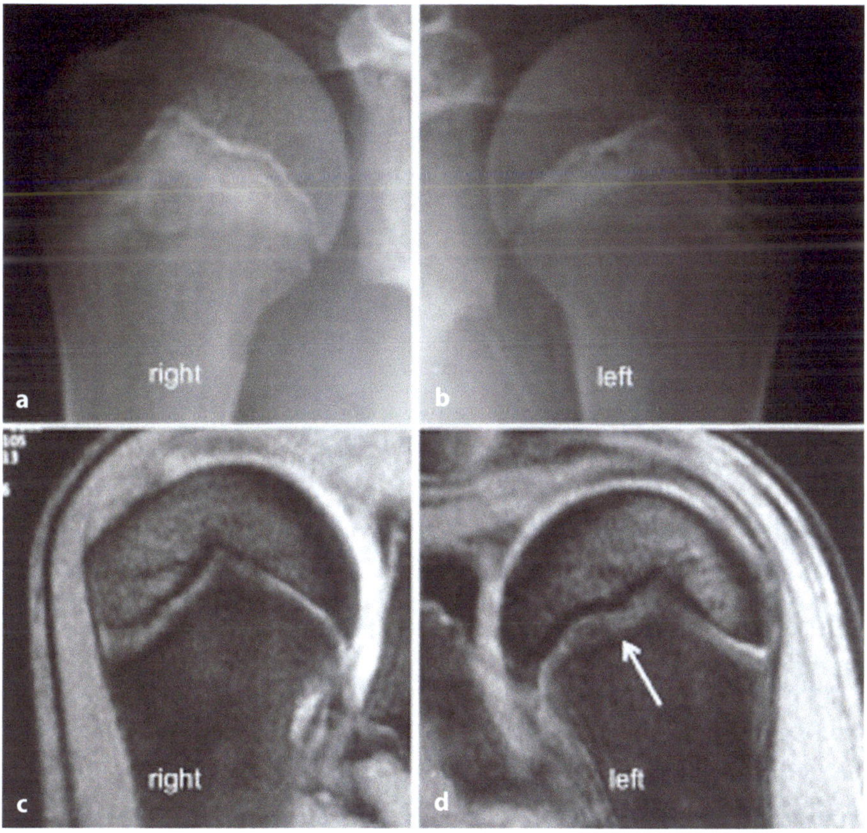

Fig. 6.8 Left painful "little league shoulder" in a 12-year-old boy. a, b The AP view on plain-film was equivocal for growth plate damage. c, d Comparative gradient-echo coronal MRI allowed detection of a type I Salter-Harris fracture of the left humeral growth plate, evidenced by widening of the physeal line on the internal aspect (*arrow*)

5. Acquire good knowledge of pediatric trauma imaging. To err is human, but human error is avoidable by practicing the three Cs (culture, caution, and care of proper procedures). Remember that one recognizes only what one knows. Understanding the mechanism of injury and the expected fracture pattern helps the radiologist supervising the examination to decide which additional views may be needed;
6. In doubtful cases, take an accurate history and perform a physical examination (Fig. 6.9).

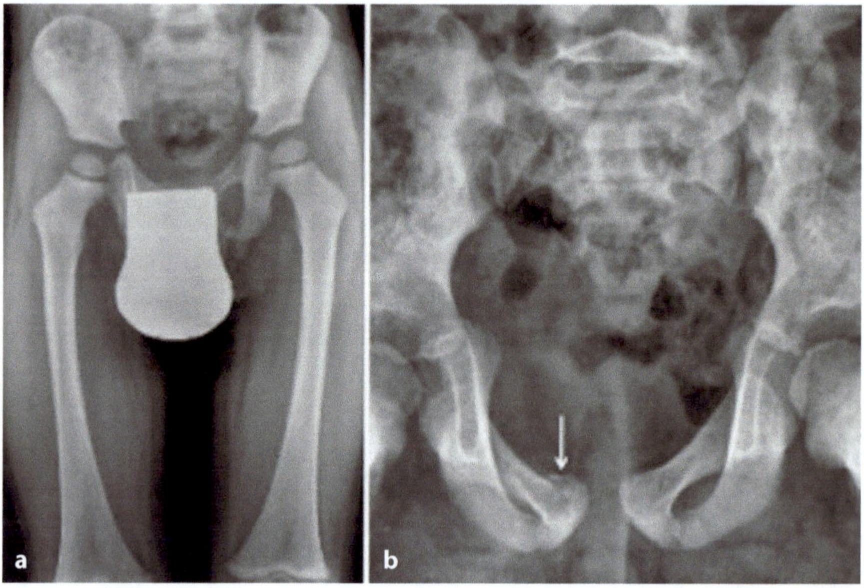

Fig. 6.9 a Radiography of an injured pelvis performed with gonadal protection, which obscures the ischiopubic arch of the painful side. After a physical examination of the child, the radiologist decided to perform an additional X-ray (**b**) without gonadal protection, which highlighted the missed fracture (*arrow*)

References

1. Berlin L (2001) Defending the ''missed'' radiographic diagnosis. AJR 176:317-322
2. Swischuk LE, Hernandez JA (2004) Frequently missed fractures in children (value of comparative views). Emerg Radiol 11:22-28
3. Perron AD, Miller MD, Brady WJ (2002) Orthopedic pitfalls in the ED: pediatric growth plate injuries. Am J Emerg Med 20:50-54
4. Della-Giustina K, Della-Giustina DA (1999) Emergency department evaluation and treatment of pediatric orthopedic injuries. Emerg Med Clin NA 17:895-922
5. Worlock P, Stower M, Barbor P (1986) Patterns of fractures in accidental and non-accidental injury in children: a comparative study. Br Med J (Clin Res Ed) 293:100-102
6. Hernandez JA, Swischuk LE, Yngve DA, Carmichael KD (2003) The angled buckle fracture in pediatrics: a frequently missed fracture. Emerg Radiol 10:71-75
7. Wardrope J, Chennells PM (1985) Should all casualty radiographs be reviewed? Br Med J (Clin Res Ed) 290:1638-1640
8. Furnival RA, Woodward GA, Schunk JE (1996) Delayed diagnosis of injury in pediatric trauma. Pediatrics 98:56-62
9. Petinaux B, Bhat R, Boniface K, Aristizabal J (2011) Accuracy of radiographic readings in the emergency department. Am J Emerg Med 29:18-25
10. Berlin L, Hendrix RW (1998) Perceptual errors and negligence. AJR 170:863-867
11. Berbaum KS, El-Khoury GY, Ohashi K et al (2007) Satisfaction of search in multitrauma patients: severity of detected fractures. Acad Radiol 14:711-722

12. Guly HR (2001) Diagnostic errors in an accident and emergency department. Emerg Med J 18:263-269
13. Pinto A, Brunese L (2010) Spectrum of diagnostic errors in radiology. World J Radiol 2:377-383
14. Brook OR, O'Connell AM, Thornton E et al (2010) Quality initiatives: anatomy and pathophysiology of errors occurring in clinical radiology practice. Radiographics 30:1401-1410
15. Crowe J, Swischuk LE (1977) Acute bowing fractures of the forearm in children: a frequently missed injury. AJR 128:981-984
16. Close BJ, Strouse PJ (2000) MR of physeal fractures of the adolescent knee. Pediatr Radiol 30:756-762
17. Carey J, Spence L, Blickman H, Eustace S (1998) MRI of pediatric growth plate injury: correlation with plain film radiographs and clinical outcome. Skeletal Radiol 27:250-255
18. Wei CJ, Tsai WC, Tiu CM et al (2006) Systematic analysis of missed extremity fractures in emergency radiology. Acta Radiol 47:710-717
19. Jadhav SP, Swischuk LE (2008) Commonly missed subtle skeletal injuries in children: a pictorial review. Emerg Radiol 15:391-398
20. Smith BG, Rand F, Jaramillo D, Shapiro F (1994) Early MR imaging of lower-extremity physeal fracture-separations: a preliminary report. J Pediatr Orthop 14:526-533
21. May DA, Disler DG, Jones EA, Pearce DA (2000) Using sonography to diagnose an unossified medial epicondyle avulsion in a child. AJR 174:1115-1117
22. Hubner U, SchlichtW, Outzen S et al (2000) Ultrasound in the diagnosis of fractures in children. J Bone Joint Surg Br 82:1170-1173
23. Williamson D, Watura R, Cobby M (2000) Ultrasound imaging of forearm fractures in children: a viable alternative? J Accid Emerg Med 17:22-24
24. Cho KH, Lee SM, Lee YH, Suh KJ (2010) Ultrasound diagnosis of either an occult or missed fracture of an extremity in pediatric-aged children. Korean J Radiol 11:84-94

Plain Film or MDCT as a First Diagnostic Tool in Patients with Cervical Spine Injury: Critical Issues

7

Gianluigi Guarnieri, Roberto Izzo, and Mario Muto

7.1 Introduction

Spinal trauma is a very frequent injury that differs in severity and prognosis, varying from an asymptomatic condition to temporary neurological dysfunction, a focal deficit, or even a fatal event. Cervical spine injuries are estimated to occur in 2–10% of such cases, with more than 10,000 new cases each year. The major causes of spinal trauma are high- and low-energy falls, traffic accidents, sport-related, and blunt impact. In all such cases, the associated costs of these injuries are high [1]. Clinical evaluation involves different specialties, including emergency medicine, trauma surgery, orthopedics, neurosurgery, and radiology or neuroradiology [2].

Management depends on the patient's clinical status: conscious, unconscious, sedated and intubated, or non-cooperative. An accurate and rapid diagnosis of the injuries is important because a delayed or undiagnosed unstable injury can lead to severe morbidity and mortality. Among all patients with cervical trauma, 5–10% will show a deterioration of their neurological functions during their Emergency Department admission because of a delay in diagnosis or inadequate spinal immobilization [3].

The rationale of imaging is: (1) to diagnose the traumatic abnormality and characterize the type of injury; (2) to estimate the severity, potential spinal instability or damaged stability, and the presence or absence of associated neurological lesions, in order to avoid neurological worsening and thus potentially medical legal issues; and (3) to evaluate the state of the spinal cord and surrounding structures (MRI is the gold standard technique).

G. Guarnieri (✉)
Department of Diagnostic Radiological Imaging, Neuroradiology Service,
"A. Cardarelli" Hospital,
Naples, Italy

7.2 Plain Film X-Ray vs. Computed Tomography

A common question in patients with spinal trauma is whether there is still a role for plain film X-ray examination, or whether CT has become the first-line modality. Controversy persists regarding the most efficient and effective method of cervical spine evaluation after trauma: cervical standard X-ray (CSR) with three projections (anteroposterior, lateral, and open-mouth odontoid views), multi-detector CT (MDCT), or a combined technique.

Radiography is generally reserved for evaluating patients with suspected cervical spine injury and those with injuries of the thoracic and lumbar areas when suspicion of injury is low. There are as yet no randomized controlled trials but due to the high quality and performance of MDCT and its software (multi-planar-reconstruction and 3D-volume rendering), the superiority of cervical-CT (CCT) over CSR for the detection of clinically significant cervical spine injury is well demonstrated. In fact, based on its improved ability, rapidity, and accuracy in excluding injury and on its high local availability, CCT is replacing CSR for the initial evaluation of patients at any risk for injury [4].

Moreover, given the high sensitivity and specificity of MDCT, trauma patients in many centers are examined only by this modality. However, despite its widespread use, the increased radiation exposure of must be considered, especially in patients who are not at high risk of a lesion, in which case this approach is not justified. Indeed, the abuse of MDCT to search for cervical injury subjects the patient to an unnecessarily high radiation dose to the thyroid, lens, and breast [5].

In order to reduce exposure, it is important to determine exactly which patients would benefit from imaging, based on the clinical evaluation and the probability of a cervical spine injury. Thus, MDCT should be reserved only for appropriate patients, resulting in more cost-effective screening [6].

7.3 Criteria for Patient Selection in MDCT

Choosing the appropriate imaging modality relies on the answers to two questions: (1) Which patient requires imaging and when? (2) Which type of imaging will provide the necessary information?

The rationale of selecting patients for CSR vs. CCT should be based on several criteria. First of all, it is necessary to distinguish the degree of trauma. Patients considered to have a *minor trauma* are stable, mentally alert, not under the influence of alcohol or other drugs, and have no history or physical findings suggesting a neck injury. Patients with *major and severe trauma* include those with multiple traumas, as well as those who are unstable, with a simple temporary neurological dysfunction, focal neurological deficit, or a history or mechanism of injury sufficient to have caused the physiologic range of motion to be exceeded.

Second, it is important to establish whether *trauma risk factors* are present, such as: (a) violent trauma, i.e., a high-energy fall (high risk) vs. one that is of low energy (low risk); (b) the age of the patient: < 5 years old, > 65 years old;

(c) associated lesions, involving the head, chest, abdomen (multi-trauma), etc; and (d) clinical signs, such as Glasgow Coma Scale (GCS), neurological deficit, and vertebral deformation. Combining these elements will allow a decision as to whether a patient is at low risk or high risk for cervical injury. The first group comprises patients who are awake (GCS 15), alert, cooperative, non-intoxicated, and without any distracting injury. The second group consists of those who are unconscious, sedated, intoxicated or non-cooperative or those with a distracting injury or altered mental state (GCS < 15). These patients are considered to have at least a 5% chance of cervical spine injury [3, 6].

7.4 Performance of CCT vs. CSR

Evidence exists that CCT significantly outperforms CSR as a screening test for patients at very high risk of cervical spine injury (major or multi-trauma) and should therefore be used in the initial evaluation. On the other hand, there is insufficient evidence to suggest that CCT should replace CSR as the initial screening method for less injured patients, i.e., those who are at low risk for cervical spine injury (minor trauma) but still require a screening radiographic examination [7].

Two studies were developed as the basis for clinical prediction in minor-trauma, low-risk patients: the National Emergency X-Radiography Utilization Study (NEXUS) and the Canadian Cervical Spine Rule (CCSR).

In 2000, the NEXUS study, after analyzing the data of 34,069 patients, established low-risk criteria to identify patients with a low probability of cervical spine injury who therefore did not need cervical spine imaging [2, 8-12]:

- No tenderness at the posterior midline of the cervical spine;
- No focal neurological deficit;
- Normal level of alertness;
- No evidence of intoxication;
- No clinically apparent, painful injury that might distract the patient from the pain of a cervical spine injury.

If all of these criteria are met, then a radiographic examination should not be performed because the patient has only a low probability of a cervical spine injury, based on a sensitivity of 99% and a specificity of 12.9% [2, 13] (Fig. 7.1).

In 2001, the CCSR study developed three high-risk criteria:

- Age ≥ 65 years;
- Dangerous mechanism;
- Paresthesias in the extremities;

in addition to five low-risk criteria:

- Simple rear-end motor vehicle collision;
- Sitting position in emergency department;
- Ambulatory at any time;
- Delayed onset of neck pain;
- Absence of midline cervical spine tenderness.

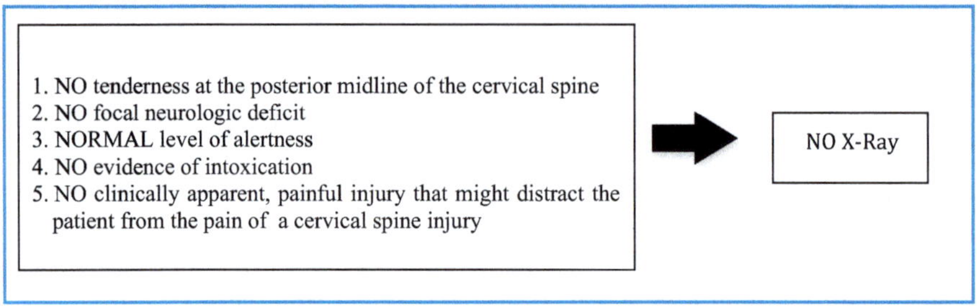

Fig. 7.1 NEXUS low-risk criteria

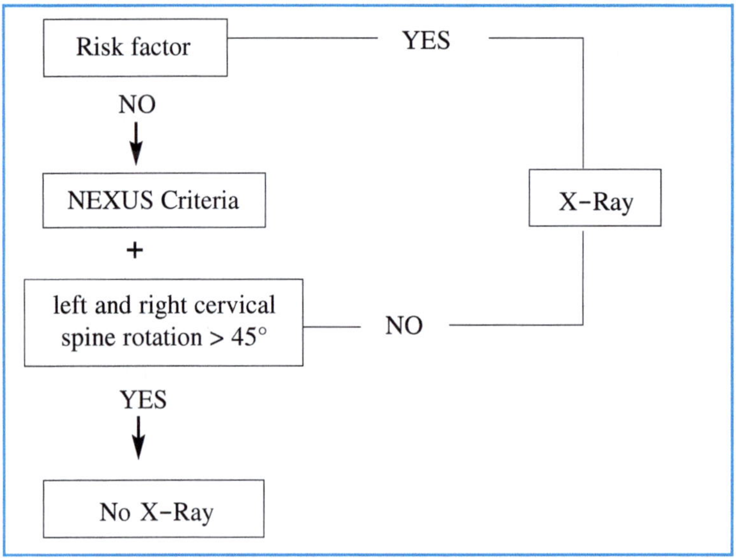

Fig. 7.2 CCSR clinical criteria

These are considered together with the ability of the patient to actively rotate his or her neck in order to determine the need for cervical spine radiography. In practice, if one of these risk factors is present, the patient should undergo imaging evaluation. However, in the absence of these risk factors, the NEXUS criteria should be applied along with a functional evaluation of the cervical spine (left and right cervical spine rotation > 45°). If this functional evaluation is possible, imaging is unnecessary. If cervical movement is determined to be incomplete, then the patient should undergo imaging. The results of that study showed the criteria to have a sensitivity of up to 100% and a specificity as high as 42.5% [12] (Fig. 7.2). If these clinical criteria cannot be applied, a CCT must be performed.

According to the authors, assessing the fulfillment of these criteria prior to cervical spine imaging resulted in a decrease in the number of negative CCTs by about 23.9%. Application of the more liberal NEXUS criteria, including the presence or absence of pain, limited range of motion, or posterolateral cervical spine tenderness, resulted in a decrease of up to 20.2% in the number of negative studies [2].

Both sets of criteria have been accepted by the American College of Radiology (ACR) [14] and by the British Trauma Society in their Appropriateness Guidelines, as a means of screening patients before imaging of the cervical spine. The latter organization recommended fusing the NEXUS criteria with those of the CCSR [15].

The Eastern Association for the Surgery of Trauma (EAST), in a retrospective review of 848 consecutive trauma patients studied by CSR, observed that plain film radiographs were inadequate to fully evaluate the cervical spine and a supplemental CT was commonly required in 72.2% of cases. The study concluded that the NEXUS criteria are inaccurate compared with CT to diagnose cervical-spine fractures and recommended performing a CCT even if the criteria were met [16-18], since a complete cervical spine CT is available, efficient, and accurate.

Blackmore and Hanson developed a set of high-risk criteria to identify trauma patients at high risk of cervical-spine injury who would benefit from CT scanning as the primary radiological investigation. Major and severe traumas justify a direct CCT screening, especially as there may be associated lesions [19, 20].

7.5 Evaluating the Abilities and the Limits of CSR

The same limits encountered with CCT also apply to CSR, and despite these criteria, especially in minor-trauma patients, there are injuries that can be potentially missed. Indeed, false-negative interpretation occurs at a rate of 15–30% and typically includes the following injuries (Figs. 7.3, 7.4):

- A non-displaced fracture of the transverse process of C1 with extension to a lateral mass;
- Type III odontoid fracture of the axis;
- Isolated non-displaced fracture of the transverse process and lamina of C7;
- Fracture of the lamina of C6;
- Isolated fracture of the anterior process of C1.

In these situations, an integrated CCT should be requested [21, 22].

7.6 Conditions Frequently Resulting in False-negative CSRs

The pitfalls of CSR consist of *false-negative* and *false-positive interpretation*, both of which necessitate MDCT integration. False-negative misinterpreta-

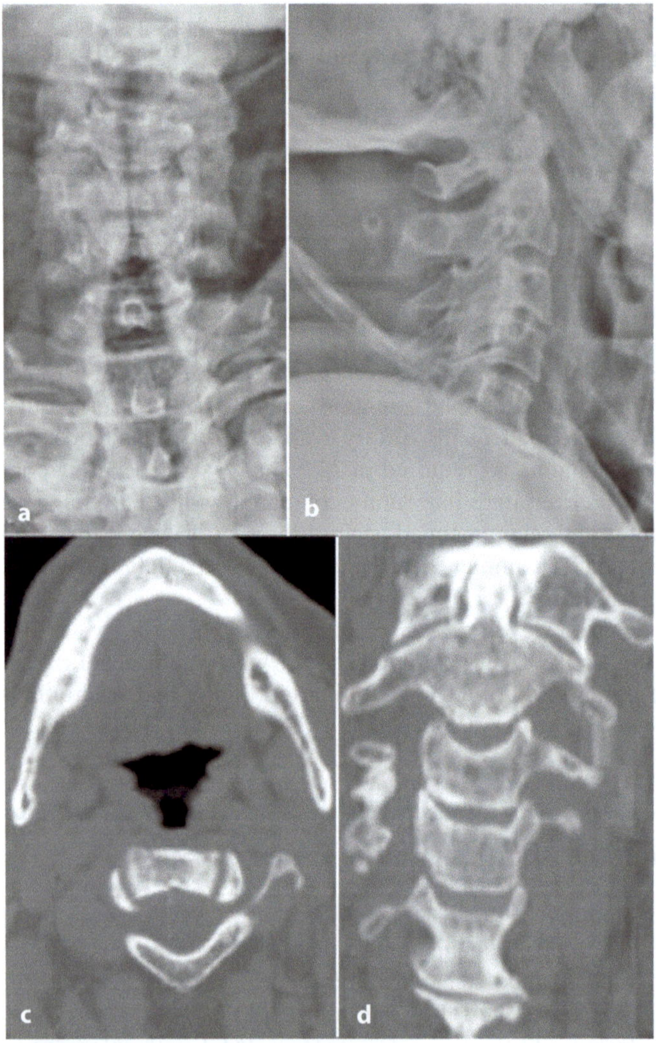

Fig. 7.3 A 60-year-old male who suffered a minor trauma, with neck pain but without neurological deficit. **a, b** The AP and lateral cervical X-ray images did not indicate fracture. The vertebrae were visible up to C6 on the lateral view and a CT integration was required. **c, d** MDCT with axial, coronal and sagittal (not shown) MPR reconstructions revealed a fracture of the C2 vertebral body

tions often involve the cranio-cervical junction as well as at the articular pillars, pedicles, and ligamentous injuries. Hyperflexion ligamentous injury, missed by CSR, should nonetheless be suspected when on the lateral X-ray a focal narrowing of the anterior portion of the intervertebral disc space, focal kyphosis with splaying of the interspinous distance, chip fracture of the anterior cortex of the vertebral body, and subluxation are present. Hyperextension

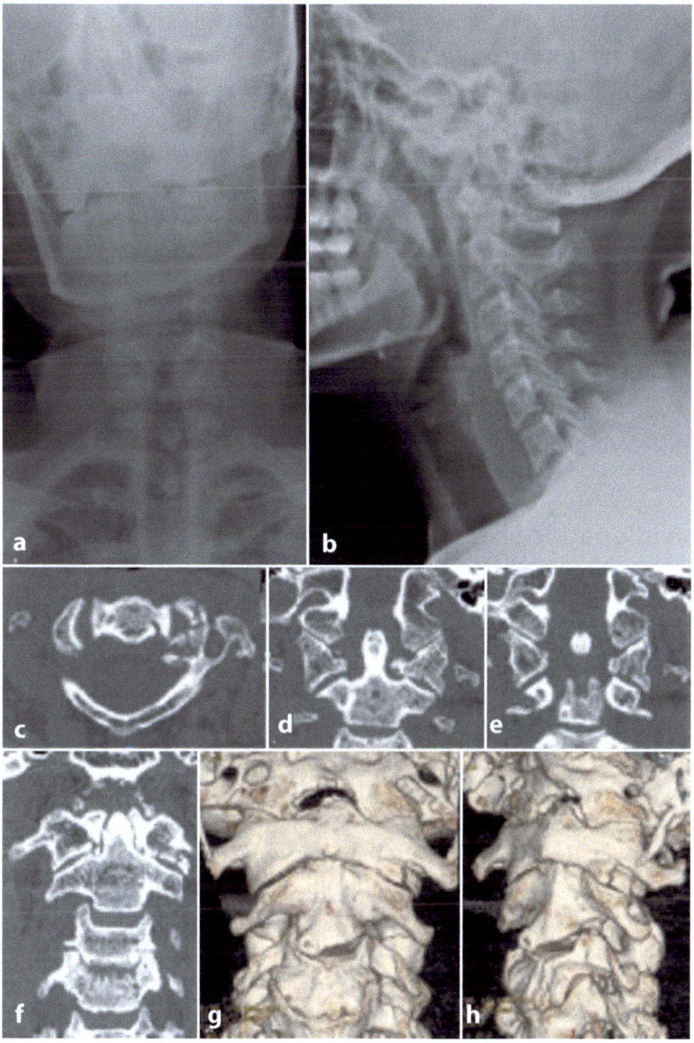

Fig. 7.4 A 40-year-old male who suffered a minor trauma without neurological deficit. **a**, **b** The AP and lateral cervical X-ray images did not indicate fracture. Since the patient complained of a stiff neck, CT integration was required. **c-h** MDCT with axial, coronal, and sagittal (not shown) MPR reconstructions and 3D-volume r

injuries should be suspected if anterior disc space widening, focal lordosis, chip fractures of the anterior vertebral body cortex, and subluxation are seen on the CSR [21].

The articular pillars and the facet joint must be carefully scrutinized on X-ray and then on CT to evaluate whether there are pedicular and laminar fractures. These injuries are caused by extension and slight bending or rotation and they often are non-displaced at the time of presentation, with facet subluxation developing later. Articular pillar injuries are often subtle and they frequently are unstable. Pedicular and laminar fractures are more readily and better seen on coronal MPR MDCT than on AP or lateral radiographs [23]. A focal kyphosis of more than 11° on a static radiograph can suggest a spinal instability and a CCT should be requested [24].

False-negatives are more frequent in patients over the age of 65, as in this group CSR is generally of poor quality or it is done with the patient on his or her back, with a limited view (of at least the first vertebrae) on three-view X-ray films and without any cooperation from the patient. There may also be pre-existing diseases, such as Forestier disease (diffuse idiopathic skeletal hyperostosis, DISH), ankylosing spondylitis (AS), degenerative spondylosis, cervical myelopathy and cervical-occipital stiffness. These can overlap such that a cervical injury is missed.

7.6.1 Diffuse Idiopathic Skeletal Hyperostosis

This common disorder of unknown etiology is characterized by exuberant hyperostosis of the anterolateral aspect of the spinal column, causing bone ankylosis, and by ossification of extraspinal entheses. The enthesopathy leads to ossification of the anterior and posterior longitudinal ligaments of the spine and to the formation of osteophytes and thus, in some cases, stenosis of the medullary canal [25]. In patients with DISH, even slight trauma can result in injuries of the cervical spine that are often difficult to detect by CSR. In fact, plain film radiographs are neither sensitive nor specific in such cases and are inadequate to fully evaluate the cervical spine in these patients. The anatomically modified spine is particularly vulnerable to occult fractures an intense search for injuries by CCT and in some patients by MRI. The poor quality of CSR in DISH patients is due to the exuberance of the bone matrix, the stiffness of the cervical spine, the inability to perform a correct exam, the difficulty in detecting a posterior element injury, the fracture of bridging osteophytes, and hypertrophy of the facet joints, which can produce instability [26-29].

7.6.2 Ankylosing Spondylitis

Ankylosing spondylitis is an inflammatory disorder that, like DISH, is of unknown etiology. In AS, the characteristic ossification of the spinal ligaments, joints, and disks places the patient at maximal risk of suffering a fracture due to a minor trauma, such as represented by a physical load, because of the spine's poor elasticity (so-called bamboo spine) [30]. Hyperextension is the most frequent cause of fracture in the cervical spine of AS patients (81.2%), and the diagnosis may be delayed because the CSR is initially misinterpreted [31]. On plain radiography, problems frequently occur in obtaining lateral-projection radiographs of the lower cervical spine, with failure to visualize this portion o the spine in its entirety. Due to the rigidity of the AS spine, a swimmer's view is also obtained with difficulty, in addition to potentially being a neurologically hazardous maneuver. Generally, given the poor quality of the X-ray images or incorrect technique, articular-process injuries, atlanto-occipital joint fractures, fractures of the C2 laminae, and transverse-process fracture may go undetected on CSR [32].

7.6.3 Pre-existing Degenerative Disease

The most common condition (39.6%) to be misinterpreted as an acute traumatic subluxation or fracture of the cervical spine is pre-existing degenerative disease. For example, degenerative subluxation can be misinterpreted especially when motion is limited at the level of the narrowed disk space [33]. The facet joints above or below this level are subject to increased stress and develop degenerative changes along with stretching of the ligaments and capsular structures. This leads to forward subluxation (anterolisthesis) of a vertebra in relation to the one below it. The disk space at the level of the anterolisthesis is usually preserved. Differential features from a traumatic subluxation are the absence of fracture, the presence of disk space narrowing above or below, facet arthrosis, and other degenerative changes such as spur formation of the vertebral bodies and vacuum disk phenomena.

CSR is unable to distinguish degenerative antero- or retrolisthesis from ligamentous injury in patients with severe degenerative disk disease and facet arthritis, such that an injury may be missed or resulting in a false-positive interpretation. As noted above, every case of anterolisthesis is associated with narrowing of the intervertebral disk spaces below or above the level of the slippage but the intervertebral disk space at this level is always preserved. The degenerative changes are manifested by narrowing or widening of the joint space, sclerosis, spur formation, and a ribbon-like attenuation of the facets with the joint surfaces parallel to each other. A horizontal lucent line seen in the lateral view over the vertebral body produced by uncovertebral joint degeneration may be mistakenly diagnosed as a linear fracture. The uncinate processes are hypertrophic and sclerotic, potentially mimicking an injury. Degenerative ossification in the anterior longitudinal ligament at the lower cervical spine could be misinterpreted as an avulsion fracture. Generally, spondylotic spurs and flattening deformity of the adjacent anterior corner of the vertebral body are present.

Spondylotic retrolisthesis is most commonly seen in the mid-cervical region and is to be differentiated from traumatic extension injury. In spondylotic retrolisthesis, disk-space narrowing, end-plate irregularity, sclerosis, and spur formation are always present at the level of the slippage. In acute traumatic extension injury, the disk space is widened anteriorly in extension. There may also be an accompanying avulsion fragment and associated soft-tissue swelling. Retrolisthesis is also associated with hyperflexion tear-drop fracture. Fractures in the vertebral body and posterior elements, widening of the facet joint spaces, and pre-vertebral soft-tissue swelling may occur in traumatic hyperflexion injury. Degenerative flattening of the vertebral body (platyspondylia) is sometimes misinterpreted as a compression fracture. Features that may serve to differentiate from an acute traumatic compression fracture include osteophyte formation, disk-space narrowing, and other degenerative changes such as vacuum phenomena or ossification of the anterior longitudinal ligament . Again, uncovertebral joint degeneration may produce a horizontal lucent line on the lateral view of the cervical spine, which may be confused with a fracture. In these cases, advanced degenerative changes such as osteophytes and disk-space narrowing are always present. Degenerative ossification in the anterior longitudinal ligament may involve the anterior aspect of the vertebral body. Spondylotic spurs or a flattening deformity of the anterior corner of the adjacent vertebral body are always present in degenerative ossification and might be confused with an avulsion fracture [21].

In patient 65 years and older, cervical-occipital joint injury can be missed on CSR if the patient is non-cooperative such that an open-mouth odontoid view cannot be obtained, resulting in the ability to identify degenerative spondylosis and stiffness of the spine. To avoid this pitfall, a direct CCT should be performed.

7.6.4 Congenital Anomalies

Plain radiographs are particularly limited for the evaluation of the pediatric population because children are less likely to develop fractures, and more likely to have ligamentous and spinal cord injuries without radiographic abnormality (SCIWORA). A pre-existing congenital anomaly is the second most common condition (17.2%) that is confused with acute injuries. For example, in congenital block vertebrae no facet arthrosis or intervertebral disk space narrowing is present and the subluxed vertebral body is buttressed by a spur from the vertebral body below [33].

Congenitally absent cervical pedicle syndrome, characterized by an absent pedicle, abnormal transverse process, and displaced articular segment, is poorly understood but it can mimic cervical injury. The plain film shows the absent pedicle with elongation of the neuroforamen extending from the pedicle above to the pedicle below, mimicking a fracture. CCT can confirm this congenital lesion, showing the absence of the pedicle, the abnormal transverse process and displaced articular segment with well-corticated and smooth margins [34].

Recognition of an asymmetry of the atlantoaxial facets supports the diagnosis of anomalous development of the base of the odontoid. The os odontoideum should be easily differentiated from acute fractures of the dens. The os is rounded and does not match up with the body of the dens, as is true in an odontoid fracture. Additionally, shortening of the sagittal diameter of the ring of the atlas or the overdevelopment or absence of the anterior arch of the atlas may be present with os odontoideum.

7.7 Common Sources of Error in MDCT

Errors can also occur in MDCT imaging. Although the technique is highly sensitive and specific for bony injuries, there are some conditions that can mimic or reduce the sensitivity for the detection of acute spinal injuries. These can be classified as *anatomical variants, imaging artifacts*, and certain *underlying spinal pathologies* [35].

Anatomical variants include block vertebrae, hemivertebrae and spina bifida. Suspected lesions with either well-corticated or smooth margins, as seen on MPR, must be further evaluated to distinguished between a normal finding and a true line fracture. The vascular channels formed by the venous plexuses and nutrient arteries within the vertebra may be mistaken for fractures. Prominent venous channels (Hahn's channels) are recognized by their centrally traversing linear lucency, which is fairly regular and uniform at the equatorial zone of the vertebra.

Motion-related and beam-hardening artifacts during image acquisition may lead to unsharpness from image blur and misregistration artifacts. The former may obscure injuries, while the latter can mimic injuries such as spondylolisthesis and fractures. Generally, an artifact can be suspected if the lucent line is too straight and extends beyond the margin of the vertebral body. A repeat scan should be performed if there is any uncertainty.

As for CSR, on MDCT underlying spinal pathologies (such as DISH, ossification of the posterior longitudinal ligament, AS, and osteoporosis) can be deceptive and lead to fracture misinterpretation. In fact, discontinuous ossification in any of these conditions may mimic vertebral fractures. Conversely, a non-displaced fracture at the level of the end-plates may be mistaken for discontinuous ossification. In an osteoporotic spine, the loss of normal trabeculae may render fracture lines less perceptible and cortical discontinuity may be the only sign.

7.8 Conclusions

The management of cervical spine injuries remains complex and controversial. Clinical status, the type of trauma, and the various trauma risk factors are important elements that must be considered in the choice of an imaging modality. The continued development of high-performance and fast CT with the possibility of low-dose radiation will allow the screening of all patients with suspected lesions.

References

1. Leucht P, Fischer K, Muhr G, Mueller EJ (2009) Epidemiology of traumatic spine fractures. Injury 40:166-172
2. Griffith B, Bolton C, Goyal N et al (2011) Screening Cervical Spine CT in a Level I Trauma Center: Overutilization? AJR 197:463-467
3. Saltzherr TP, Fung Kon Jin PH et al (2009) Diagnostic imaging of cervical spine injuries following blunt trauma: A review of the literature and practical guideline. Injury 40:795-800
4. Bailitz J, Starr F, Beecroft M et al (2009) CT should replace three-view radiographs as the initial screening test in patients at high, moderate, and low risk for blunt cervical spine injury: a prospective comparison. J Trauma 66:1605-1609
5. Chan PN, Antonio GE, Griffith JF et al (2005) Computed tomography for cervical spine trauma. The impact of MDCT on fracture detection and dose deposition. Emerg Radiol 11:286-290
6. Hanson JA, Blackmore CC, Mann FA, Wilson AJ (2000) Cervical spine injury: a clinical decision rule to identify high-risk patients for helical CT screening. AJR 174:713-717
7. Holmes JF, Akkinepalli R (2005) Computed tomography versus plain radiography to screen for cervical spine injury: a meta-analysis. J Trauma 58:902-905
8. Hoffman JR, Wolfson AB, Todd K, Mower WR (1998) Selective cervical spine radiography in blunt trauma: methodology of the National Emergency X-Radiography Utilization Study (NEXUS). Ann Emerg Med 32:461-469
9. Tins BJ, Cassar-Pullicino VN (2004) Imaging of acute cervical spine injuries: review and outlook. Clin Radiol 59:865-880
10. Dickinson G, Stiell IG, Schull M et al (2004) Retrospective application of the NEXUS low-risk criteria for cervical spine radiography in Canadian emergency departments. Ann Emerg Med 43:507-514
11. Stiell IG, Clement CM, McKnight RD et al (2003) The Canadian C-Spine Rule versus the NEXUS low risk criteria in patients with trauma. N Engl J Med 349:2510-2518
12. Stiell IG, Wells GA, Vandemheen KL et al (2001) The Canadian C-spine rule for radiography in alert and stable trauma patients. JAMA 286:1841-1848
13. Hoffman JR, Mower WR, Wolfson AB et al (2000) Validity of a set of clinical criteria to rule out injury to the cervical spine in patients with blunt trauma. National Emergency X-Radiography Utilization Study Group. N Engl J Med 343:94-99
14. Appropriateness Criteria American College of Radiology Website American College of Radiology: ACR Appropriateness Criteria. Clinical condition: suspected spine trauma. www.acr.org/SecondaryMainMenuCategories/ qualitysafety/appcriteria/pdf/ExpertPanelonNeurologic Imaging SpineTrauma Published 1999 Updated 2009
15. British Trauma Society (2003) Guidelines for the initial management and assessment of spinal injury. British Trauma Society, 2002. Injury 34:405-425
16. Duane TM, Mayglothling J, Whelan JF et al (2011) National Emergency X-Radiography Utilization Study criteria is inadequate to rule out fracture after significant blunt trauma compared with computed tomography. J Trauma 70:829-831
17. Ghanta MK, Smith LM, Polin RS et al (2002) An analysis of Eastern Association for the Surgery of Trauma practice guidelines for cervical spine evaluation in a series of patients with multiple imaging techniques. Am Surg 68:563-567
18. Gale SC, Gracias VH, Reilly PM, Schwab CW (2005) The inefficiency of plain radiography to evaluate the cervical spine after blunt trauma. J Trauma 59:1121-1125
19. Berne JD, Velmahos GC, El-Tawil Q et al (1999) Value of complete cervical helical computed tomographic scanning in identifying cervical spine injury in the unevaluable blunt trauma patient with multiple injuries: a prospective study. J Trauma 47:896-902
20. Blackmore CC, Emerson SS, Mann FA, Koepsell TD (1999) Cervical spine imaging in patients with trauma: determination of fracture risk to optimize use. Radiology 211:759-765
21. Crim JR, Moore K, Brodke D (2001) Clearance of the cervical spine in multitrauma patients: the role of advanced imaging. Semin Ultrasound, CT MR 22:283-305

22. Theocharopoulosa N, Chatzakisc G, Karantanasc A et al (2010) CT evaluation of the low severity cervical spine trauma: When is the scout view enough? Eur J Radiol 75:82-86
23. Mower WR, Oh JY, Hoffman JR for the NEXUS group (2001) Occult and secondary injuries missed by plain radiography of the cervical spine in blunt trauma patients. Emerg Radiol 8:200-206
24. White III A, Panjabi M (1990) Clinical biomechanics of the spine, 2nd edn. JB Lippincott, Philadelphia
25. Colina M, Govoni M, De Leonardis F, Trotta F (2006) Diffuse idiopathic skeletal hyperostosis (D.I.S.H.). Reumatismo 58:104-111
26. Hendrix RW, Melany M, Miller F, Rogers LF (1994) Fracture of the spine in patients with ankylosis due to diffuse skeletal hyperostosis: clinical and imaging findings. AJR Am J Roentgenol 162:899-904
27. Sreedharan S, Li YH (2005) Diffuse idiopathic skeletal hyperostosis with cervical spinal cord injury -a report of 3 cases and a literature review. Ann Acad Med Singapore 34:257-261
28. Strohm PC, Zwingmann J, Bley TA et al (2006) Injuries of the cervical spine with Forestier's disease. Problems in the diagnostic and surgical management Unfallchirurg 109:905-909
29. Harrop JS, Sharan A, Anderson G et al (2005) Failure of standard imaging to detect a cervical fracture in a patient with ankylosing spondylitis. Spine 30:417-419
30. Einsiedel T, Schmelz A, Arand M et al (2006) Injuries of the cervical spine in patients with ankylosing spondylitis: experience at two trauma centers. J Neurosurg Spine 5:33-45
31. Westerveld LA, Verlaan JJ, Oner FC (2009) Spinal fractures in patients with ankylosing spinal disorders: a systematic review of the literature on treatment, neurological status and complications. Eur Spine J 18:145-156
32. Koivikko MP, Kiuru MJ, Koskinen K (2004) Multidetector computed tomography of cervical spine fractures in ankylosing spondylitis. Acta Radiol 7:751-759
33. Kim KS, Rogers LF, Regenbogen V (1986) Pitfalls in plain film diagnosis of cervical spine injuries: false-positive interpretation. Surg Neurol 25:381-392
34. Gurpinar EI, Dross P (1999) Imaging of the congenitally absent cervical pedicle: avoidance of misdiagnosis in a setting of trauma Emerg Radiol 6:307-309
35. Khoo JN, Chong le R, Chan EH, Poh AC (2011) Pitfalls in multidetector computed tomography imaging of traumatic spinal injuries. Emerg Radiol 18:551-562

Errors in Sonography

8

Roberto Farina and Amelia Sparano

8.1 Introduction

Ultrasound (US) is particularly subject to errors, more than any other diagnostic imaging technique; indeed, the misinterpretation of images should be considered as a significant risk in US-based diagnosis [1]. Ultrasonography is highly operator-dependent, making it essential that the sonographer is properly trained in order to be able to implement the full diagnostic capabilities of the technique. The skill of the operator is based on the ability to maximize the diagnostic information available and to properly interpret the images.

As a preliminary step in proper US scanning, the sonographer should first evaluate the patient in terms of physical constitution and the presence of conditions potentially limiting the examination, such as obliged positions, scars, etc. Correct choices regarding the transducer, the setting of the technical equipment, and the amount of sonographic gel are fundamental to obtain usable diagnostic images [2]. At the same time, the need to modify one or all of these parameters during the examination, according to the different conditions that may be encountered, must be recognized, as the proper adjustment(s) could make the difference between a good US exam and a non-diagnostic one.

Modern US equipment is pre-loaded with "pre-sets," a set of pre-determined parameters related to the different organs and type of patient. While such pre-sets are useful as screening images or as an initial approach, they almost always need to be adjusted to the particular clinical situation and pathology.

To demonstrate these concepts, the following cases are representative:

A. Sparano (✉)
Department of Diagnostic Radiological Imaging, "A. Cardarelli" Hospital, Naples, Italy

1. A patient complains of right flank pain. Abdominal US scanning should be initially performed using a convex probe. If an acute appendicitis is suspected based on clinical or diagnostic appearances, the US examination should be integrated with further scanning using a high-frequency linear probe (7–10 Mhz rather than 10–13 Mhz). Rhythmic compression can be exerted on the abdominal wall at the location corresponding to the appendix to check for the presence of Blumberg's sign [3];
2. A woman complains of acute pain in the lower abdomen. Pelvic US scanning should be initially performed with a convex probe to evaluate the pelvic anatomy and any signs of pathology. If a gynecological pathology is suspected, the US examination should be integrated with transvaginal or transrectal scanning. Transvaginal sonography better evaluates the morphology, structure, and vascularization of the pelvic organs. Its findings might be more specific than those obtained with computed tomography (CT) and are even as informative as those obtained with magnetic resonance imaging (MRI) [4].

These examples emphasize the importance of completing the exam with a second probe. Failure to do so may compromise the ability to make a diagnosis, regardless of sonographer experience. Evaluation of the diagnostic hypothesis, formed by integrating the US images with the clinical history, epidemiology, and possible differential diagnosis, will lead to the most appropriate treatment planning.

There is considerable evidence showing that the first source of "error" in ultrasonography depends on the technical skill of the operator. Obtaining a good diagnostic exam is directly related to operator skill, training, and experience. A sonographer's responsibilities include maximal use of the capability of US, the knowledge of what to look for, and the ability to interpret the appearances on the image, based on an understanding of the physiology and pathological changes of the examined organs (Fig. 8.1).

Another source of misinterpretation in US concerns artifacts, which together with faulty interpretation of the image in an US-based diagnosis can lead to incorrect and potentially harmful treatment. Both may depend on the physical pitfalls of US imaging or the inadequate quality of the equipment, due to its low technical standards and/or poor maintenance. The operator should know how to obtain the most useful and relevant images from the US device at hand and to avoid the pitfalls of scanning. Physical artifacts are mostly due to the physical properties of US waves and the environment in which they are propagated. Accordingly, the appropriate procedures and imaging methods must be applied in order to reduce or even eliminate this source of error. The ability to recognize and, as far as possible, to remedy US artifacts will improve image quality and ultimately patient care. Nonetheless, under certain conditions artifacts may not be prevented and the weight of their negative impact on a correct final diagnosis is totally dependent on the experience and knowledge of the sonographer. In fact, artifacts can provide clues as to tissue composition and even aid in the diagnosis. For example, one of the greatest limits in

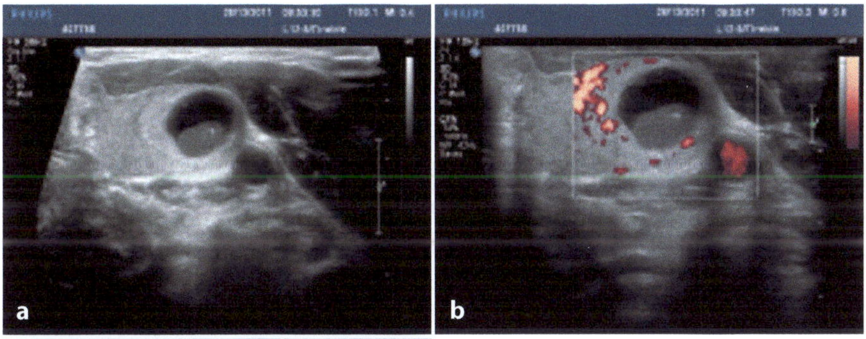

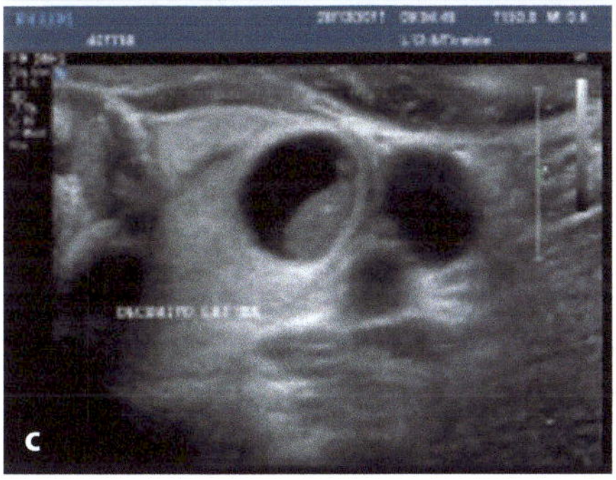

Fig. 8.1 a This patient was brought to our attention for fine-needle aspiration cytology (FNAC) of a complex nodule in the left lobe of the thyroid gland, with endoluminal papillary-like proliferation. **b** Color-Doppler did not detect any vascular signal. **c** By varying the decubitus of the patient the endoluminal proliferation changed position as well, thus demonstrating its necrotic nature. The FNAC was no longer needed

abdominal US is gastrointestinal meteorism. While there are a few technical tricks that can be used to limit the associated noise and thereby to obtain better diagnostic images, sometimes the distribution of the intestinal gas can also guide the diagnosis; for example, pneumoperitoneum depending on a blown viscera, bowel dislocation by an expansive mass, etc.

In a pelvic US examination, expansion of the bladder will raise the bowel, allowing better evaluation of the pelvic organs.

Sometimes, a repeat US examination, after proper intestinal premedication (laxatives, fasting, semi-liquid diet, etc.), can help in resolving diagnostic doubts.

Certain artifacts, such as shadowing and enhancements, can be useful for determining the nature of masses and can lead to a diagnosis, such as acoustic shadowing in breast nodules, the gallbladder, or renal lithiasis, glimmering in renal intracaliceal stones, color-Doppler jet flow in a ureteral jet, etc.

Optimization of the US image also depends on the skill of the operator, who should be able to distinguish a noisy image, as the product of an inadequate setting and/or the overlap of artifacts, from the expression of a complex disease. As examples [1, 2, 5]: In a gallbladder presenting echogenic content, is it corpusculated bile (Fig. 8.2)? Is an ovarian cyst with echoes scattered throughout its lumen a corpus luteum or mucinous cysts? And an echogenic renal cyst, is it a complicated cyst or a cystic tumor (Fig. 8.3)?

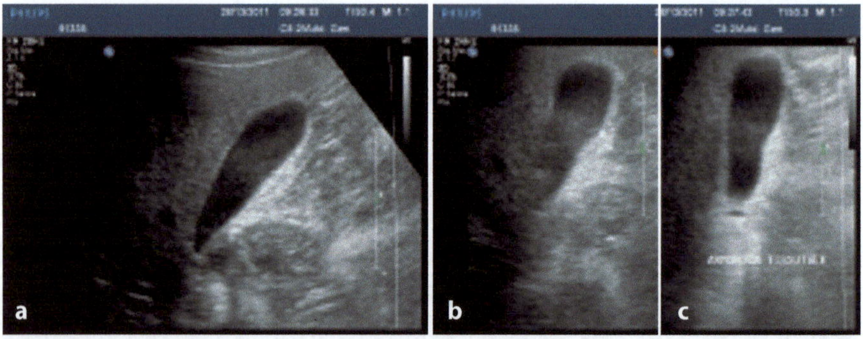

Fig. 8.2 **a** Painful cholecystitis with corpusculated material in the lumen of the gallbladder. **b** The gallbladder contains inhomogeneous content: thickened bile? **c** Rather than a speckle noise suppression filter, which was considered too strong, a "tissue harmonic imaging" filter was employed, revealing an actual corpusculated content. The artifact was reduced without eliminating the fine echoes

Furthermore, there are circumstances in which exaggerated pre- or post-processing of the images, so-called noise reduction, could eliminate many signs of potential diagnostic value. It should be kept in mind that the best US image, from an iconographic point of view, is not always the most diagnostic one.

A skilled sonographer should always request a repeat examination after hours or days, as and when needed. An early US evaluation of an acute pancreatitis may not find any specific pattern, while a few hours later there may be sufficient ultrasonographic evidence, such as parenchymal edema or a peripancreatic fluid collection. Similarly, in the evaluation of an ovarian complex cyst, repetition of the exam a few days later, depending on the patient's menstrual cycle, could help in differentiating a corpus luteus from a mucinous cyst or other pathology. An echogenic ovarian cyst detected in the second phase of the ovarian cycle remains unchanged in size and appearance after several days when it is a mucinous cyst, while it will evolve within a few days, showing thin intraluminal fibrin septa (the "fishing net" sign) or strangely shaped, coarse clots (sailing, star, etc.), until it undergoes a complete spontaneous involution when it is a hemorrhagic corpus luteum. An ectopic pregnancy provides little information during an early US examination while it can be diagnosed if a tubal sac is present between the ovary and uterine horn, indicating the presence of a tubal pregnancy [6]. Similarly, in the early evaluation of abdominal trauma, splenic or hepatic lesions may be missed and detected only after a few hours.

Advances in modern US equipment have significantly improved the diagnostic power of sonography. Features that allow better image quality or the elimination of imaging defects reduce the risk of image misinterpretation and their proper use is of utmost importance. In addition, there are numerous methods by which the different manufacturers of US devices allow compromises to be made during the scanning process in order to improve image quality and

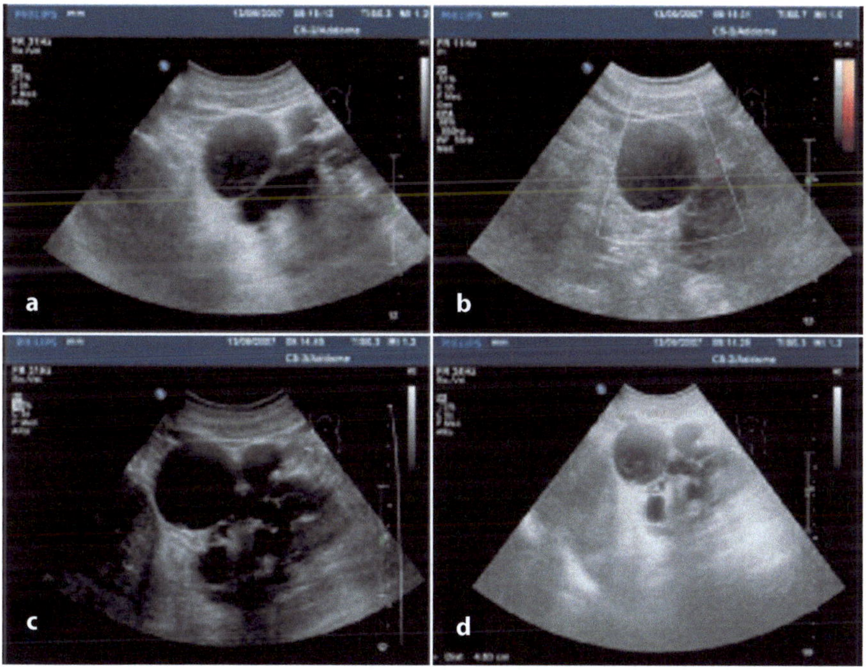

Fig. 8.3 Adult polycystic kidney. **a** Visibility of irregular echoes in the lumen of a major cyst. **b** Detail of the complex cyst. **c** Post-processing "correction" of the possible error with filters. The cysts are now entirely non-echogenic and well defined. **d** Excessive filtering of the image caused a diagnostic error: a proliferative component (cystic tumor) was evident in the major cyst but disappeared in the filtered image

enhance diagnostic information, such as the introduction of contrast medium [7], pre- and post-processing elaboration (i.e., 3D volume rendering), and highly sensitive color-power-Doppler [8, 9].

Ultrasound imaging has become an important diagnostic tool for an increasing number and range of clinical conditions, such as the detection of abdominal masses or as the first evaluation of trauma or a non-traumatic acute abdomen. In many cases, imaging can even be performed at bedside. Additional strengths of US imaging are its safety, non-invasive nature, and comparatively low cost, which support its use as a first-line diagnostic test in many different clinical scenarios. US also significantly contributes to minimally invasive therapy and to more complex diagnostic procedures, increasing diagnostic accuracy and enabling a greater range of treatment options to be offered to patients.

Nevertheless, a scan that is properly executed with low-quality equipment by a knowledgeable and well-trained operator is far better than a poorly performed scan obtained with the latest high-tech machine. A good sonographer will get the best out of even the lowliest scanning device and produce a result that will promote correct patient management. A misleading result from a top-of-the-line scanner can be highly damaging as, at the very least, it will delay correct treatment but, far more serious, it may direct incorrect management. The operator should be aware of the limitations of the technique and take them into account, communicating them where necessary and asking for other diagnostic imaging options (CT, MRI, angiography, etc.) when appropriate [10]. The ability to make these types of evaluations represents part of the skill of the sonographer and allows the definition of shared diagnostic protocols.

8.2 Optimizing B-mode Ultrasound Scanning

- Perform one or more preliminary wide scans.
- Focus the attention on the disease or at least on the detected anomaly.
- Use multifrequency probes and choose the highest frequency one for the region of interest.
- Use the lowest frame rates and the greatest line density.
- Enlarge the image by using depth rather than zooming.
- Put the focal zone on the affected area or immediately below it.
- If there are multiple focal zones, use the fewest of them on the region of interest.
- Perform the initial basic scans without using correction software.
- Use correction software only after having identified the clinical condition.
- Modify the gain and the contrast of the images comparatively on double images.
- Gradually compress to remove artifacts and evaluate the modifiability of the lesion.
- Turn on the color-power-Doppler only after having obtained a successful image optimization in B-scan.
- Use the most advanced methods (contrast agents ultrasound, CT, MRI) only after a basic ultrasound scan.
- Do not hesitate to ask for a second opinion by consulting another colleague.

8.3 Optimizing Color-Power-Doppler Ultrasound Scanning

- Perform a preliminary B-mode ultrasound scanning.
- Optimize the B-scan image.
- Compare color-power-Doppler and B-scan images on double images.
- Use the highest frequency.
- In the evaluation of paired organs (such as testicles), set the color-power-Doppler parameters on the healthy organ.
- Change the PRF (pulse repetition frequency) and the ROI (region of interest) to evaluate low- or high-speed flow.
- Note that the Doppler effect is dependent on the angling of the probe; cor-

rectly put set the probe on the patient's skin to ensure an angle of insonation < 60°.

- To evaluate very low flows or when a proper angle of insonation cancould not be ensured, use the power, which is more sensitive.

8.4 Common Sources of Error in Sonography

- Lack of knowledge of the technical equipment.
- Inadequate optimization of the image.
- Use of inappropriate probes.
- Lack of attention to the clinical history and examination.
- Lack of communication with the patient, who may be afraid or uncooperative.
- Lack of knowledge of the possible clinical disorders and their complications.
- Lack of knowledge of the possible differential diagnoses.
- Over-estimation of one's own skill and failure to suggest other investigative techniques, such as CT or MRI.
- Inadequacy of the diagnostic report, too terse or verbose.
- Poor clinical evaluation of the detected pathology and its possible evolution.
- Failure to suggest further ultrasound examinations or to recognize their proper timing.

References

1. Feldman MK, Katyal S, Blackwood MS (2009) US artifacts. Radiographics 29:1179-1189
2. Yeh HC (2001) Some misconceptions and pitfalls in ultrasonography. Ultrasound Q 17:129-155
3. Vissers RJ, Lennarz WB (2010) Pitfalls in appendicitis. Emerg Med Clin North Am 28:103-118
4. Ozdemir S, Celik C, Emilik D et al (2009) Assessment of myometrial invasion in endometrial cancer by transvaginal sonography, Doppler ultrasonography, magnetic resonance imaging and frozen section. Int J Gynecol Cancer 19:1085-1090
5. Mostbeck GH, Mallek R (1993) Possibilities of error and pitfalls in sonography of the gallbladder and bile duct. Radiologe 33:19-26
6. Gurel S, Sarikaya B, GurelK, Ahata D (2007) Role of sonography in the diagnosis of ectopic pregnancy. J Clin Ultrasound 35:509-17
7. Dietrich CF, Ignee A, Hocke M et al (2011) Pitfalls and artefacts using contrast enhanced ultrasound. Gastroenterol 49:350-356
8. Rubens DJ, Bhatt S, Nedelka S, Cullinan J (2006) Doppler artifacts and pitfalls. Radiol Clin North Am 44:805-835
9. Kruskal JB, Newman PA, Sammons LG, Kane RA (2004) Optimizing Doppler and color flow US: application to hepatic sonography. Radiographics 24:657-75
10. Sparano A, Acampora C, di Nuzzo L et al (2006) Color power Doppler US and contrast-enhanced US features of abdominal solid organ injuries. Emerg Radiol 12:216-222

Errors in Color Doppler Ultrasonography

9

Ciro Acampora, Fabio Pinto, and Giuseppe De Magistris

9.1 Introduction

Artifacts are encountered daily in routine clinical sonography. They may be observed in B-mode gray-scale imaging, spectral pulsed Doppler imaging, and color Doppler imaging. In the context of imaging, the word " artifact" is taken to mean components of the image that are generated in the imaging process but which are not properly indicative of the structures studied. Being aware of an artifact's typical location and appearance helps to avoid misinterpretation and can actually be exploited diagnostically. Doppler artifacts can be grouped into three broad categories [1]:

1. Artifacts related to inappropriate settings, including Doppler gain setting errors, incorrect Doppler angle setting, velocity scale errors, and aliasing;
2. Anatomically related artifacts, including mirror image artifacts and "pseudo-flow" patterns;
3. Instrument-related artifacts, including directional ambiguity, twinkle artifacts, and vascular parietal calcifications.

9.2 Artifacts Related to Inappropriate Settings

9.2.1 Doppler Gain Setting Errors

Doppler gain controls the amplitude of the color display in color or power Doppler mode and the spectral display in pulse Doppler mode; it is critical in Doppler processing for the accurate depiction of flow characteristics. As with

---

C. Acampora (✉)
Department of Diagnostic Radiological Imaging, "A. Cardarelli" Hospital,
Naples, Italy

any ultrasound system, it is prudent to use the lowest gain or power setting that allows the recording of adequate signal.

For spectral Doppler, the tracing should be continuous and easy to visualize, without any low-level noise band above and below the baseline. Excess spectral gain in pulse-wave Doppler produces noise that may be misinterpreted as flow. For color imaging, the color gain is set by turning it up until noise is encountered and then backing off until the noise just clears from the image.

A machine setting related to gain for color and power Doppler is the color-write priority [2]. This allows the user to select a gray-scale cut-off value above which all color information is suppressed. In contrast to the larger vessels, which require a low setting of color-write priority, the small vessels, such as those of the testes, do not have a resolvable anechoic lumen on gray-scale sonography; as a result, color information can be easily suppressed by inappropriate adjustment of the color-write priority. If the color -write-priority settings are too low, the color may not be enrolled in the image of the testis, even when it has been successfully detected by the device (Fig. 9.1).

The color Doppler gain setting is particularly important in situations in which color Doppler ultrasound is often the only useful imaging method, as in the case of torsion. Testicular torsion is a true urological emergency and must be differentiated from other complaints of testicular pain because a delay in diagnosis and management can lead to loss of the testicle.

Rapid diagnosis is important in order to salvage a viable testis with prompt surgery. The testicular salvage rate is 80–100% if surgery is performed within 5–6 h, but the rate decreases to approximately 20% if detorsion is performed more than 12 h after the onset of symptoms [3].

Testicular torsion is characterized, using the appropriate settings at color Doppler imaging, by the absence of arterial flow in the twisted vessel segment (compared to the contralateral side) (Fig. 9.2). In partial testicular torsion, with only disturbed venous outflow, spectral waveform analysis will demonstrate a characteristic reversal of the diastolic plateau on the affected side [4] (Fig. 9.3).

9.2.2 Incorrect Doppler Angle Setting

In diagnostic ultrasound, the Doppler effect is used to measure blood flow velocity. In general, for vascular applications, the arterial or venous interfaces are best detected when the ultrasound beam is displaced perpendicular to them. Unfortunately, this imaging configuration is unacceptable for Doppler imaging. In the Doppler equation, the blood flow velocity may be calculated from the Doppler frequency shift occurring at a given transmitted frequency and angle of incidence. This is the angle between the path of the Doppler pulses and the direction of flow in the vessel. When this angle is 90° (perpendicular to moving blood cells), there is no frequency shift and the flow direction cannot be determined. This is reflected in the color duplex scan by the absence of

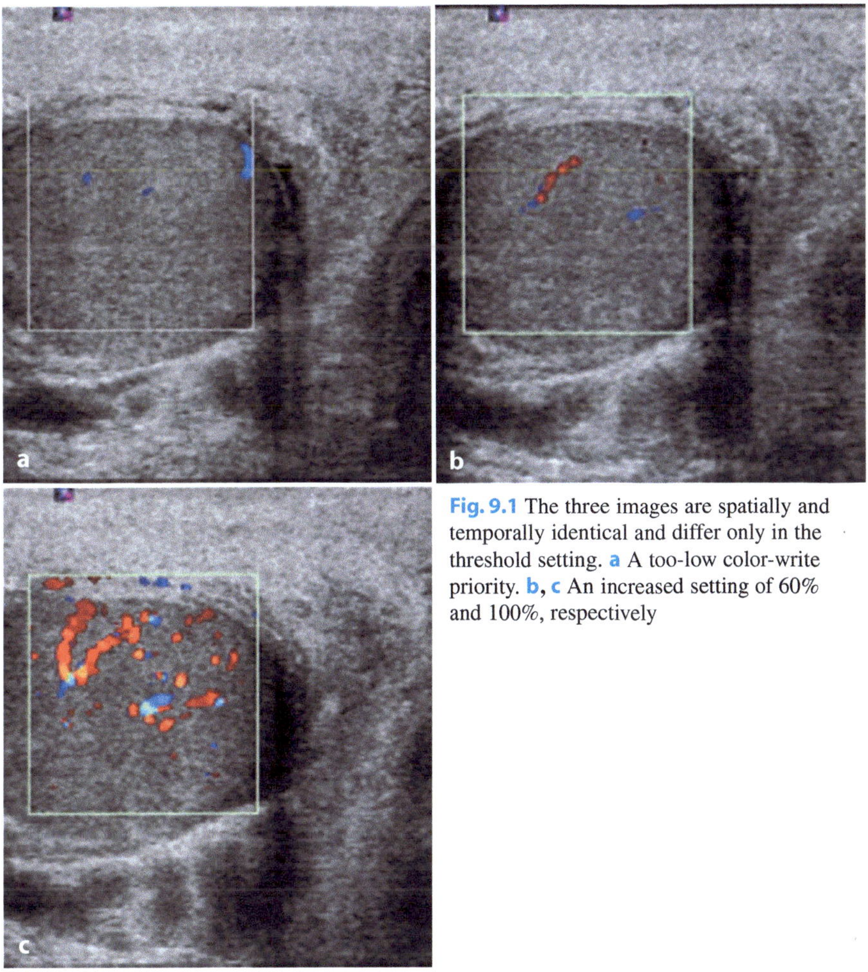

Fig. 9.1 The three images are spatially and temporally identical and differ only in the threshold setting. **a** A too-low color-write priority. **b, c** An increased setting of 60% and 100%, respectively

color flow signals, although flow is present. When this angle decreases, the Doppler shift increases as well. Ideally , a small angle should be used (< 60°).

The usual procedure is to first try and achieve a perpendicular beam angle for morphologic evaluation of the vessel wall and to then sample the Doppler information, with either activation of beam steering (lateral beam deflection) or a smaller insonation angle (Fig. 9.4). This is relevant only in the velocity mode and not in power mode, as the latter is virtually independent from the Doppler angle. As with any imaging modality, the success of duplex ultrasonography depends mostly on a careful technique.

Color Doppler imaging is by far the most common imaging examination performed worldwide in the diagnosis of carotid disease and, in most cases, is

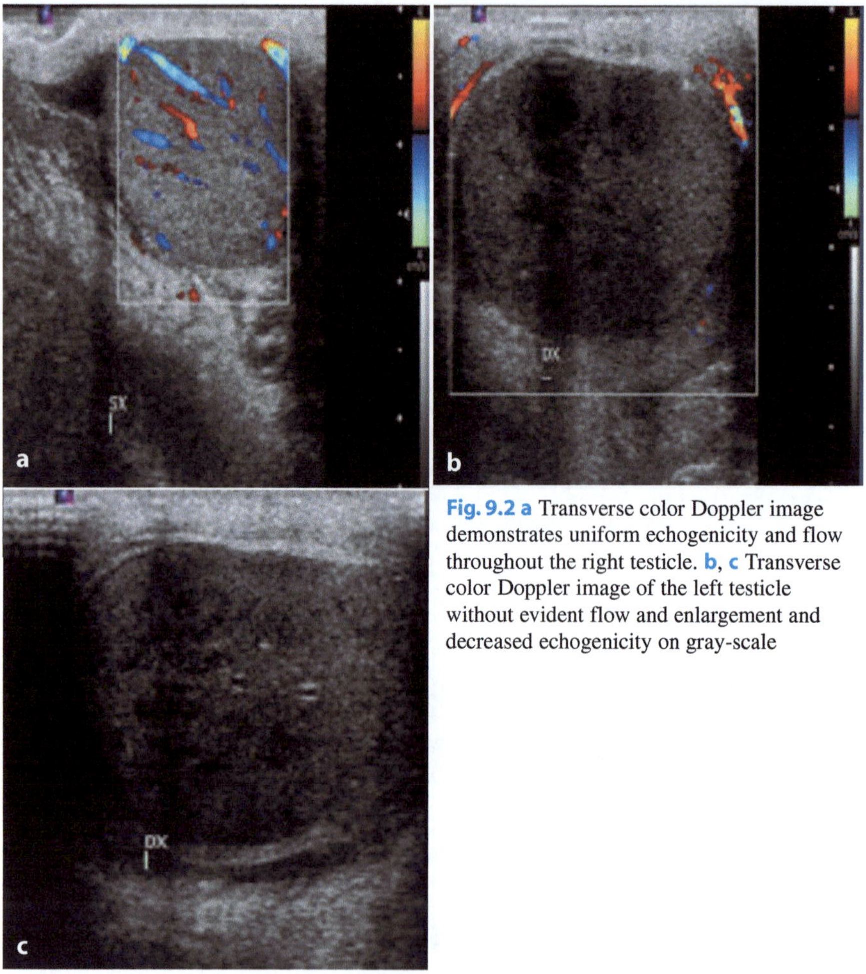

Fig. 9.2 a Transverse color Doppler image demonstrates uniform echogenicity and flow throughout the right testicle. **b, c** Transverse color Doppler image of the left testicle without evident flow and enlargement and decreased echogenicity on gray-scale

the only preoperative imaging study performed before carotid endo-arterectomy [5]. Flow velocity is the main parameter to diagnose a hemodynamically significant vessel stenosis (> 60%) [6]. Velocity measurements are a more reliable indicator than morphologic measurements, in which the narrowest portion of the residual lumen is compared with the original lumen in the same area or with the normalized lumen distally (ESCT or NASCET method) [7] (Fig. 9.5).

Errors in positioning the Doppler gate and in accounting for the Doppler angle are common in current clinical practice. Since interpretative criteria for carotid stenosis are heavily based on Doppler velocities, errors in Doppler position and angle correction will lead to serious errors in diagnosis. To minimize errors in the calculation of blood flow velocity and in other quantitative

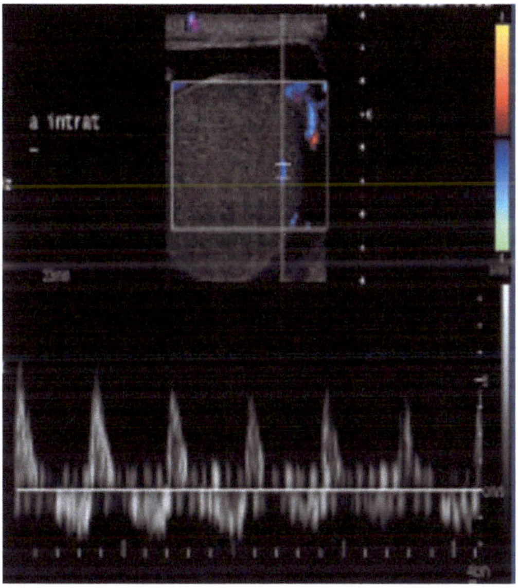

Fig. 9.3 When torsion is partial or in progress, arterial flow, visualized with the appropriate spectral Doppler gain setting, may still be present but with variably reduced, absent, or reversed diastolic flow

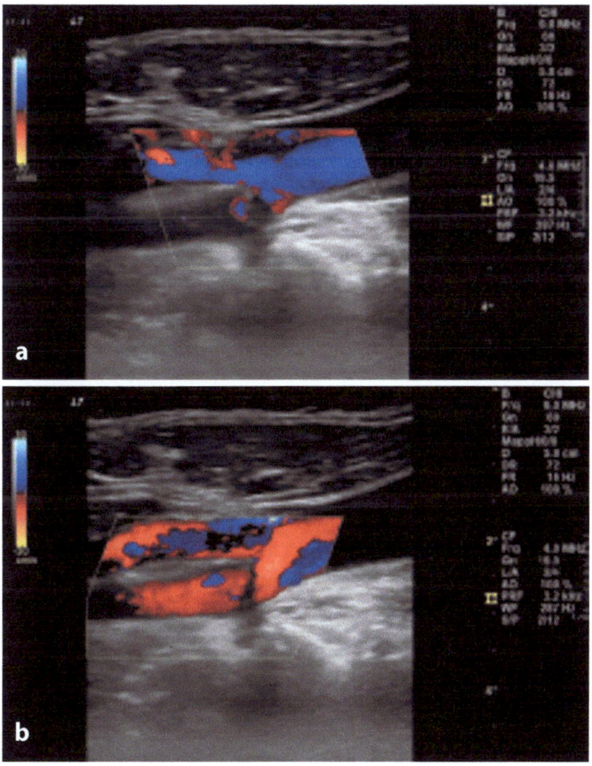

Fig. 9.4 a Effect of beam steering of the Doppler in color mode at the carotid bifurcation: color signal is absent in the external carotid artery because the angle of insonation is perpendicular to the vessel. **b** Changing the beam steering direction allows visualization of the color flow signal in the vessel (angle < 60°)

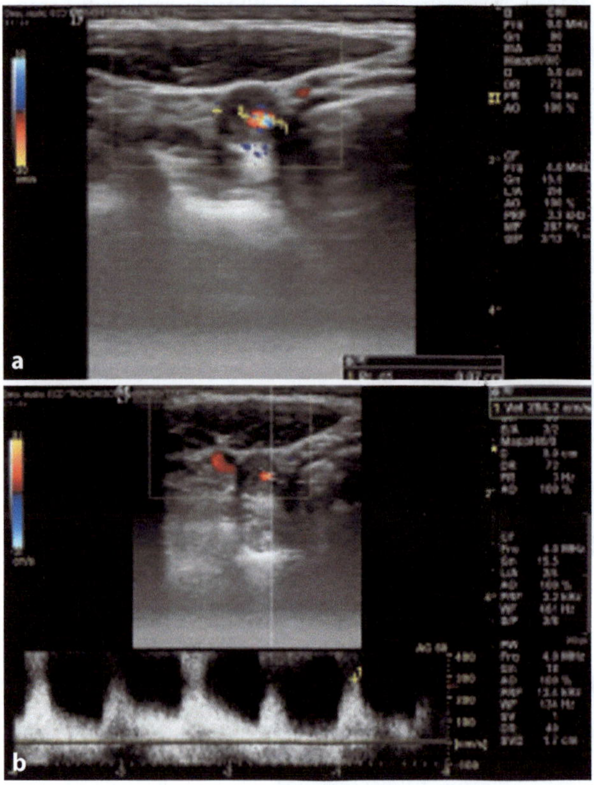

Fig. 9.5 a Cross-section color image (ECST method) demonstrating the percentage of the area of stenosis (56%). **b** Same case: color Doppler frequency analysis shows a high peak systole and diastole, indicative of a hemodynamically significant stenosis (> 70%)

determinations, the angle must be as small as possible and should not exceed 60°. An angle setting error of ±5° causes a 20% error in the velocity measurement at a Doppler angle of 60°. A larger angle of incidence leads to a rapid progression in the magnitude of the error [8].

9.2.3 Velocity Scale Errors and Aliasing

The velocity scale controls the range of frequencies displayed and is critical in color and spectral Doppler imaging. The color velocity scale is an operator-defined range of velocities that requires adjustment , analogous to the window width and level of a gray-scale image. If the scale setting is too high, color signals may not be displayed in a vessel, thus leading to an incorrect diagnosis of vessel occlusion, particularly in low-flow vessels, such as in a near-occlusion of the internal carotid artery. The distinction of near versus total occlusion is clinically extremely important, as patients with near occlusion may be surgical candidates, while those with total occlusion are not.

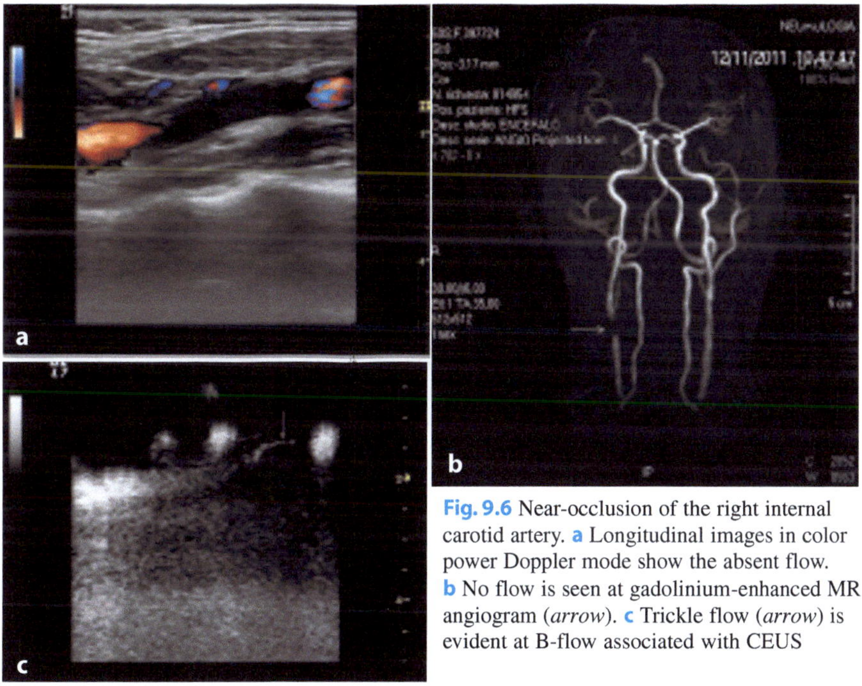

Fig. 9.6 Near-occlusion of the right internal carotid artery. **a** Longitudinal images in color power Doppler mode show the absent flow. **b** No flow is seen at gadolinium-enhanced MR angiogram (*arrow*). **c** Trickle flow (*arrow*) is evident at B-flow associated with CEUS

In case of near occlusion of the internal carotid artery, the velocity parameters may not apply, since velocities may be undetectable, resulting in a false-positive for occlusion. In this setting, the area of interest should be re-evaluated using very low color velocity settings (< 15 cm/s), power Doppler, or B-flow to enhance the detection of trickle flow in a near-occlusion [9]. At ultrasound standard imaging, if the absence of flow signal is revealed, contrast-enhanced imaging (CEUS, CT-angiography, MR-angiography, or conventional angiography) may be required to differentiate near versus complete occlusion (Fig. 9.6).

If the velocity scale setting is too low, the dynamic range will not able to display the high-velocity signals accurately and aliasing results. Aliasing is one of the most significant artifacts in Doppler examinations because it tends to occur when blood is moving fast: this is often associated with pathology. Aliasing is an incorrect and paradoxical display of color spectral Doppler velocity that occurs when the velocity range exceeds the range scale. This phenomenon is related to the fact that spectral Doppler and color flow utilize pulsed sound beams and the maximum velocity scale is limited by the number of ultrasound pulses per second that can be transmitted and received by the transducer (i.e., the pulse repetition frequency, PRF). If the Doppler shift is higher than PRF/2 (Nyquist limit), an ambiguous or aliased signal will be pro-

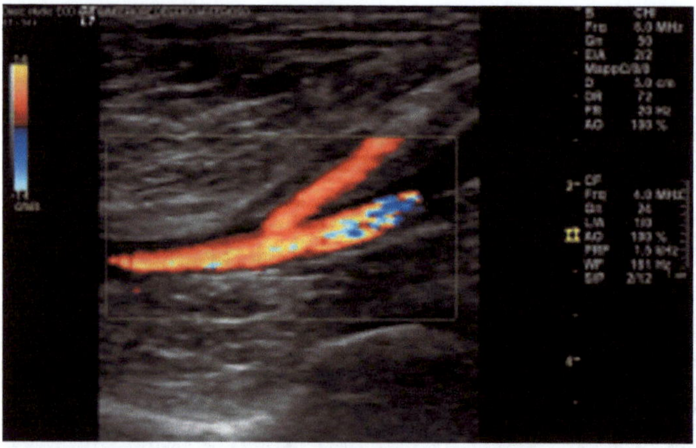

Fig. 9.7 Examination of the popliteal artery. There is aliasing because the Doppler shift frequencies are set above the Nyquist limit. Aliasing is seen in the color Duplex image as a color change from light red, through yellow, to blue

duced [10]. If the scale is too small, a large shift will exceed the available range and be displayed as multiples of a small shift. Practically, the display "wraps around" the scale and overwrites the existing data.

For spectral Doppler flow toward the transducer, the velocity peak is cut off at the top of the scale and the missing portion is written from the lowest portion of the scale back toward the top.

For color Doppler aliasing within a vessel, the color signal is displayed as adjacent colors from red to yellow to light blue to dark blue (Fig. 9.7).

Aliasing can be advantageously used to demonstrate high or low flow and turbulence. If the color velocity scale is set below the mean velocity of blood flow, aliasing throughout the vessel lumen makes it impossible to identify the high-velocity turbulent color jet associated with a tight stenosis. Conversely, if the color velocity scale is set significantly higher than the mean velocity of blood flow, aliasing may disappear, resulting in a missed stenosis .The tortuosity of the carotid arteries due to kinking can cause erroneously high velocities associated with aliasing (Fig. 9.8). Finally, aliasing can be useful because it quickly identifies the highest velocity region within a vessel and readily reveals an abnormal high-velocity vessel; both are often missed on gray-scale (i.e., artero-venous fistula) (Fig. 9.9).

To avoid spectral aliasing , several options are available; increasing the Doppler angle (with decreased Doppler shift), increase the velocity scale (which also increases the PRF), changing the baseline setting, or using a lower ultrasound frequency (Fig. 9.10).

In case of color Doppler aliasing, it will be necessary to increase the velocity scale and reduce the frequency.

Power Doppler avoids aliasing because it has no directional or velocity component [11].

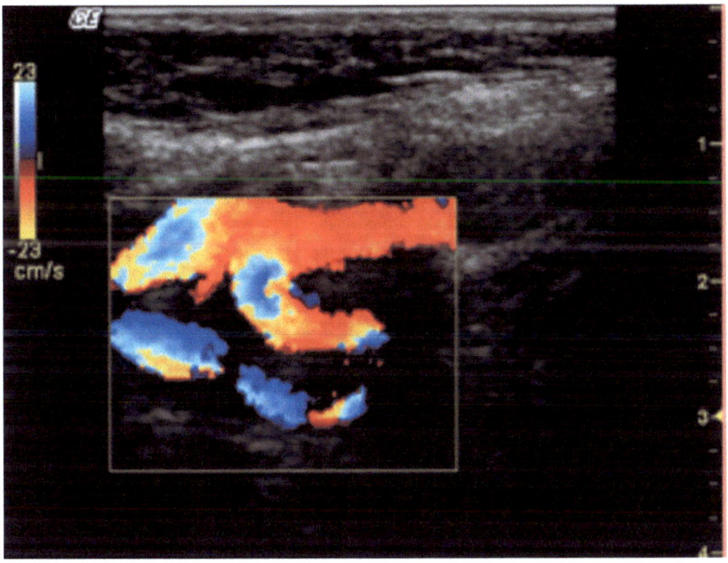

Fig. 9.8 Tortuosity of the internal carotid artery. The change in the artery's color depiction is not due to a change in blood flow velocity but instead indicates the changing direction of blood flow relative to the Doppler angle of incidence

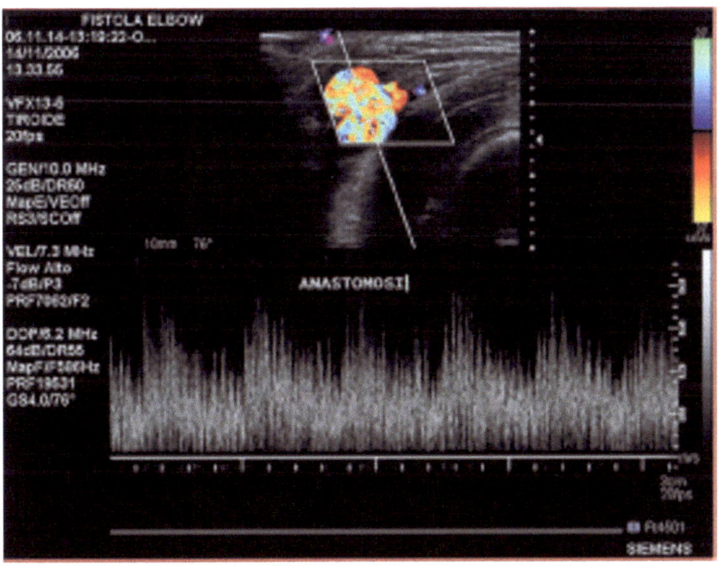

Fig. 9.9 Fistula at the elbow. Aliasing in color Doppler mode as a sign of turbulent flow at the critical vein-graft anastomosis and in spectral mode with high peak systolic flow velocity (> 500 cm/s)

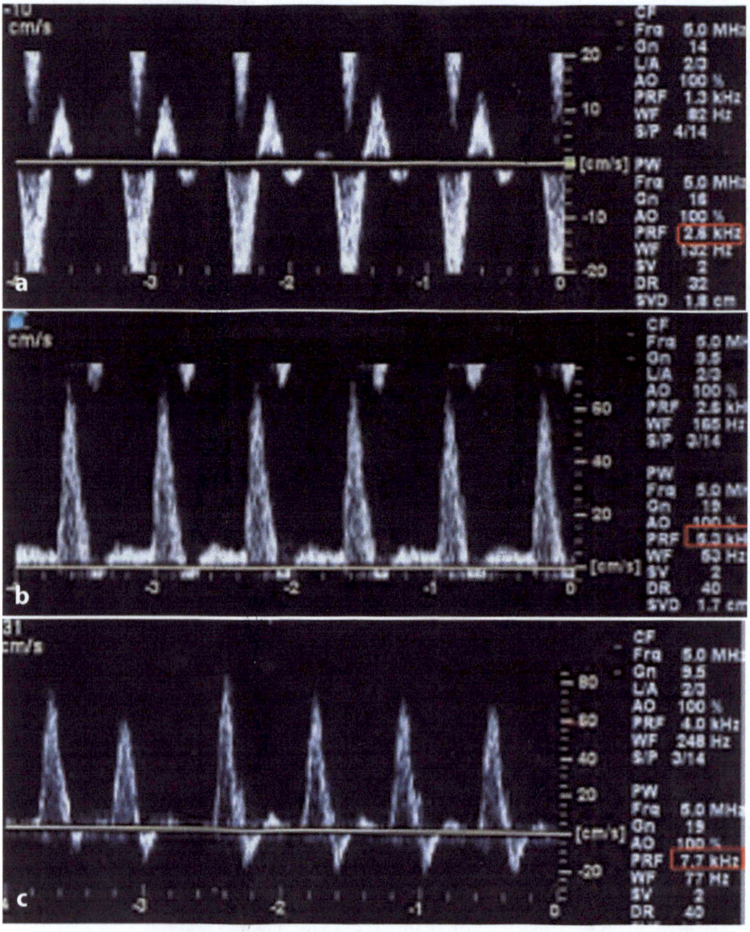

Fig. 9.10 a-c The effect of a progressive increase in the pulse repetition frequency (PRF) on an aliased spectral signal (as highlighted in the *red box*)

9.3 Anatomically Related Artifacts

9.3.1 Mirror-image Artifacts

A mirror-image artifact is created by the reflection of the sound beam against an interface between zones of high and low acoustic impedance such that an object is displayed on both sides although it is located on only one side. Mirror-image artifacts are commonly observed at conventional B-mode imaging, particularly with strongly reflecting surfaces (e.g., the portion of the liver behind the diaphragm) [12]. A similar artifact can occur with color Doppler

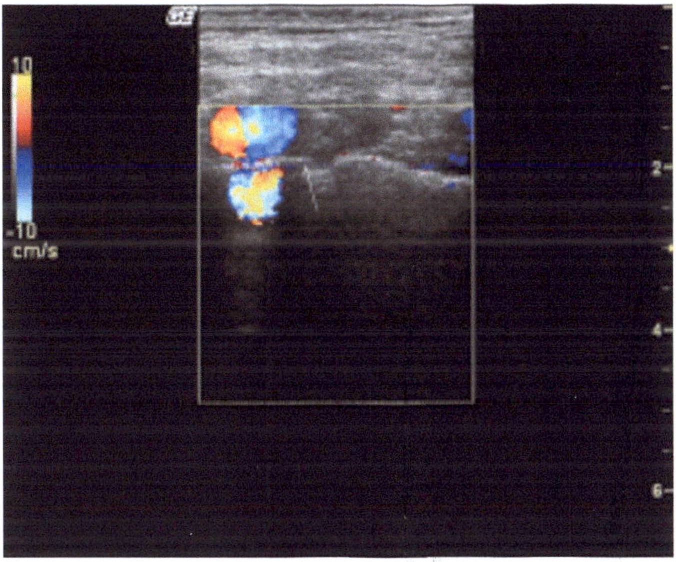

Fig. 9.11 Image of the supraclavicular region shows two apparent subclavian veins. The more anterior vessel is the true vein. The deeper vessel below the pleura (*arrow*) is actually an artifactual mirror image caused by a reflection off the lung apex

imaging of any vessel adjacent to a highly reflective surface, such as the lung.

The supraclavicular region is the most notorious for this artifact. Reflection of the pleura causes an apparent duplication of the subclavian artery or vein; the phantom vessel is always projected deeper in the image (Fig. 9.11).

Mirror-image artifacts will disappear when the reflector is scanned with oblique orientation [13].

9.3.2 Pseudo-flow Artifacts

Pseudo-flow is related to motion and appears similar to real blood flow at color or power Doppler ultrasound, but in the absence of a vascular structure [14]. The color or power Doppler images are artifactually represented since the fluid motion continues. These artifacts may be misinterpreted as flow unless Doppler analysis is used, as spectral Doppler will reveal flow that is atypical for a normal vessel.

Spontaneous pseudo-flow may be caused by the motion of ascites, amniotic fluid, and urine (ureteral jet). The ureteral jet identifies the ureteral orifice and is useful to exclude complete obstruction or to denote asymmetric ureteral emptying in the case of partial obstruction [15] (Fig. 9.12).

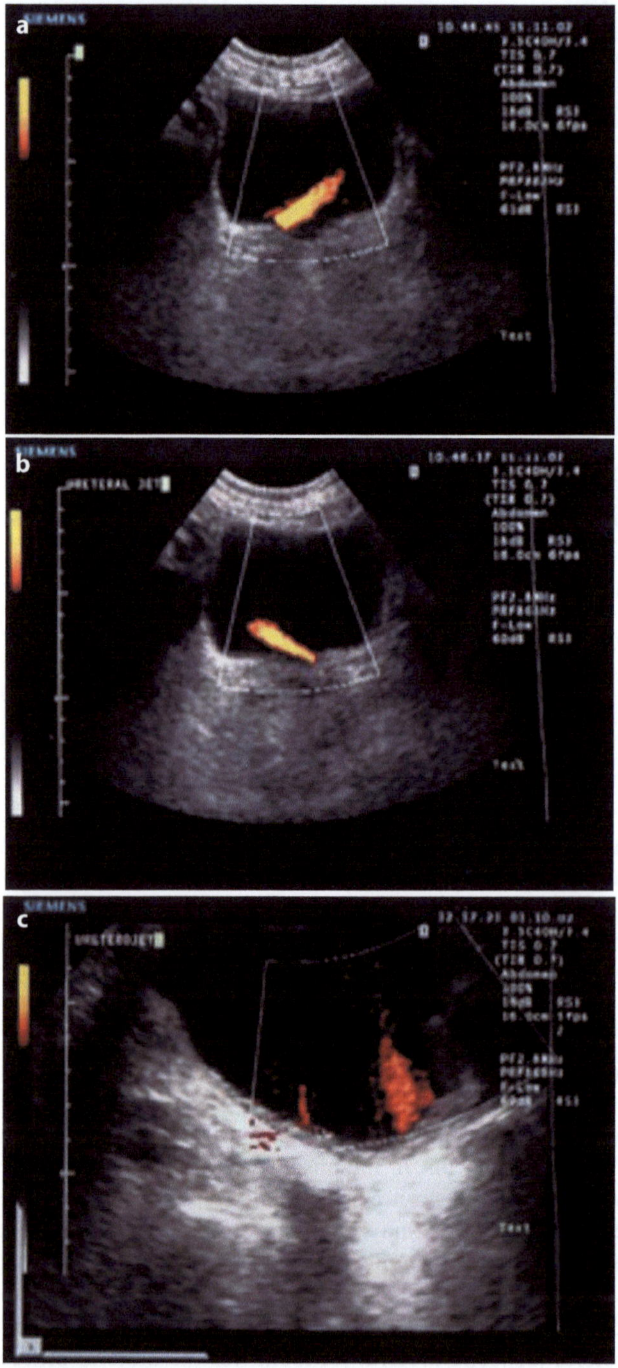

Fig. 9.12 Pseudo-flow caused by bladder jets. **a**, **b** Transverse ultrasound image of the bladder showing a jet of urine flowing from the right and left ureters. This finding indicates that the ureters are not obstructed. **c** Transverse image showing a full jet of urine only from the left ureter, whereas on the right side a tiny ureteral jet is revealed, indicating partial, but not complete, obstruction secondary to ureteral calculus

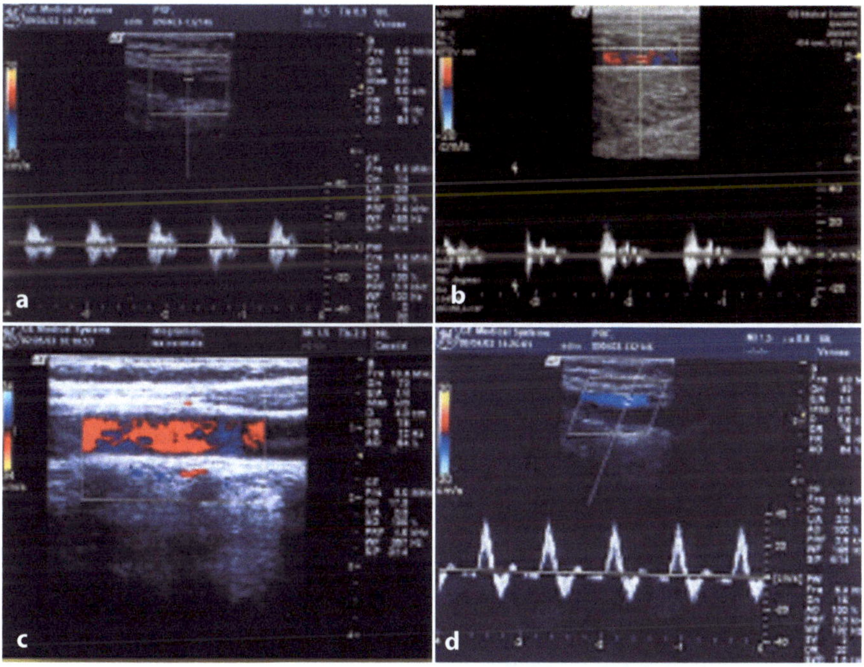

Fig. 9.13 Directional ambiguity. a, b An inverted image of the Doppler spectrum can occur if the Doppler angle is near 90°, with signal displayed in the upper and the lower spectral channels. c In the color image, the fluctuating, often random allocation of reds and blues can give the impression of flow reversal. d The ambiguity is easily corrected when the interrogating beam direction is shifted to an angle at either side of 90°

9.4 Instrumental-related Artifacts

9.4.1 Directional Ambiguity

The Doppler effect measures a shift or a difference in frequency between the transmitted and the received ultrasound pulse generated by motion of either the source or the detector. The greatest difference or strongest signal is achieved when the motion is parallel to the ultrasound beam, and no signal is generated when the motion is perpendicular to it, unlike in gray-scale US imaging whereby the best image is obtained perpendicular to the beam.

When the angle between the axis of the ultrasound beam and the blood vessel is 90°, a signal is detected because of the geometric divergence of the beam, but it is displayed both above and below the spectral baseline and is most common in small vessels, especially those that may be traveling in and out of the image plane [16].

In the color image, the fluctuating, often random location of reds and blues can give the impression of flow reversal. The ambiguity is easily corrected when the interrogating beam direction is shifted to an angle at either side of 90°(Fig. 9.13). However, directional ambiguity should not be confused with

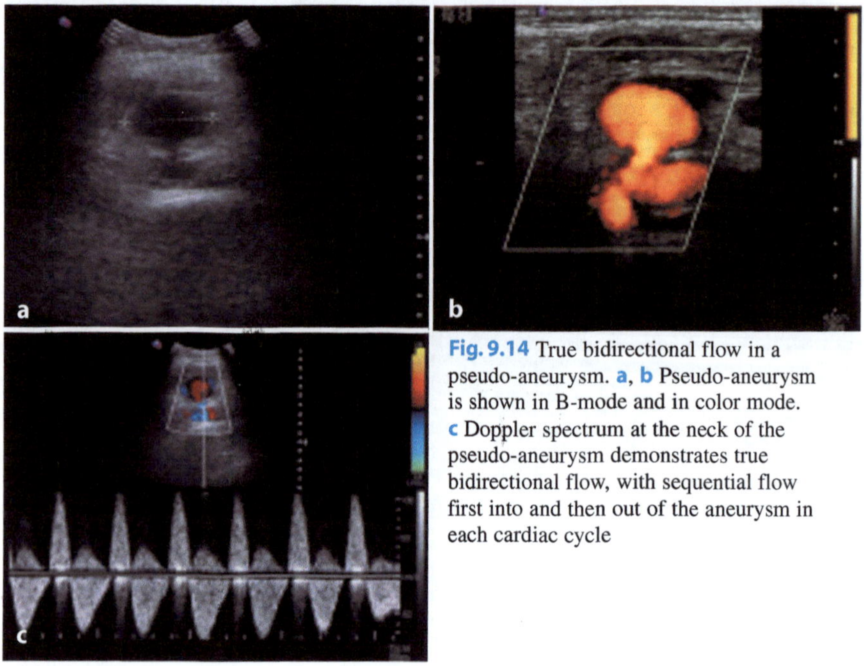

Fig. 9.14 True bidirectional flow in a pseudo-aneurysm. a, b Pseudo-aneurysm is shown in B-mode and in color mode. c Doppler spectrum at the neck of the pseudo-aneurysm demonstrates true bidirectional flow, with sequential flow first into and then out of the aneurysm in each cardiac cycle

true bidirectional flow. In the latter, blood actually flows in two directions, such as in the neck of a pseudo-aneurysm (Fig. 9.14). The clue here is that the flow is first in one direction, then in the other, all within the cardiac cycle, and is never simultaneously symmetric above and below the baseline [17].

9.4.2 Twinkling Artifact

Twinkling artifact is described as color Doppler signals that imitate motion or flow behind a stationary strongly reflecting interface. This artifact can be noted behind small, focal, hyperechoic areas made up of individual reflectors, such as urinary tract stones, renal calculi, and bladder calcifications. A twinkling artifact appears as a rapidly alternating red and blue color Doppler signal located deep to a stationary echogenic reflector, which gives the appearance of movement (Fig. 9.15). However, the Doppler spectrum is absolutely flat, a finding that is characteristic of noise [18].

The presence of a twinkling artifact may aid in stone detection, especially if the stone lacks a strong echo or discrete shadowing. A calcified carotid plaque with twinkling can be differentiated from a potentially ulcerated plaque with flow in the ulcer cavities.

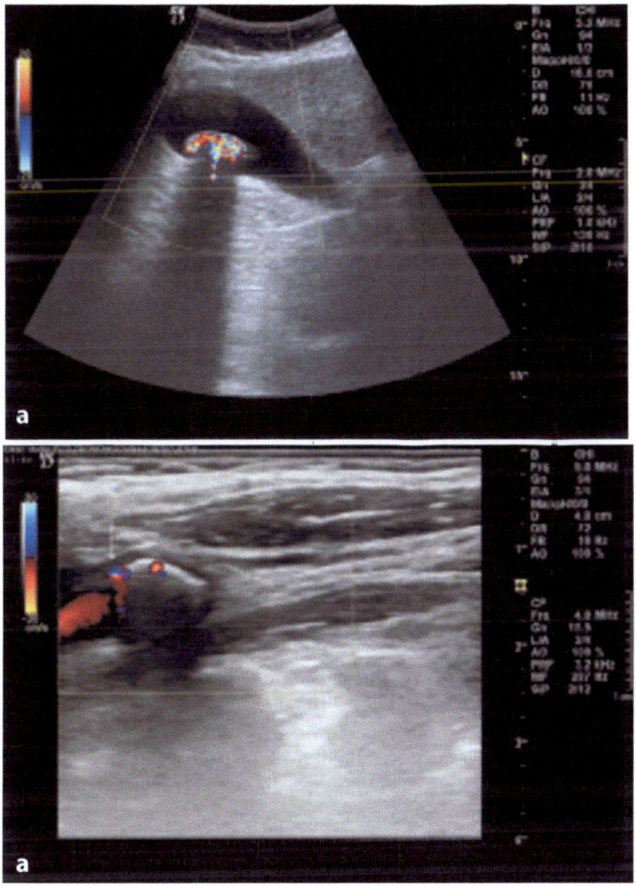

Fig. 9.15 a Twinkling artifact due to gallstones. **b** A twinkling artifact is seen behind the calcifications (*arrow*) in an atherosclerotic plaque, not to be misinterpreted as ulceration

9.4.3 Vascular Parietal Calcifications

The presence of vascular parietal calcifications can potentially limit the diagnostic accuracy of color Doppler ultrasound because in these situations the color image will be limited in its ability to display the vessel lumen. Heavily calcified plaques may act as a barrier to the ultrasound waves and cause posterior acoustic shadowing. This shadow makes the involved segment inaccessible to gray-scale or Doppler examination.

In the presence of a hard calcified plaque, flow patterns immediately distal to the lesion should be observed: if flow remains normal or is only moderately disturbed, there is unlikely to be significant stenosis (> 50%) behind the shadowing segment (Fig. 9.16). Damped or turbulent flow distal to the plaque should raise suspicion of a tight stenosis, which should be confirmed with another imaging modality [19].

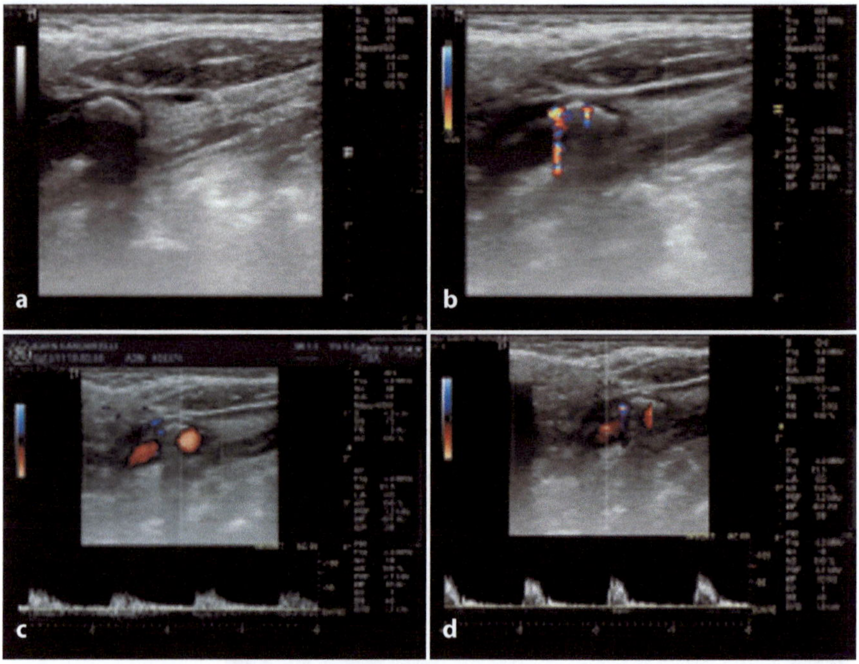

Fig. 9.16 a, b A heavily calcified plaque, at the origin of the internal carotid artery, leading to wide posterior shadowing in B-mode, without evidence of color Doppler flow signals in the involved segment. Note the twinkling artifact at the level of the hard plaque. **c, d** A color Doppler image obtained immediately proximal and distal to a circumferential shadowing plaque shows no sign of turbulence; the peak systolic velocity is within normal limits. Therefore, a significant stenosis behind the calcified plaque is unlikely

References

1. Campbell SC, Cullinan JA, Rubens DJ (2004) Slow flow or no flow? Color and power Doppler US pitfalls in the abdomen and pelvis. Radiographics 24:497-506
2. Zweibel WS, Pellerito JS (2005) Basic concept of Doppler frequency spectrum analysis and ultrasound blood flow imaging. Introduction to vascular ultrasonography. Elsevier Saunders, Philadelphia
3. Fitzgerald SW, Erickson S, De Wire DM et al (1992) Color Doppler sonography in the evaluation of the adult acute scrotum. J Ultrasound Med 11:543-548
4. Dogra VS, Sessions A, Mevorach RA, Rubens DJ (2001) Reversal of diastolic plateau in partial testicular torsion. J Clin Ultrasound 29:105-108
5. Nederkoorn PJ, Mali W,Eikelboom BC et al (2002) Preoperative diagnosis of carotid artery stenosis: accuracy of noninvasve testing. Stroke 33:2003-2008
6. Eisman BH, Legemate DA, van der Heyden et al (1996) The use of color-coded duplex scanning in the selection of patients with lower extremity arterial disease for percutanous trans luminal angioplasty: a prospective study. Cardiov Intervent Radiol 19:313-316
7. Browman MW, Cooperberg PL, Harrison PB et al (1995) Duplex ultrasonography criteria for internal carotid stenosis of more than 70% diameter: angiographic correlation and receveir operating characteristic curve analysis. Can Assoc Radiol J 46:291-295

8. Gaitini D, Soudak M (2005) Diagnosing carotid stenosis by Doppler sonography: state of the art. J Ultrasound Med 24:1127-1136
9. El Saden SM, Grant EG, Hathout GM et al (2001) Imaging of the internal carotid artery: the dilemma of total versus near total occlusion. Radiology 221:301-308
10. Taylor KJ, Holland S (1990) Doppler US. Part.I. Basic principles, instrumentation, and pittfalls. Radiology 174:297-307
11. Torp-Pedersen ST, Terslev L (2008) Settings and artefacts relevant in colour-power Doppler ultrasound in rheumatology. Ann Rheum Dis 67:143-149
12. Lewandowski BJ,Winsberg F (1983) Echographic appearance of the rigth hemidiaphragm. J Ultrasound Med 2:243-249
13. Charboneau JW, Cooperberg PL (1990) Color and spectral Doppler mirror-image artifact of the subclavian artery. Radiology 174:41-42
14. Campbell SC (2004) Doppler Ultrasound artifacts. Elsevier, Philadelphia
15. Deyoe LA, Cronan JJ (1995) New techniques of ultrasound and color Doppler in the prospective evaluation of acute renal ostruction. Do the replace the intravenous urogram? Abdom Imag 20:58-63
16. Burns PN (1993) Principles of Doppler and color flow. Radiol Med 85:3-16
17. Abu-Yosef MM, Wiese JA, Shamma AR (1988) The "to and fro" sign: Duplex Doppler evidence of femoral artery pseudoaneurysm. AJR 150: 632-634
18. Rahmouni A, Bargoin R, Herment A, Bargoin N (1996) Color Doppler twinkling artifact in hyperecoic regions.Radiology 199:269-271
19. Strandness DE Jr (1993) Duplex scanning in vascular disorders. Raven, New York

Errors in MDCT Angiography 10

Roberto Dore, Adele Valentini, and Emilio Bassi

10.1 Introduction

Recent technological developments in MDCT scanner have resulted in the improvement and optimization of CT angiography (angioCT) in the evaluation of the small and large arteries. Faster scanning speeds and better isotropic spatial resolution provide detailed depictions of the vascular anatomy and related pathologies. Imaging is further enhanced by the use of contrast agents containing high concentrations of iodine, which lower both the energy requirement and the radiation exposure of the patient.

Anomalies in the distribution of contrast medium (CM) in the lumen of the great vessels, whether due to local extravascular or vascular diseases or to alterations in cardiac output, may result in errors in the visualization of CM within central or peripheral vessels. Other sources of error in vessel imaging derive from certain pitfalls, which lead to incorrect interpretations of transverse images. These topics are discussed below.

10.2 Errors Due to Patient-related Factors

Cardiac output, body weight, and central venous retention are the main patient factors causing the attenuation of contrast agent in the vessel of interest.

R. Dore (✉)
Institute of Radiology, Foundation IRCCS "San Matteo" University Hospital, Pavia, Italy

10.2.1 Variations in Cardiac Output

Global cardiac function critically determines both the time and the magnitude of contrast attenuation in the vessel lumen [1]. The pulmonary and systemic arteries enhance with different delay times and with different degrees of contrast enhancement according to cardiac performance.

Reduced cardiac output. A depression of the ejection fraction is characteristic of dilated cardiomyopathy, congestive cardiopathy, and in the elderly. Angio-graphically, it manifests as the slow progression of CM and blood in the great vessels such that the target artery enhances and is visualized after a conspicuous delay. In addition, the concentration of iodine within the vessels is typically very high.

Common errors in angioCT studies in patients with depressed cardiac output arise from incomplete contrast enhancement along the entire length of the vessel. While at the beginning of the scan the contrast agent is well-concentrated in the vessel, during scanning it becomes progressively less evident. This is particularly the case when the scan direction is cephalocaudal and scanning is faster than blood flow. Errors in angioCT are more often associated with studies of the pulmonary arteries, but they may also occur during angioCT of the thoraco-abdominal aorta. Images generated with the aid of maximum-intensity projections (MIPs) and volume rendering technique (VRT) are usually altered by errors related to reduced cardiac output (Fig. 10.1).

To avoid and reduce the incidence of these errors, whether in a patient with a depressed ejection fraction or in an elderly patient, the following strategies are recommended:

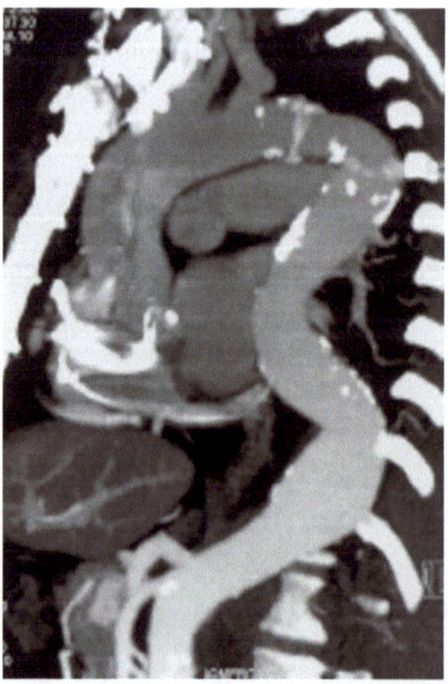

Fig. 10.1 CT angiography of the thoracic and abdominal aorta in a patient with depressed cardiac output. The distribution of contrast enhancement in the aorta is inadequate, because the scan was faster than the slow blood flow. The same result is obtained when the delay time is too short

- Bolus tracking should originate in the distal segment of the artery (in the distal abdominal aorta for studies of the entire aorta);
- A bolus test should be carried out in order to predict contrast attenuation times;
- The injection flow rate should be reduced from 5 to 3–4 ml/s and the scan duration to 10–12 s;
- The injection duration should be approximately 20 s.

Accelerated cardiac output. In patients with a large ejection fraction, the flow of CM and blood through the arteries is very rapid. Consequently, intravascular iodine is quickly diluted; the vessels are enhanced for a much shorter duration, and by the time the scan is started the contrast bolus is in the late phase. Thus, at the beginning of the scan the vessel lumen only slightly enhances and as scanning continues enhancement is progressively reduced, such that the vessel is not adequately depicted or is visualized only partially. This pattern occurs in some physiologic states, such as during pregnancy and in young athletes, but also as a result of certain pathological conditions, such as tachycardia, arteriovenous fistula, and shunt. Thus, in angioCT studies of these patients, errors of visualization are possible.

Errors related to a high ejection fraction can be avoided or minimized with the following measures:

- The scan duration should be no longer than 6–7 s;
- The flow rate injection should be > 5 ml/s;
- The iodine concentration should be > 350 mgI/ml.

10.2.2 Errors Due to Body Weight

The magnitude of vascular contrast enhancement depends also on the patient's body weight [2]. Since blood volume is larger in a heavy patient than in a slim one, the same amount of contrast agent will become progressively diluted with increasing body weight. In addition, the vessel lumen may enhance very poorly in overweight patients, defined as those with a body mass index (BMI) > 190. Insufficient enhancement becomes significant in small arteries such as the coronary, renal, and cerebral arteries, and in branching arteries such as the pulmonary arteries [3].

These errors may be avoided by a concomitant increase in the injection flow rate and the amount of iodine administered (increasing the amount of contrast agent or increasing the iodine concentration, respectively).

10.2.3 Influence of Peripheral Venous Access

In angioCT studies of thoracic systemic arteries, pulmonary arteries, and coronary arteries, the presence of contrast agent in the brachiocephalic vein and superior vena cava may cause numerous imaging problems and reduce the quality of imaging, potentially resulting in diagnostic errors. Specifically, if intravenous contrast agent containing a high iodine concentration enters these veins, artifacts will occur in the surrounding structures, such as the supra-aortic vessels, the ascending and transverse aorta, and right pulmonary arteries.

In the superior vena cava, CM coming from one brachiocephalic vein is non-homogeneously mixed with blood flow coming from the other brachiocephalic vein; these two opposite blood channels enhance the likelihood of artifacts on angioCT.

In the right atrium, CM coming from the superior vena cava meets blood flow coming from the inferior vena cava, without CM; as a result, contrast enhancement in the right cardiac chambers is very inhomogeneous and complicates evaluation of the cardiac cavities and wall, but also of the right coronary artery.

A common error in chest angioCT is performing the scan during transit of the CM bolus through the superior vena cava; this can generate several artifacts around the vena cava that may be the source of diagnostic errors. For example, the paratracheal lymph nodes or the subclavian artery may be obscured, resulting in a misinterpretation or overlooked diseases. In addition, these artifacts can lead to imaging anomalies that mimic the appearance of aortic dissection or aortic intramural hematoma (Fig. 10.2). They may also hide aortic lesions, especially acute ones, or a thrombus in the right pulmonary artery and its ascending branch. Finally, they can mimic or distract attention from a mass or embolus in the right cardiac atrium and ventricle (Fig. 10.3).

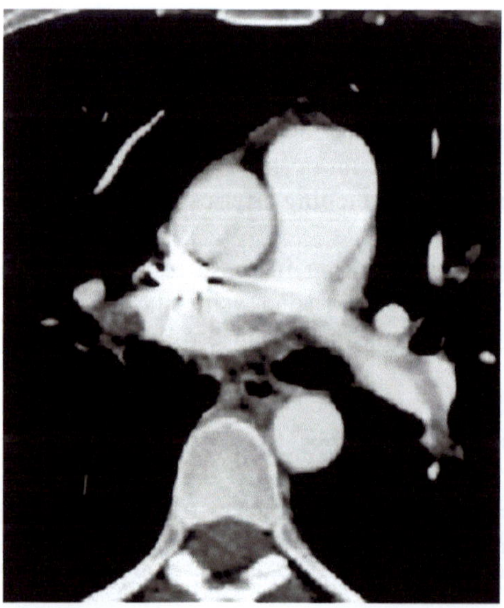

Fig. 10.2 Pulmonary angioCT in a patient with an acute pulmonary embolism. Streak artifacts, due to excessive contrast agent in the superior vena cava, generate false images or aortic dissection in the ascending aorta. Artifacts are recognized because they are linear and extend outside the aorta

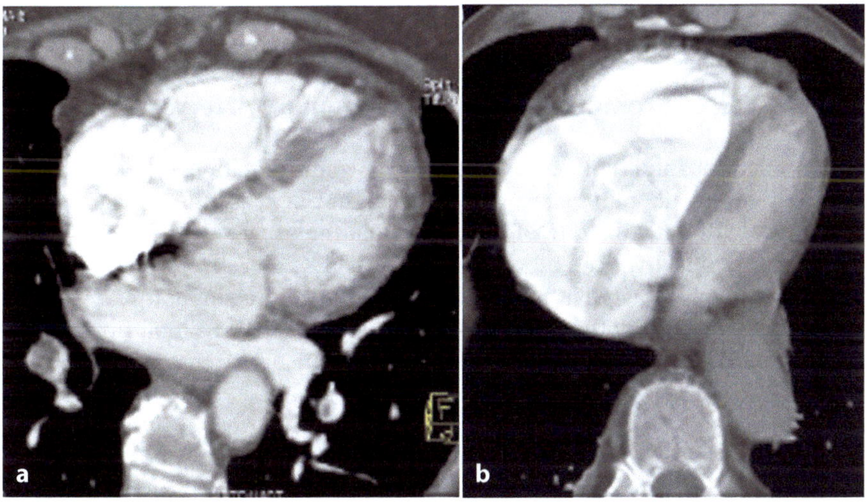

Fig. 10.3 During thoracic angioCT, contrast enhancement in the right atrium is always very inhomogeneous, due to the inflow of contrast medium from the superior vena cava and blood from the inferior vena cava. a Acute pulmonary embolism with false images of an atrial mass or thrombus. b Massive acute pulmonary embolism in another patient; surgery confirmed a long acute thrombus in the right atrium and ventricle

To avoid and reduce the incidence of these errors in chest angioCT several CM injection strategies are recommended:

- A second bolus, made up of ~50 ml of saline solution, should follow the first CM bolus, at the same flow rate; this is useful to reduce CM in superior vena cava during scan;
- Alternatively, a second bolus may consist of CM with a reduced iodine concentration (≤ 50% than the first CM bolus);
- The delay time between the beginning of the i.v. injection and the beginning of the scan should allow the scan to be started during transit of the saline or second CM bolus in the superior vena cava. This may be difficult because the common routine is to start the angioCT scan at the preselected threshold of contrast enhancement in the aorta or pulmonary artery. Nevertheless, an excess in the delay time in angioCT of the pulmonary artery may be problematic if the scan starts during the phase of descending CM enhancement;
- Smaller volumes of CM are often more effective and the injection time should not be too much longer than the scan time; for instance, if the scan time is about 10 s, the injection time must not be longer than 14–15 s, with a threshold of about 120 HU at the start of the scan (with bolus tracking or the appropriate software).

10.3 Errors and Pitfalls in CT Angiography of the Pulmonary Arteries

10.3.1 False Thrombus in the Main Pulmonary Artery

Large pleural fluid collections, pulmonary consolidation, pneumothorax, compression of the pulmonary parenchyma, and increased pulmonary vessel resistance will slow the rate of blood flow on the same side as the pleural or lung lesion, thus diverting blood flow towards the contralateral side. The CM bolus will travel slowly but immediately into the contralateral artery, while in the homolateral artery the CM bolus mixes with the native blood flow, resulting in a defect of CM enhancement inside the main artery that mimics thrombus (Fig. 10.4).

This defect occurs only in one main pulmonary artery in unilateral lung transplantation (in the homolateral artery in the native lung), in extensive pulmonary consolidation or atelectasis, and in larger pleural collections, but never in descending and segmental arteries. Thus, in patients with unilateral lung transplantation, pulmonary atelectasis, and extensive pleural effusion, the following steps are recommended:

- A 3- to 4-s increase in the delay time and a reduction in the amount of contrast medium;
- Positioning the ROI in the main pulmonary artery on the same side of the pleural or pulmonary lesion.

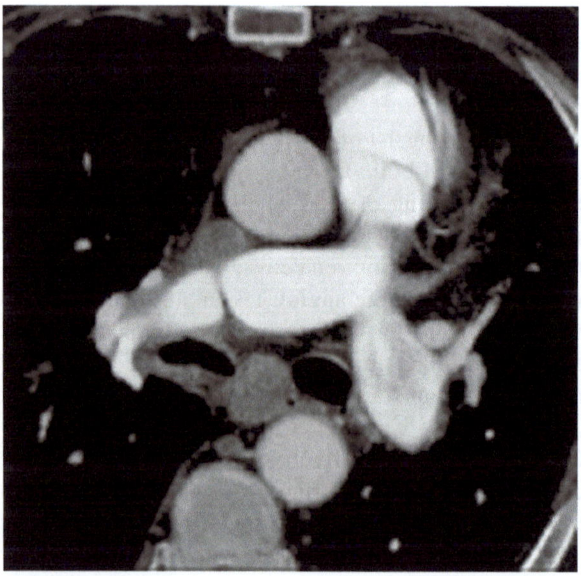

Fig. 10.4 Pulmonary angioCT of a transplanted right lung in a patient with pulmonary fibrosis. A false thrombus is present in the left pulmonary artery. Blood and contrast flow is rapid in the right pulmonary artery but slow on the left side because of the high vascular resistance, resulting in an inhomogeneous distribution of contrast bolus in the left main pulmonary artery and mimicking thrombus

10.3.2 Other Intra-arterial Masses Mimicking Thrombotic Disease in the Main Pulmonary Arteries

Here, one must first consider all the rare arterial tumors, such as sarcomas (Fig. 10.5). The clinical diagnosis of sarcomas of the pulmonary arteries is often difficult. In some patients, echocardiography will reveal pulmonary hypertension, with angioCT performed mainly to define or exclude pulmonary chronic embolic disease or to search for signs of venous-occlusive or diffuse pulmonary disease. However, on angioCT arterial tumors can mimic chronic thrombus, since both may partially or totally occlude the lumen of the main pulmonary artery. Several CT signs are helpful to distinguish tumor from thrombus:

- Chronic thrombus is never situated in the common pulmonary artery;
- Sarcomas may lie in the common trunk or in one main pulmonary artery;
- Sarcomas enlarge the vessel while chronic occlusive thrombi cause arterial retraction;
- The proximal aspect of the sarcoma is convex while that of a thrombus is generally concave;
- Both may contain calcifications;
- A comparison of an unenhanced scan with a contrast-enhanced one or with a second, later scan will often show that intra-arterial tumors enhance while a thrombus does not;
- In chronic embolic disease, any of the following may be detected in both lungs: intravascular webs, stenosis, vessel occlusions of segmental or subsegmental arteries, ground glass opacification with mosaic perfusion, and post-infarction scars. None of these signs are observed bilaterally in pulmonary artery sarcomas.

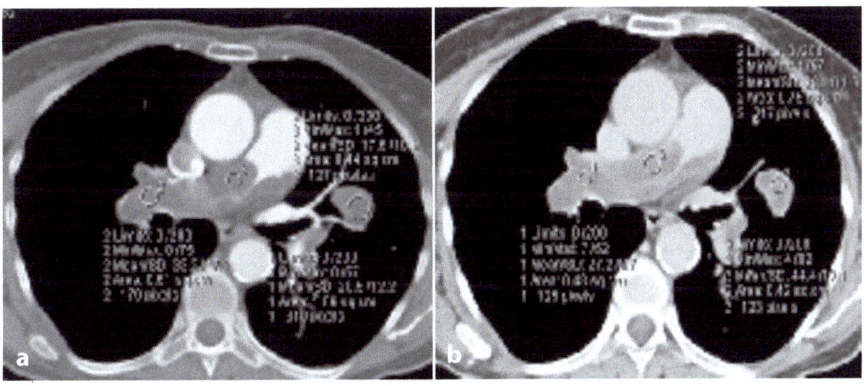

Fig. 10.5 Pulmonary angioCT in a patient with pulmonary hypertension. In the first spiral scan, the intra-arterial bilateral mass mimics a huge thrombus (**a**); in the late scan (**b**) contrast enhancement of the mass is suggestive of tumor (sarcoma of the pulmonary arteries)

Thus, confusion between an arterial tumor and a chronic thrombus can be avoided by using either a non-enhanced or a second scan to identify contrast enhancement of an arterial tumor. In addition, a thorough and expert CT evaluation will allow the parenchymal signs of a tumor to be distinguished from the vessel signs of chronic embolic disease.

10.3.3 False Thrombus in Segmental and Subsegmental Arteries

If the convolution image filter is too hard, the "edge effect" will generate a false hyperdense annular ring corresponding to the arterial wall and mimicking a thrombus in the lumen (Fig. 10.6). This error can be avoided by instead evaluating images obtained with a soft rather than a hard (for instance, high-resolution images) convolution filter.

Artifacts may also arise due to partial-volume effects on bronchial images, which can produce false images of a thrombus in the contiguous artery. The segmental and subsegmental pulmonary arteries are in contact with the corresponding segmental or subsegmental bronchus. When the CT slice is too thick, partial-volume artifacts mimicking emboli or thrombi may occur in vessels with an oblique orientation with respect to the axial scan plane. To avoid this error, it is important to evaluate the segmental and subsegmental pulmonary arteries on thin slice thickness images.

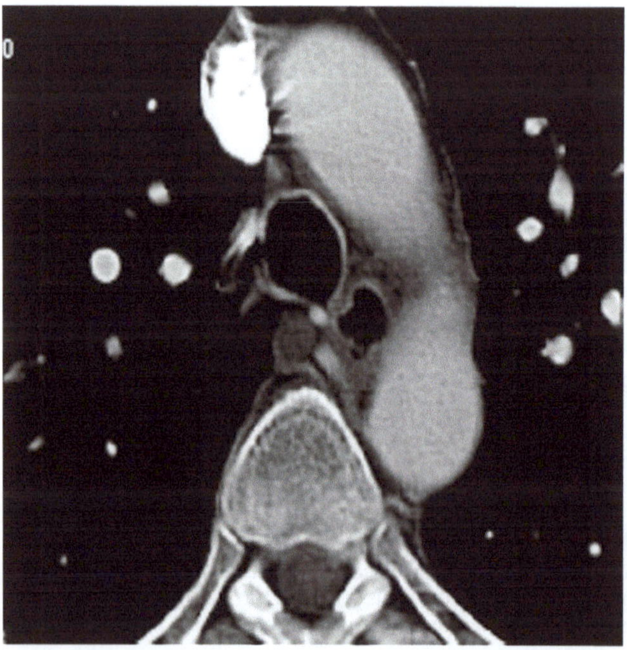

Fig. 10.6 Pulmonary angioCT. Axial image reconstructed with a hard convolution filter that enhances the contours of the vessels especially those of the arterial system, mimicking vessels containing thrombus

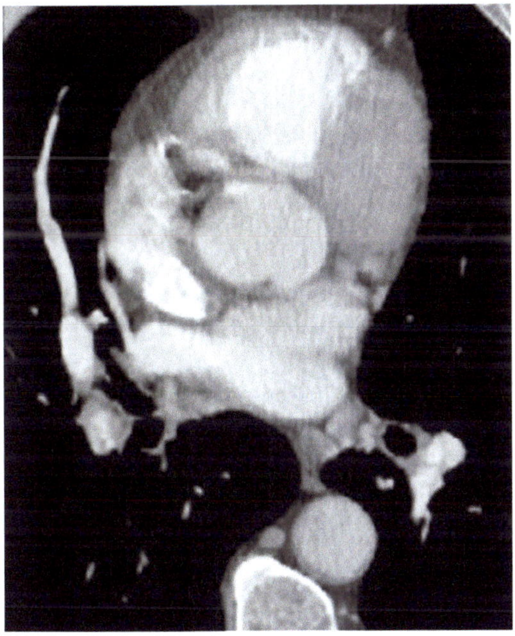

Fig. 10.7 Pulmonary angioCT in a patient with pulmonary hypertension. Bilateral defects in the arteries of the lower lobes are due to intravascular webs or bands, typical in chronic embolic disease. They are linear, thin, and differ from the round and thick defect characteristic of acute emboli

10.3.4 Chronic vs. Acute Pulmonary Embolic Disease

Chronic and acute pulmonary thrombo-emboli differ not only in the clinical setting but also on cardiac ultrasonography and CT. Nevertheless, CT imaging of chronic thrombo-embolic disease must be performed correctly in order to recognize this entity and distinguish it from acute embolism. In daily practice, it is not a rare radiological error to confuse chronic with acute thrombo-embolic disease.

In both conditions, endoluminal defects are the main diagnostic CT signs, with involvement of the main, segmental, and subsegmental arteries. However, there are also several chronic finding that can mimic endoluminal defects such as acute emboli:

- Endoluminal "webs" are short and linear flaps generally located in the distal part of the descending pulmonary branch, or in the proximal part of the segmental arteries. They are considered to be the result of an incomplete and poor re-canalization in chronic thrombo-embolic disease. In some patients, they serve as unique signs of chronic embolic disease on axial CT images, but they also can be confused with acute emboli. However, endoluminal webs differ from emboli in that the webs are septal, thin, linear, and short while acute emboli are round, thick, and generally extend along the entire length of the segmental or subsegmental vessel. Webs divide the vessel lumen into two channels, while emboli reduce the lumen to a peripheral ring (Fig. 10.7);

- Total occlusion of the pulmonary arteries can occur in both acute and chronic embolic disease, and is therefore another source of confusion. Several morphological CT features can help in the differential diagnosis: acute occlusions enlarge the native vessel diameter, while chronic occlusions reduce and retract the vessel. In acute disease, totally occluded vessels are synchronous with partially occluded ones showing the acute typical aspect of a ring of CM surrounding the embolus, between it and the vessel wall.

10.4 Errors and Pitfalls in CT Angiography of the Aorta

The main diagnostic indication in angioCT of the thoracic aorta is the detection and diagnosis of an acute lesion (dissection, intramural hematoma, atherosclerotic penetrating ulcer) [4]. On the one hand, a variety of pitfalls can cause the CT image of a lesion to mimic aortic dissection while, on the other hand, different factors may result in the false-negative diagnosis of aortic dissection.

10.4.1 Technical Factors in the False-negative Diagnosis of Aortic Dissection

On angioCT, a variety of technical factors can result in a false-negative diagnosis of aortic dissection:

- Insufficient contrast enhancement of the aortic lumen (secondary to a slow injection rate or to improper timing of CM administration) complicate visualization of the intimal flap. To avoid this error, a high iodine concentration and/or low radiation energy are necessary when venous peripheral access is difficult;
- If the delay time between CM injection and the start of the scan is too short, a false lumen, without CM, may appear, mimicking thrombus in cases of aneurysm or dissection (Fig. 10.8). To avoid this error in patients with a clinically suspected acute aortic lesion, two consecutive volumetric scans are recommended—with the option of extending the scan over the entire aorta—without delay between them;
- When dissection causes the internal mural layer to peel 360°, the intimal flap may migrate distally, potentially retracting into a thrombus-like lesion. The false lumen then disappears such that the dissection becomes difficult to recognize (Fig. 10.9);
- Wall motion in the proximal ascending aorta can obscure images of a completely or incompletely dissected intimal flap.

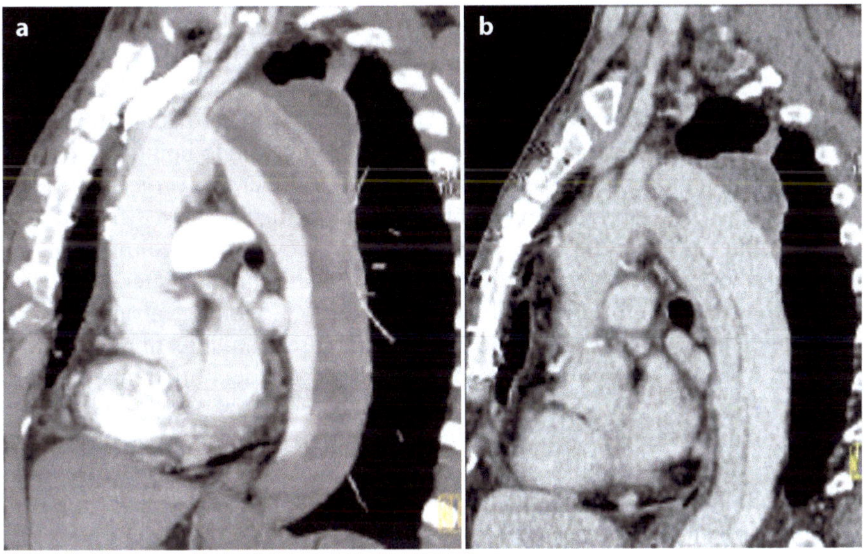

Fig. 10.8 False thrombus in the false lumen of a type B dissection after surgical repair of the ascending aorta. a In the first scan, during contrast enhancement of the true lumen, contrast medium is not seen in the false channel, a situation mimicking thrombus. b In the second scan, taken immediately after the first, contrast enhancement is seen in both the true and the false channel, without any evidence of thrombus in the latter

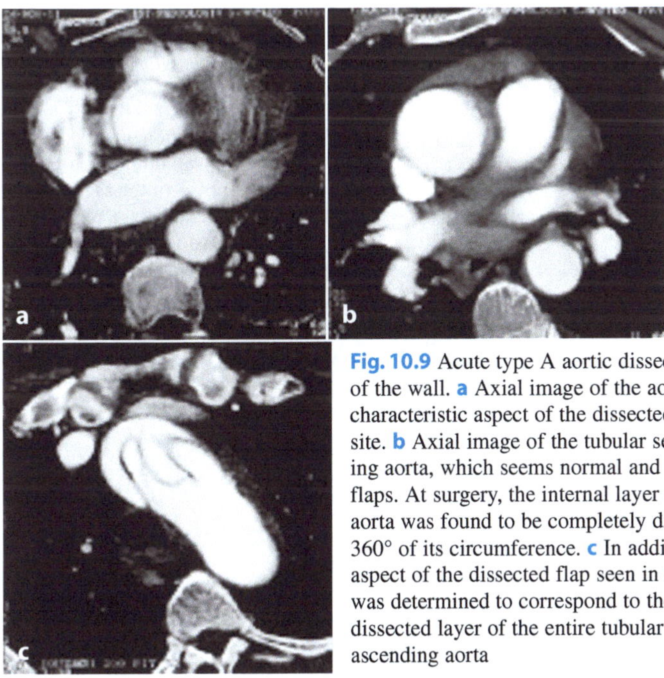

Fig. 10.9 Acute type A aortic dissection involving 360° of the wall. a Axial image of the aortic root with the characteristic aspect of the dissected flap in the typical site. b Axial image of the tubular segment of the ascending aorta, which seems normal and without any dissected flaps. At surgery, the internal layer of the ascending aorta was found to be completely dissected, around all 360° of its circumference. c In addition, the invaginate aspect of the dissected flap seen in the transverse aorta was determined to correspond to the retraction of the dissected layer of the entire tubular segment of the ascending aorta

10.4.2 False-positive Diagnosis of Aortic Dissection

- Streak artifacts_are caused by high-attenuation materials (surgical staples, calcifications, pacemaker leads, CM) associated with cardiac motion. They appear as straight parallel lines, or radiate from a single point. The CM in the left brachiocephalic vein may produce an artifact that projects over the aortic arch and supra-aortic branches. Streak artifacts can be differentiated from true intimal flaps because they extend beyond the confines of the aorta whereas aortic lesions are restricted to the aortic diameter. Strategies to avoid this type of error include the injection of CM into a right antecubital vein, scan acquisition in a caudocranial direction, injection of a saline bolus after the CM bolus, and optimization of the delay time and amount of CM.
- Especially in non-ECG-gated examinations, aortic wall motion during cardiac systole and diastole will produce curvilinear artifacts in the proximal ascending aorta, mainly at the aortic root. These artifacts occur at opposite aspects of the aortic circumference, at the left anterior and right posterior walls, and mimic intramural hematoma or dissection (Fig. 10.10). They can be recognized because they occur along two opposing walls of the aorta, whereas a true acute aortic lesion involves only one aspect of the wall, generally the right anterior one. This error is avoided by performing every angioCT of the thoracic aorta with ECG-gated modalities. Indeed, this precaution can be considered mandatory.

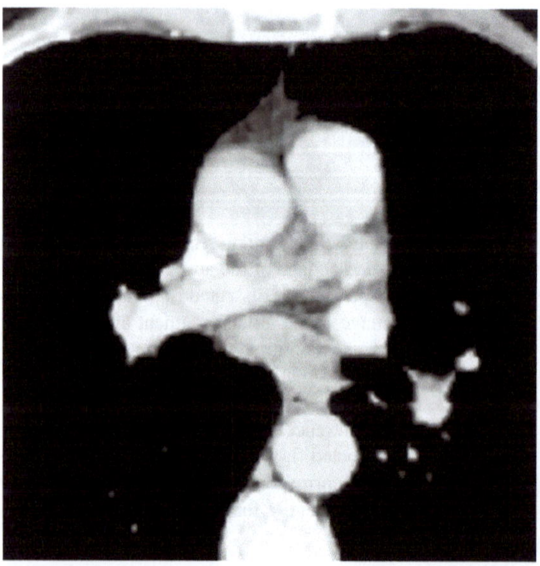

Fig. 10.10 Motion artifacts in the aortic root wall during non-ECG-gated angioCT of the ascending aorta. The axial image reproduces both the diastolic and the systolic aspect of the aortic wall, mimicking an acute lesion (dissection or intramural hematoma). The same artifact is evident in the superior vena cava and right pulmonary artery

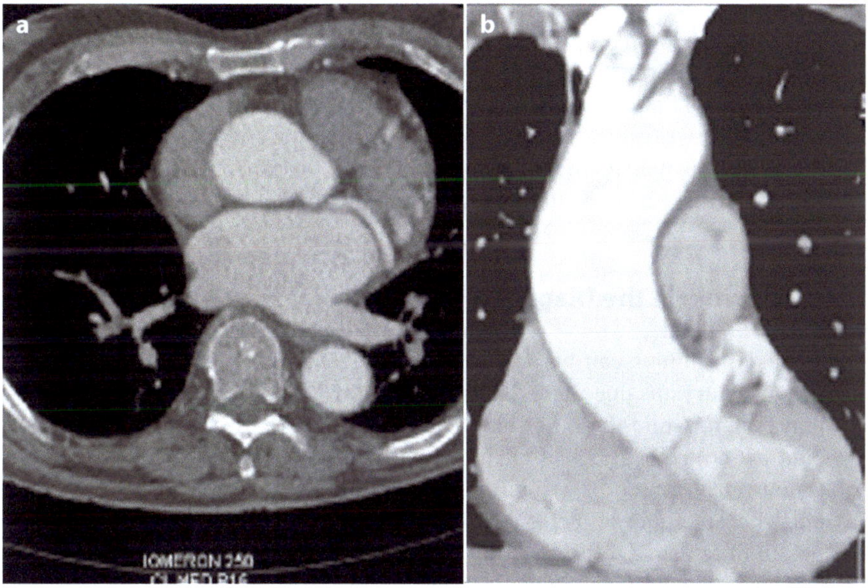

Fig. 10.11 **a** In this axial image taken during ECG-gated angioCT of the thoracic aorta, the left coronary sinus simulates an eccentric "blister like" dilation or false aneurysm of the aortic root. **b** The para-coronal reformatted image of the same case better demonstrates the normal coronary sinus, without any sign of aneurysm

- The normal left coronary sinus in the aortic root may simulate an intimal flap or an eccentric aneurysm on axial images. Thus, the aortic root, sinuses of Valsalva, and coronary ostia are better evaluated on multiplanar reformation (MPR) and 3D images than on transverse images (Fig. 10.11). The normal coronary sinuses are visualized with the corresponding proximal coronary artery, and typically show a blister-like aspect.
- Both normal vessels and peri-aortic structures may be misinterpreted as representing a double lumen or intimal flaps. In the ascending aorta, a type A dissection may be mimicked by the superior pericardial recess, the transverse pericardial sinus, residual thymus, a venous coronary bypass, and the right atrial appendage. In the aortic arch, confusion may arise with the superior intercostal vein. In the descending aorta, dissection can be mimicked by pleural thickening, atelectasis, a left inferior pulmonary vein juxtaposed with the aorta in the presence of an enlarged left atrium, or when the lower pulmonary lobe is retracted. These interpretive errors can be avoided by accurate knowledge of the normal vascular anatomy, by recognition of the vessel on contiguous images or on MPR images, and by recognition of air-bronchograms and vessels involved in segmental atelectasis.
- Congenital aortic diverticulum typically occurs at the aortic isthmus in the concave aspect of the arch. It can mimic aortic pseudoaneurysm and penetrating atherosclerotic ulcer. MPR images help in the differential diagnosis.

- Kinking of an elongated and dilated descending aorta can mimic intimal flaps on single or multiple axial images. The use of MPR and 3D images avoids this interpretive error.
- Penetrating atherosclerotic ulcer results in an intramural hematoma in the acute phase or in aortic dissection in the chronic phase. Surgical or endovascular management is more extensive for atherosclerotic ulcer than for aortic dissection or intramural hematoma.

10.4.3 Errors in the Diagnosis of Abdominal Aortic Aneurysms

- A false thrombus can be produced in some extremely large and eccentric aortic aneurysms due to the laminar flow of CM in only half of the aneurysmal lumen, while the other half remains without CM. This happens as the contrast bolus begins its transit through the aneurysm and is due to the different rates of blood flow within the aneurysmal lumen. It becomes apparent when the delay time is too short. Strategies to avoid this error include positioning the ROI for the bolus test distal to the aneurysm, setting a delay time of 7–8 s after the density threshold of bolus-tracking, or by performing a second scan without delay.
- Inflammatory tissue in the peri-aortic spaces, in retroperitoneal fibrosis, or in inflammatory aortic aneurysms can mimic aortic thrombus on angioCT scans. In these diseases, aortic wall calcifications are present along the inner aspect of the peri-aortic tissue, while in aortic aneurysms calcifications are located along the peripheral aspect of the thrombus. A second delayed scan is recommended for the evaluation of contrast enhancement in the inflammatory peri-aortic tissue in retroperitoneal fibrosis and in inflammatory aortic aneurysm.

References

1. Bae KT, Hieken JP, Brink JA (1998) Aortic and hepatic contrast enhancement at CT. Part II: effect of reduce cardiac output in a porcine model. Radiology 207:657-662
2. Kormano M, Partanen K, Soimakallio S et al (1983) Dynamic contrast enhancement of the upper abdomen: effects of contrast medium and body weight. Invest Radiol 18:364-367
3. Kirchner J, Kickuth R, Laufer U et al D (2000) Optimized enhancement in helical CT: experience with a real-time bolus tracking system in 628 patients. Clin Radiol 55: 368-373
4. Batra P, Bigoni B, Mannin J et al (2000) Pitfalls in the diagnosis of thoracic aortic dissection at CT angiography. Radiographics 20:309-320

Errors in MDCT Coronary Angiography 11

Vitaliano Buffa, Carlo Nicola De Cecco, and Vittorio Miele

11.1 Introduction

Multidetector computed tomography (MDCT) coronary angiography is an accurate, cost-effective, and safe imaging technique in coronary evaluation. An increasing amount of evidence supports the role of MDCT in cardiac protocols, especially with the broad availability of a new generation of scanners. The improved accuracy and safety of MDCT has reduced the need for catheter-based coronary angiography, which in addition to patient-safety benefits is likely to achieve overall cost savings in the diagnostic pathway.

MDCT allows direct visualization of the vessel wall and atheromatous plaques, unlike coronary angiography which is essentially luminography. The sensitivity and specificity of MDCT in coronary stenosis assessment have increased over time, following technological advancements in detector number and spatial resolution. Moreover, increments in computational power have allowed the development of dedicated post-processing software such that multiplanar reformations and volume-rendering can now be obtained, yielding a more accurate representation of the coronary vessels and cardiac structures. The technological standard for coronary evaluation is 64-row MDCT; however, newer scanners, with 256- and 320-rows or two X-ray tubes (dual-source CT) have since been commercialized. These machines allow faster acquisition and are less sensitive to heart rate and motion artifacts. The temporal resolution obtained with a dual-source scanner is very low, about 83 ms, but still higher than that of coronary angiography. In coronary CT using conventional MDCT systems, a heart rate of < 65 beats per minute (bpm) is usually recommended. By using dual-source CT, even patients with an elevated heart rate

V. Buffa (✉)
Department of Cardiovascular Radiology, "San Camillo-Forlanini" Hospital,
Rome, Italy

can undergo coronary evaluation, resulting in images of good diagnostic quality. An extremely high spatial resolution, with a voxel dimension of 0.4 mm, and high contrast resolution are features of the latest scanners, which can be used to accurately depict the coronary arteries. Spatial and temporal resolution are critical factors in cardiac imaging since the coronary arteries are small structures, from 5 mm to less than 3 mm, and they are constantly in motion. Accordingly, heart rate is the most important parameter to obtain high-quality images. An irregular or elevated heart rate can severely hamper image quality, producing a non-diagnostic examination or images plagued by radiological pitfalls. Another confounding element is represented by calcifications, which impair lumen visualization and thereby hinder accurate stenosis assessment.

In coronary CT, radiation dose is a challenging issue. In order to visualize small structures in rapid movement, such as the coronary arteries, it is necessary to synchronize cardiac motion with the acquisition; for this purpose, a retrospective or prospective trigger can be used. In a retrospective trigger, the entire cardiac cycle is acquired using an extremely low pitch (0.2–0.3), resulting in data oversampling with a significant increase in radiation dose administration. Moreover, the need to obtain an elevated signal-to-noise ratio (SNR) is related to a larger radiation exposure. In prospective gating, however, only a small part of the cardiac cycle is sampled, which significantly reduces the radiation dose. Other technical improvements, such as automatic dose modulation, are also fundamental in radiation dose reduction. Tailoring the acquisition to the patient‘s characteristics will avoid unnecessary irradiation; for example, lower kV and mA values can be applied in a young patient or in individuals with a low body mass index, whereas these parameters must be increased in the obese patient to maintain a sufficient SNR.

Post-processing techniques play a fundamental role in image analysis and the radiologist should be properly trained to elaborate high-quality reconstructions. Radiological reporting, as the conclusive act of the examination, is strongly influenced by image quality.

Several errors committed during image acquisition can affect image generation and quality, leading to an erroneous evaluation. In this case, further unnecessary investigations might be performed or the patient may undergo an erroneous surgical or medical procedure. Radiological errors in coronary CT concern technical limitations, incorrect acquisition, or incorrect image analysis. Moreover, the extensive use of post-processing software imposes on the radiologist a strong technological dependence on image interpretation, especially in assessments of the degree of stenosis. For this reason, thorough knowledge of the hidden errors in the post-processing phase is required.

11.2 Acquisition Technique

As noted above, two different acquisition techniques, retrospective and prospective cardiac gating, can be used in coronary CT. In the retrospective modality, a spiral acquisition with low pitch (0.2–0.3) is used to acquire the entire cardiac cycle. With this modality, the phase with the best image quality can be chosen, thus largely avoiding artifacts and pitfalls. The main disadvantage is the patient's high radiation dose, related to the low pitch and oversampling. Modulation dose algorithms, ECG pulsing, and acquisition parameters should be tailored to the patient's characteristics in order to reduce the total exposure.

In the prospective modality, only a small part of the cardiac cycle is acquired, using a sequential scan. Consequently there is a significant reduction in the radiation dose; however, only a small number of cardiac phases are available such that in case of artifacts it is not possible to increase the image quality by choosing a different reconstruction interval.

As with other parameters, the acquisition technique should be selected according to the patient's characteristics in order to reduce the radiation dose. The prospective modality can be used in young individuals with a low heart rate, and the retrospective modality in patients with an unstable, elevated heart rate and diffuse calcified plaques. A common procedural error is to not adopt the proper acquisition technique, thus exposing the patient to an unnecessarily high radiation dose.

11.3 CT Technique Artifacts

Coronary vessels and atheromatous plaques are small structures; accordingly, high spatial and temporal resolutions are the main requirements to adequately evaluate them with MDCT. Using the latest scanners, images with a slice thickness of 0.625–0.75 mm and a 0.4 mm voxel size can be acquired. Intravenous contrast medium administration is necessary to evaluate the coronary lumen. Good vessel opacification is obtained using contrast medium with a high iodine concentration injected at high velocity. Bolus tracking is used to visualize the contrast injection and to choose the correct acquisition time.

Calcified plaques can hamper lumen visualization due to a "blooming" effect; in this case, beam hardening caused by a high-density structure can be visualized as a hypodense streak near the calcified lesion, mimicking a fibrolipidic plaque; this situation represents a frequent interpretation pitfall. A convolution filter with a high resolution and low SNR can reduce the blooming effect such that calcifications are represented in their true dimensions. This modality can also be used in stent evaluation, in which the beam-hardening artifact is also present.

Heavily calcified coronary vessels are poorly evaluated with coronary CT, necessitating a preliminary quantification of the calcium burden with a calcium score study. If a significant amount of calcified plaque is detected, the patient should be referred for another imaging modality, such as coronary angiography, or a stress test.

Motion artifacts related to cardiac movement represent the main problem in coronary CT evaluation. In this case, artifacts during scan acquisition are the

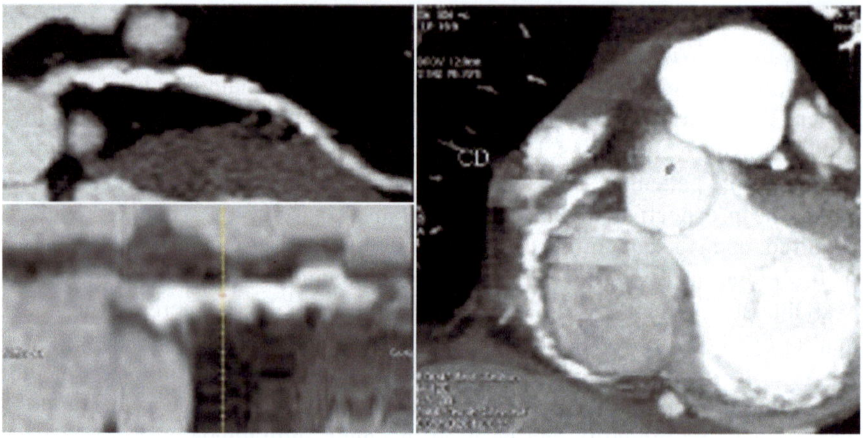

Fig. 11.1 Calcifications and typical cardiac motion artifacts due to arrhythmia result in inadequate depiction of the vessel lumen

result of poor temporal resolution and partial-volume effects due to cardiac motion and arrhythmia (Fig. 11.1). Temporal resolution is the critical factor in coronary CT acquisition. The temporal resolution obtained with a 64-row CT operating with one X-ray tube is 165–150 ms; the patient's heart rate should be < 65 bpm to avoid significant artifacts. In this setting, pre-medication of the patient with beta-blocker drugs is frequently required. A dual-source CT provides a temporal resolution of 83 ms, making it possible to study patients with a higher heart rate and thus to reduce the need for pre-medication.

11.4 Post-processing-related Artifacts

Acquisitions subjected to multiplanar reformation and volume rendering are fundamental in the reporting process. However, interpretation errors can be related to the application of steep opacity curves with possible over- or undersizing of lumen stenosis (Fig. 11.2).

11.5 Reporting Mistakes

The radiology report contains all the critical elements of the examination, including the technical condition and an assessment of the exam quality. In case of low exam quality, clinicians should be informed because it will allow them to appreciate the diagnostic limits of the interpretation. Extensive calcification or artifacts that can hamper lumen evaluation should also be reported. A significant stenosis as seen on coronary CT is classified as a lumen reduction > 50%, while a hemodynamically significant stenosis implies a caliber

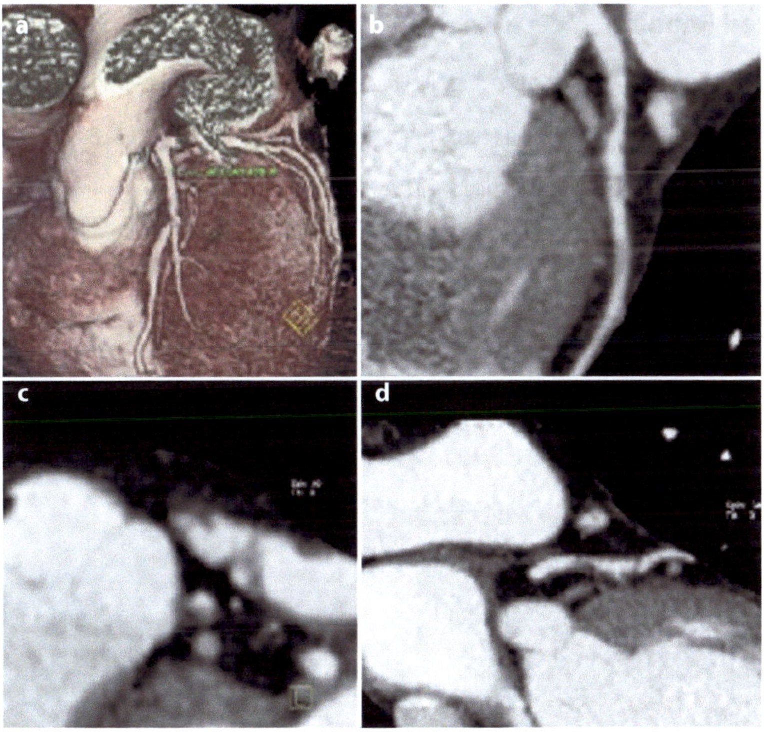

Fig. 11.2 Underestimation of stenosis on a 3D image. a The 3D image shows an apparently normal lumen. b-d Multiplanar views of the same vessel reveal an atheromatous plaque with stenosis of the lumen

reduction of > 70%. Accurate stenosis quantification plays a fundamental role in patient management and diagnostic pathway selection (stress tests or coronary angiography).

11.6 Conclusions

Coronary CT is an accurate, evolving imaging technique. Its non-invasiveness accounts for its use in an increasing number of patients requiring coronary evaluation. Nonetheless, several factors can lead to low-quality exams with no diagnostic information or to radiological pitfalls; both conditions have serious clinical and therapeutic implications or can expose the patient to further, invasive diagnostic tests. The routine application of coronary CT in clinical practice relies on the execution of a high-quality exam, proper image interpretation, and accurate reporting. In the presence of technical limitations or diagnostic incertitude, reporting should in any case suggest the subsequent diagnostic step.

Suggested Reading

Cademartiri F, Casolo G, Midiri M (2011) Clinical applications of cardiac CT, 2nd ed. Spinger-Verlag Italia, Milan

Nakanishi T, Kayashima Y, Inoue R et al (2005) Pitfalls in 16-detector row CT of the coronary arteries. Radiographics 25:425-440

De Cecco CN, Buffa V, Fedeli S et al (2011) Dual-source CT coronary angiography: prospective versus retrospective acquisition technique. La Radiologia Medica 116:178-188

Errors in the Diagnosis of Hepatic Neoplasms

12

Alfonso Ragozzino, Onofrio Catalano, and Paquale Paolantonio

12.1 Introduction

The diagnosis of hepatic neoplasms represents a challenging issue in abdominal radiology as it requires the careful analysis of multiple clinical and imaging parameters. First of all, the radiologist should have at hand precise clinical information, such as the patient's age, sex, clinical history, lab test results, and clinical presentation [1]. Then, findings of previous imaging tests should be accurately reviewed. This is followed by choosing the most accurate imaging modality allowing characterization of the (suspected) hepatic neoplasm. The imaging protocol, including acquisition parameters and contrast medium choice, needs to be tailored to the patient's case. The final, and obviously important, step is the image review. Image interpretation is strongly influenced by the radiologist's experience. It requires a systematic approach in which all imaging findings are accurately reviewed and interpreted, leading to the correct diagnosis. The latter is achieved when it has been clearly demonstrated that the lesion shows the typical findings and clinical history described in the literature. However, there will also be many cases requiring that the radiologist is aware of the limits of diagnostic imaging, as in the case of a hepatic tumor with an atypical appearance or a mismatch between the imaging findings and the clinical data. When confronted with these situations it is imperative that the radiologist not overcall a specific diagnosis but instead accurately describe the imaging findings and recommend further management (alternative imaging, biopsy, follow-up, surgery). Moreover, each step of this complex diagnostic process is a source of potential pitfalls. There are many possible sources of error that can lead to a misdiagnosis or to a missed diag-

A. Ragozzino (✉)
Department of Radiology, "Santa Maria delle Grazie" Hospital, ASL Napoli 2 Nord, Pozzuoli (NA), Italy

nosis of a hepatic lesion. Errors may be related to a lack of clinical information, an incorrect imaging modality or technical imaging protocol, and finally to the wrong interpretation of the images [1]. Even when the imaging procedure is properly chosen and the imaging studies have been performed accurately, medical mistakes can still be made, in the form of a perceptive error or an interpretative error. A perceptive error results in a failure to identify a hepatic neoplasm, such as may occur if it is subtle or is hidden by marked hepatic steatosis or a transient hepatic attenuation difference (THAD). Radiologists who are not well trained are more likely to commit perceptive errors but there are other relevant causes of perceptive error as well, represented by human factors (e.g., insufficient time available for reporting due to a crowded work-list) and by all the possible causes of medical malpractice.

Although interpretative errors also may be related to poor training of the reporting radiologist, they are most commonly due to rare hepatic tumors and neoplasms with atypical findings.

12.2 Errors in Cross-sectional Imaging

This chapter presents several cases that demonstrate the common errors that occur in cross-sectional imaging aimed at the diagnosis of hepatic neoplasm.

For example, on contrast-enhanced MDCT, there are several tricky images of the liver that may result in a misdiagnosis [2]. Specifically, a focal low-attenuation area is frequently visible during the portal-venous phase at the level of segment IV of the liver, along the periphery close to the falciform ligament (Fig. 12.1). This finding represents a liver pseudo-lesion due to venous drainage via the epigastric para-umbilical venous system. A pseudo-lesion arising from accessory venous drainage can be misdiagnosed as a hypodense lesion.

Another common diagnostic error in CT of the liver stems from the use of an inadequate CT protocol [3]. In many centers, the routine CT study protocol for oncologic patients includes an unenhanced CT scan and a portal-venous phase after intravenous injection of iodinated contrast medium. The lack of a complete dynamic study, i.e., arterial phase, portal-venous phase, and delayed (equilibrium) phase may lead to the misdiagnosis of hepatic tumors. Firstly, the lack of an arterial phase may lessen the chances of detecting a hypervascular lesion. In addition, the lack of a complete dynamic study may influence lesion characterization, even in the case of common hepatic lesions such as hepatic hemangioma. Some liver hemangiomas show an internal "slow flow" such that in the portal-venous phase they lack centripetal wash-in, instead appearing as hypodense lesions that can be easily misdiagnosed as liver metastases in oncologic patients. The use of complete dynamic studies and/or an evaluation with MRI can help to solve this diagnostic problem, easily leading to the correct diagnosis (Fig. 12.2).

Errors in the diagnosis of hepatic tumor may occur in case of suboptimal timing of a dynamic study acquisition, after the intravenous administration of

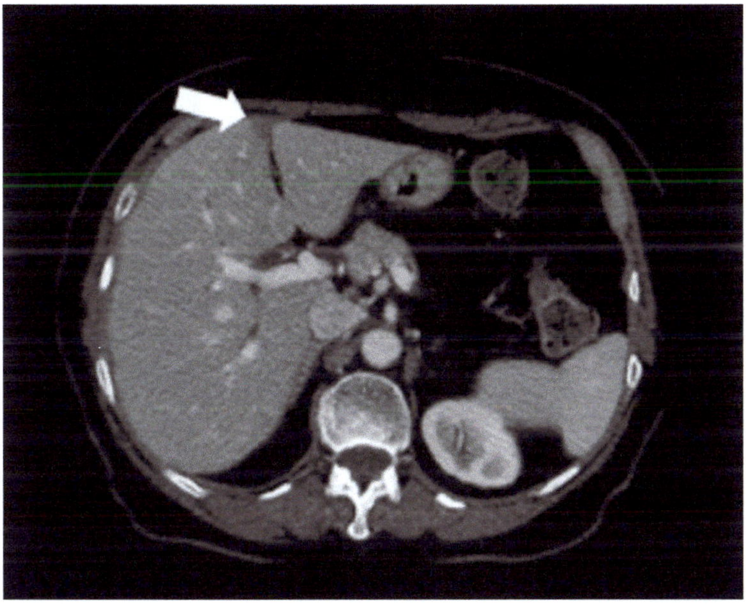

Fig. 12.1 Contrast-enhanced CT demonstrates a liver pseudo-lesion due to hepatic blood drainage via the para-umbilical venous system. A focal area of low-attenuation is seen in the liver periphery, close to the falciform ligament (*arrow*) and around the gallbladder bed. Although pseudo-lesions do not have a mass effect, in oncologic patients they can be misdiagnosed as liver metastases

iodinated contrast medium. Hepatocellular carcinoma (HCC) is identified at CT primarily on hepatic arterial-phase images, owing to the arterial feeding of these tumors. Optimizing the hepatic arterial-phase acquisition delay is crucial if an HCC is suspected. It should be kept in mind that arterial phase is influenced by many variables, such as patient cardiac output and contrast medium injection parameters. Nowadays, a test-bolus or bolus-tracking techniques can be used to optimize hepatic arterial-phase acquisition regardless of patient-dependent variables. If these techniques are not used, then the hepatic arterial phase may be acquired earlier or later than the peak in contrast enhancement of the HCC, leading to an identification error (Fig. 12.3).

Errors caused by a timing delay in hepatic- and/or portal-venous phase acquisitions as well as equilibrium-phase acquisitions may also lead to characterization errors. For instance, slow-flow hemangiomas in oncologic patients or in patients suspected of having a primitive tumor can be easily misdiagnosed as a low-attenuating liver metastasis due to the lack of adequate arterial and equilibrium phases (Fig. 12.4).

However, even if the CT protocol is correct, a challenging issue in liver imaging is the characterization of small lesions visible at CT in oncologic

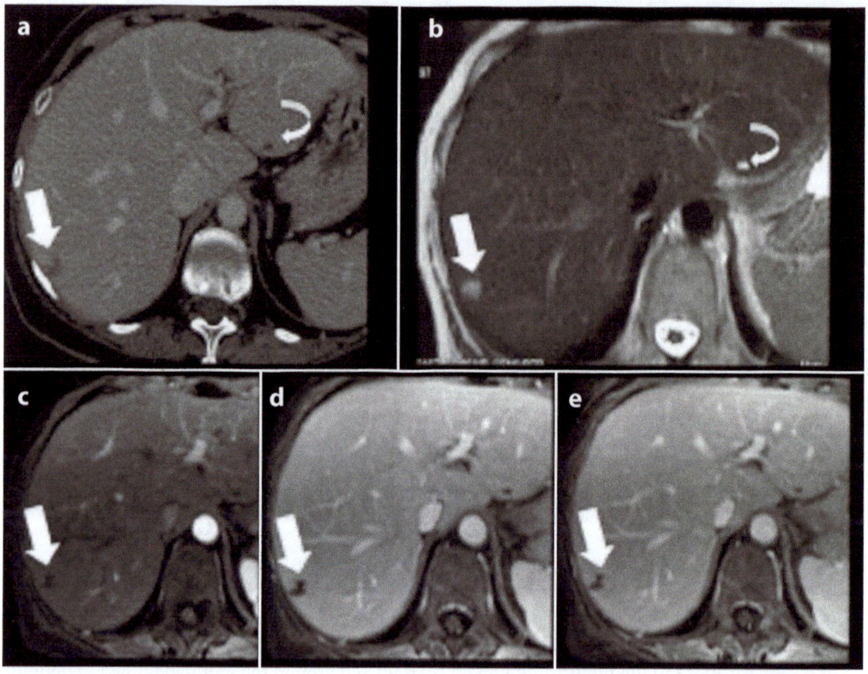

Fig. 12.2 a CT scan of the liver acquired in the portal-venous phase from a patient with colonic carcinoma. A hypodense lesion visible in segment VII (*arrow*) of the liver was misdiagnosed as a liver metastasis. MRI allowed the correct assessment of the lesion as a slow-flow hepatic hemangioma (**b-e**). The strong hyperintense signal of this lesion on T2-weighted (T2W) MRI (**b**) suggests its benign nature. The complete dynamic MRI study (**c-e**) led to the detection of areas of peripheral globular enhancement with signal intensity similar to that of arterial vessels due to the slow filling-in of the lesion with contrast material–an accurate sign of hepatic hemangioma. Another subtle sharply rounded lesion without contrast enhancement and with strong T2 signal intensity is visible in the left liver lobe (*curved arrow*); it was correctly diagnosed on both CT and MRI studies as a hepatic cyst

patients [4]. Most of these lesions are benign but the presence of a small hypodense liver lesion in a patient with cancer, or strongly suspected of having cancer, can be easily misdiagnosed as a liver metastasis. In these cases, MRI can be used as a problem-solving imaging modality, as shown in Fig. 12.5. In this patient, liver biliary hamartomas were misdiagnosed as liver metastases at CT and correctly characterized at MRI.

Moreover, the radiologist should be aware of the intrinsic limits of CT in terms of contrast resolution. It can be difficult to evaluate contrast enhancement in a lesion previously treated with lipiodol, due to partial retention of the iodized oil and subsequent beam-hardening artifacts (Fig. 12.6).

A frequent cause of misdiagnosis following US or CT is a focal liver lesion containing fat, or focal fatty liver, or focal spread in a fatty liver [5]. As shown in Fig. 12.7, at CT, a hepatic fat-containing lesion may simulate a hypovascular

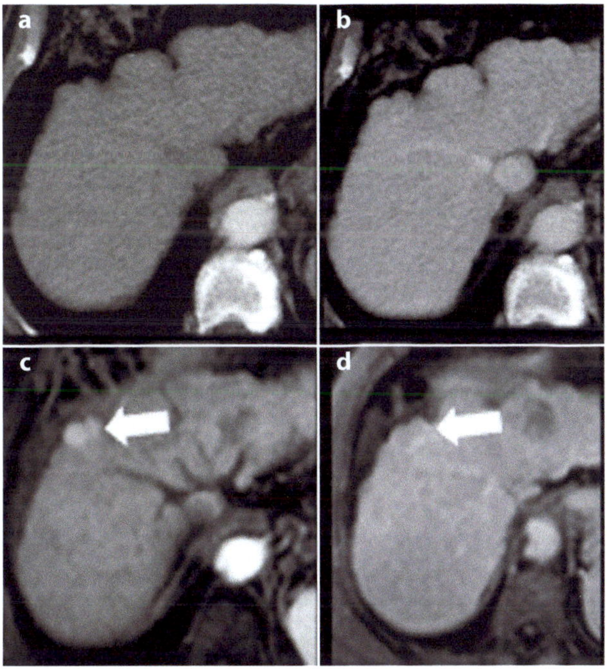

Fig. 12.3 The premature acquisition of hepatic arterial phase can result in an identification error in case of a hypervascular lesion. **a** This CT image, acquired after an early delay following contrast medium administration, shows a cirrhotic liver. No hypervascular lesions are visible because peak contrast enhancement of the hepatic tumor was missed. On portal-venous phase, HCC may appear isointense with the liver parenchyma as well (**b**). In this patient, the diagnosis was based on an MRI of the liver, correctly acquiring hepatic arterial (**c**) and equilibrium (**d**) phases. In the latter phase, HCC shows arterial enhancement with wash-out of contrast medium (*arrow*). Timing-related errors of identification can be prevented by the administration of a test-bolus or by using a bolus-tracking approach, as both allow optimal timing of the dynamic study

liver lesion, whereas at sonography focal fatty sparing in a steatotic liver may simulate a hypoechoic lesion (Fig. 12.8). MRI using chemical-shift and fat-saturated sequences offers a robust method to correctly identify focal fatty liver, focal sparing in steatotic liver, and lipomatous tumor and to distinguish these entities from liver metastasis.

Nonetheless, misdiagnosis may arise at MRI as well, as liver metastases on a fatty liver can be confused with focal steatotic spread (Fig. 12.9), and steatotic adenoma with focal fatty liver (Fig. 12.10). In both cases, an accurate review of all findings, including the contrast dynamic behavior of the lesion, allows the correct diagnosis to be made.

Even for well-trained abdominal radiologists, the atypical presentation of a liver tumor may be a possible cause of misdiagnosis. Atypical presentations reflect many different underlying conditions, such as internal bleeding, rupture,

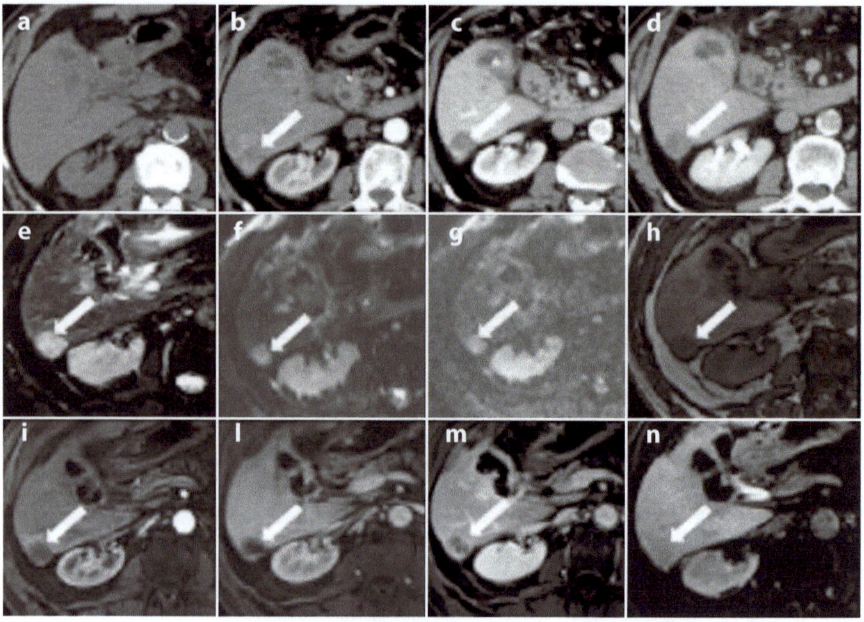

Fig. 12.4 A slow-flow hepatic hemangioma misdiagnosed at contrast-enhanced CT as a liver metastasis (**a-d**) due to incorrect timing of the dynamic study. Moreover, in this patient acute cholecystitis (*asterisk*) was misdiagnosed as gallbladder carcinoma basically due to the lack of clinical information. The liver lesion was correctly diagnosed at MRI of the liver (**e-n**). At unenhanced CT, the liver lesion (*arrow*) is isodense to the liver parenchyma (**a**). Following contrast administration, the hepatic arterial phase was acquired too early (**b**); there is no definite globular enhancement at the lesion's periphery. Due to its internal slow-flow, this hemangioma shows low attenuation even on the portal venous (**c**) and equilibrium (**d**) phases. At MRI, the lesion was correctly characterized based on its high signal intensity on T2W images (**e**). Also, the lesion's high signal on heavily diffusion-weighted imaging (DWI) (**f**) and high apparent diffusion coefficient (ADC) on the ADC map (**g**) are consistent with its T2-shine-through effect, common for benign lesions with a long T2 relaxation time. The lesion was hypointense on the unenhanced T1W image (**h**) while in the dynamic study (**i-m**) areas of strong peripheral enhancement were visible in the equilibrium phase (**m**). The hepatobiliary-phase image (**n**) does not give additional diagnostic information in the case of a hepatic hemangioma

involution, and necrotic or inflammatory changes, that can modify the classic presentation on different imaging modalities, whether enhanced or unenhanced and on dynamic studies.

As shown in Fig. 12.11, inflammatory hepatic adenoma may be difficult to distinguish from focal nodular hyperplasia (FNH) [6]. In such cases, an accurate review of all the findings is mandatory in order to correctly evaluate atypical features, such as the high signal intensity on T2-weighted (T2W) images. Moreover, the radiologist should be aware of the recent classification of adenoma subtypes as well as their pattern of enhancement using hepatobiliary

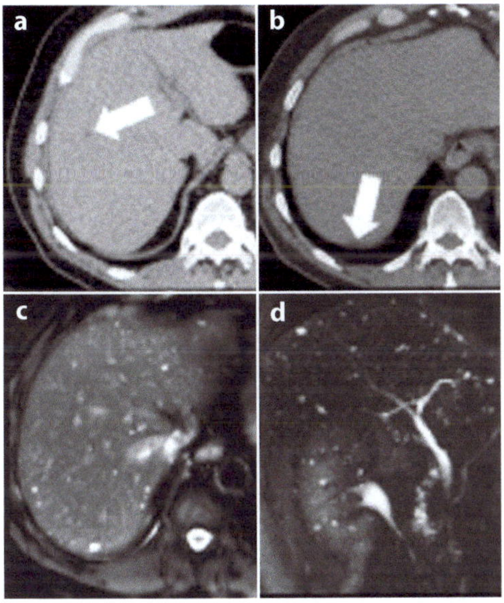

Fig. 12.5 The characterization of small hypodense lesions in oncologic patients remains a challenging issue and a possible cause of diagnostic errors based on CT findings. In this CT study of a patient with multiple biliary hamartomas and colonic carcinoma (**a**, **b**), several tiny low-attenuation lesions are poorly visible (*arrow*). Although these lesions are "too small to characterize," the radiologist overcalled the diagnosis of liver metastasis. Correct diagnosis was possible using heavily T2W MRI (**c**) and magnetic resonance cholangiopancreatography (**d**), both of which showing multiple, tiny, well-defined, and sharply rounded lesions of high signal intensity (fluid signal intensity), thus addressing the benign origin of the lesions and suggesting the correct diagnosis

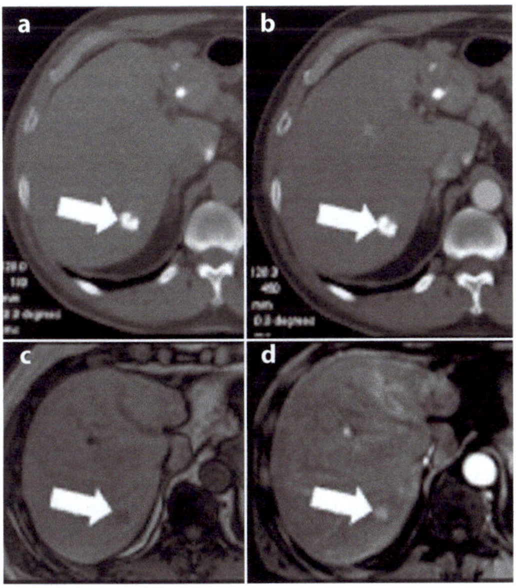

Fig. 12.6 This is a case of a small HCC recently treated by transcatheter arterial chemoembolization (TACE) using lipidol. In the follow-up CT study, blooming and bean-hardening artifacts caused by lipidiol (*arrow*) are seen on the unenhanced CT (**a**) and in the arterial-phase CT study following contrast administration (**b**), obscuring the persistence of the disease. Correct diagnosis was possible using MRI. Lipidol is hypointense on T1W images (*arrow* in **c**), such that a focus of arterial enhancement (*arrow*) clearly visible in the arterial phase allowed the correct diagnosis (**d**)

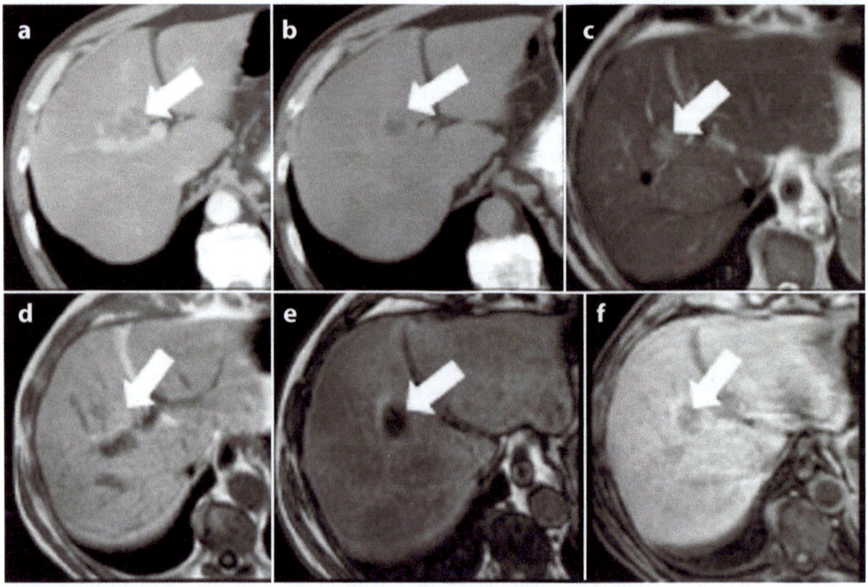

Fig. 12.7 Lipoma is an uncommon benign liver tumor that, based on its CT appearance, can be misdiagnosed as liver metastasis. In this case, a low-attenuation focal liver lesion (*arrow*) was visible on CT during the portal-venous (**a**) and equilibrium (**b**) phases. The correct diagnosis was possible at MRI, in which T2W (**c**), T1W (**d**), out-of-phase T1W (**e**), and fat-saturated T1 W (**f**) images were obtained. The typical features of a fat-containing lesion (*arrow*) are seen, such as high signal intensity on T1W images and low signal intensity on out-of-phase and fat-saturated T1W images

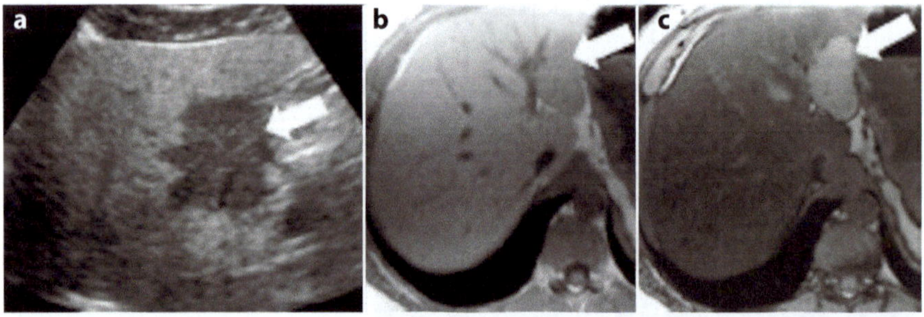

Fig. 12.8 At sonography (**a**), focal sparing in a fatty liver (*arrow*) can be misdiagnosed as a hypoechoic liver tumor. Chemical-shift MRI is a powerful tool in the assessment of liver fat content. In-phase (**b**) and out-of-phase (**c**) T1W images are shown. The diffuse fatty liver exhibits high signal intensity on the in-phase image and low signal intensity on the out-of phase image whereas in focal fatty spread (*arrow*) there is no signal drop between the two phases on T1W images

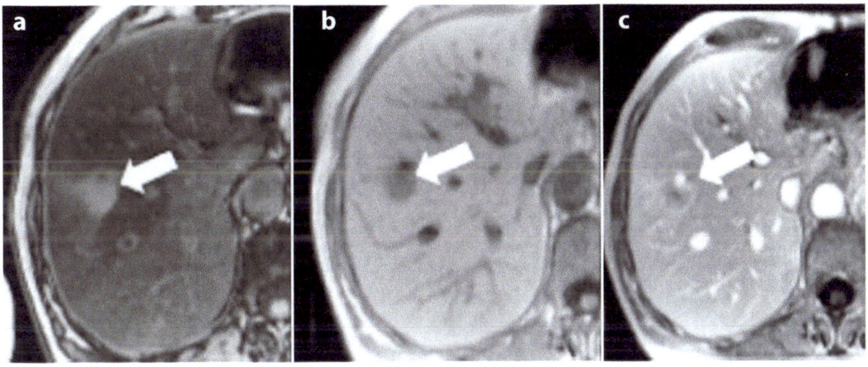

Fig. 12.9 Areas of focal sparing in the fatty liver of oncologic patients should be carefully evaluated since they are a possible cause of errors in the diagnosis of liver metastasis. Out-of-phase (**a**) and in-phase (**b**) T1W images and a contrast-enhanced MRI (**c**) evidence a liver metastasis in a steatotic liver (*arrow*)

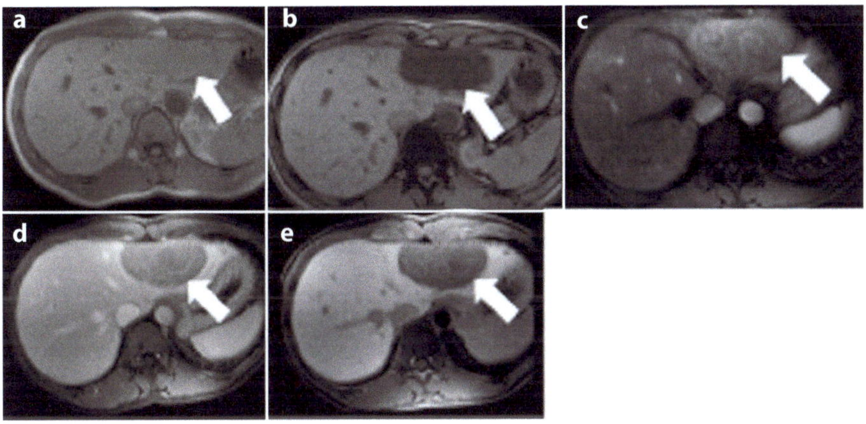

Fig. 12.10 Steatotic liver adenoma can be misdiagnosed as a focal area of steatosis. In phase (**a**) and out-of-phase (**b**) T1W images and the dynamic study with arterial (**c**), equilibrium (**d**), and hepatobiliary (**e**) phases are shown. The lesion (*arrow*) can be misdiagnosed as a focal fatty area due to the drop in signal intensity between the in-phase and out-of-phase images. However, given the mass effect of the lesion, its strong arterial enhancement, the mild wash-out on portal-venous and equilibrium phases, and the lack of enhancement on hepatobiliary phase the correct diagnosis of steatotic adenoma can be easily reached

contrast agents, as both are essential to reaching the correct diagnosis. In this particular case, it is essential to recognize that inflammatory hepatic adenomas, due to internal peliotic changes and inflammatory components, may have high signal intensity on T2W images and that these lesions show hepatobiliary enhancement using Gd-EOB-DTPA, since hepatocytes express organic-anion-

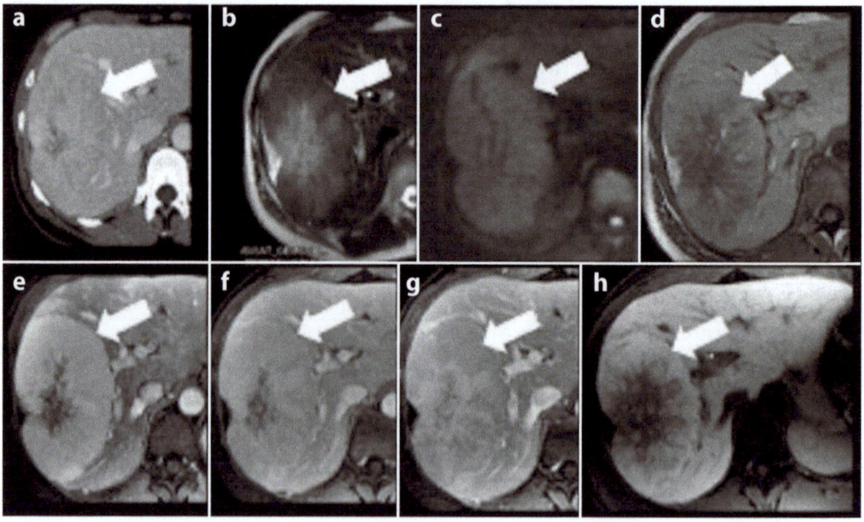

Fig. 12.11 A CT and MRI study in a 42-year-old female patient. **a** The portal-venous phase CT image shows a huge lesion in the right liver lobe (*arrow*) inhomogeneously isodense with the liver parenchyma and featuring a central scar. On MRI, the lesion is slightly and inhomogeneously hyperintense on T2W images without restriction of water molecule diffusion (**b**) as seen on DWI image (b= 800 s/mm2) (**c**). Also on DWI, tubular-shaped hypointense structures resembling engorged vessels (peliotic changes) are evident within the lesion. The lesion was inhomogeneously isointense on T1W images, with central irregular hypointense areas (**d**). The dynamic study (**e**-**g**) showed strong homogeneous arterial enhancement and a central hypointense scar. Wash-out during the portal-venous and equilibrium phases was absent. A progressive slight enhancement and a hypointense central scar are seen. During hepatobiliary phase (20 min after Gd-EOB-DTPA injection) (**h**), the lesion appears isointense to the surrounding liver parenchyma, reflecting hepatocyte expression of OATP8; an internal hypointense irregular scar is also visible. The lesion was misdiagnosed as focal nodular hyperplasia (FNH) due to the presence of arterial enhancement, the lack of wash-out, the presence of a central scar, and hepatobiliary enhancement. At follow-up, the lesion had increased in size, necessitating its surgical excision. The final diagnosis was inflammatory adenoma (in pathological series previously referred to as teleangiectasia). In this case, the radiologist did not take into account the high signal intensity on the T2W image and the capsular retraction, both of which are uncommon for FNH. Moreover, the radiologist ignored the recent subtype classification of hepatic adenomas and their behavior on Gd-EOB-DTPA study. The recent literature provides abundant reports of the biliary enhancement of inflammatory hepatic adenoma on Gd-EOB-DTPA study and of the hyperintensity on T2W images due to peliotic and inflammatory changes

ic-trasporting-peptide-8 (OATP8) on their surfaces. OATP8 is the membrane transporting protein involved in the cellular uptake of Gd-EOB-DTPA.

Hepatic tumors can be associated with anomalies of the liver's blood supply and their imaging features can be complicated by hemorrhagic changes, leading to atypical imaging presentations. In these cases, a confident diagnosis is not always possible based on imaging findings alone; instead, the radiologist should carefully consider the patient's clinical history and presentation, as well as addi-

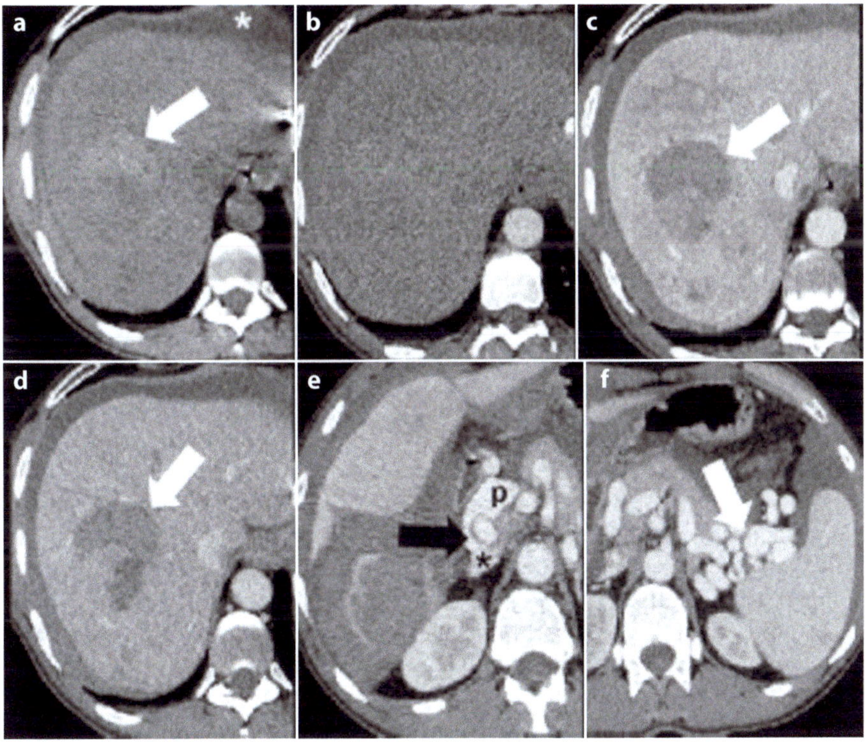

Fig. 12.12 A young patient with acute abdominal pain and hemorrhagic shock underwent an emergency CT study. On the unenhanced CT scan (**a**), a hyperattenuating liver lesion (*arrow*) with signs of hemoperitoneum (*white asterisk*) is visible, suggesting non-traumatic rupture of a liver lesion with hemorrhagic intralesional changes. In the early arterial phase (**b**), acquired to investigate the splanchnic vessels, definite enhancement of the lesion is not visible. On the portal-venous phase (**c**), the lesion is inhomogeneously hypodense. **d**, **e** There is also a vascular malformation, with portal-venous (*p*) shunting (*arrow*) into the inferior vena cava (*asterisk*) associated with splenic vein engorgement (*arrow in* **f**). This is a type II portocaval shunt following the Morgan-Superina portosystemic shunt classification system [7]. The liver is partially perfused with portal flow, leading to the development of liver lesions such as FNH and/or nodular regenerative hyperplasia (NRH). The patient underwent liver resection; the final diagnosis was hemorrhagic NRH

tional findings, such as possible disturbances in the vascular anatomy, in order to suggest patient management. This was evident in a 37-year-old male patient presenting with non-traumatic acute abdominal pain in the right upper quadrant (Fig. 12.12). Contrast-enhanced CT scan performed in the emergency department showed a hemoperitoneum due to the rupture of a hepatic lesion in a multinodular liver. Overall, the lesions were inhomogeneous due to the hemorrhagic changes that caused hyperattenuating internal areas on unenhanced CT. Moreover, the liver parenchyma showed signs of diffuse and regional perfusion alterations. A definite diagnosis based on these findings was not possible and a differential diagnosis was compiled. For a spontaneously ruptured liver lesion in a a multinodular non-cirrhotic liver the list includes hepatocellular adenoma, HCC, focal nodular hyperplasia (FNH), nodular regenerative hyperplasia (NRH), and last, but not least, liver metastasis. However in this patient a review of all images showed a vascular malformation consisting of portal-vein agenesis and portal-systemic shunt [8]. The presence of this complex anomaly of the liver blood supply was suggestive of the benign nature of the lesion. The final diagnosis at pathology after liver resection was indeed NRH.

12.3 Conclusions

In conclusion, diagnostic imaging of a liver tumor represents a complex medical process requiring that the radiologist fully understand the case based on a careful evaluation of the patient's characteristics (clinical history and presentation) and the correlation of all imaging findings with the clinical history in order to correctly assess the corresponding pathological features. Given the complexity of the liver, radiologists should follow a systematic approach in its exploration, establishing a sort of check-list that integrates all the possibilities with the findings. This approach will lead to the correct diagnosis while avoiding, as much as possible, diagnostic errors. Finally, in many complex situations a definite diagnosis of hepatic tumor is not realistic based on imaging findings alone. In these situations, perhaps the best way to avoid errors is to not limit one's conclusions to a single diagnosis but rather to address the items comprising the differential diagnosis based on a meticulous description of findings and suggesting the likelihood of the benignancy or malignancy of the lesion. This approach will be helpful in clinical dialogue and decision-making regarding correct patient management (further imaging, imaging follow-up, biopsy, or surgery).

It is important to emphasize the undeniable importance of learning from one's errors as well as those of one's colleagues. Radiologists and their institutions should be encouraged to engage in a regular practice of recording and discussing errors, such as by holding regular discrepancy/errors meetings in an "educational" interdisciplinary atmosphere.

References

1. Mankad K, Hoey ET, Jones JB et al (2009) Radiology errors: how we learn from our mistakes. Clin Radiol 64:988-983
2. Yoshimitsu K, Honda H, Kuroiwa T et al (2001) Unusual hemodynamic and pseudolesions of the noncirrhotic liver at CT. Radiographics 21:81-96
3. Rengo M, Bellini D, De Cecco CN et al (2011) The optimal contrast media policy in CT of the liver. Acta Radiol 52:467-472

4. Khalil HI, Patterson SA, Panicek DM (2005) Hepatic lesions deemed too small to characterize at CT: prevalence and importance in women with breast cancer. Radiology 235:872-878
5. Martin-Benitez G, Marti-Bonmati L, Barber C et al (2011) Hepatic lipomas and steatosis: An association beyond chance. Eur J Radiol doi.org/10.1016/j.ejrad.2011.06.018
6. Goodwin MD, Dobson JE, Sirlin CB et al (2011) Diagnostic challenges and pitfalls in MR imaging with Hepatocyte-spcific Constrast agent. Radiographics 31:1547-1568
7. Morgan G, Superina R (1994) Congenital absence of the portal vein: two cases and a proposed classification system for portasystemic vascular anomalies. J Pediatr Surg 29:1239-1241
8. Chandler TM, Heran MK, Chang SD, et al (2011) Multiple focal nodular hyperplasia lesions of the liver associated with congenital absence of the portal vein. Magnetic resonance Imaging 29:81-96

Pitfalls in Pancreatic Imaging

13

Roberto Pozzi Mucelli and Stefano Canestrini

13.1 Introduction

The diagnosis of pancreatic diseases generally requires the combined use of different imaging modalities, allowing evaluation of the pancreatic parenchyma, pancreatic ducts, and adjacent soft tissues [1]. Generally, in a clinical picture of abdominal pain and other symptoms that raise suspicion of pancreatic involvement, the first approach is represented by ultrasonography, which is relatively inexpensive and widely available. After the ultrasound (US) findings are confirmed, depending on their characteristics, investigations using computed tomography (CT) and magnetic resonance imaging (MRI) may be recommended.

The high spatial and contrast resolution of US are further increased by the use of second-generation contrast media. Thus, if correctly performed, the US exam represents the best imaging modality for diagnostic as well as therapeutic procedures, such as radiofrequency ablation. However, US is often limited by excessive meteorism, the presence of a very thick layer of subcutaneous fat, or by the alteration of anatomical planes, as occurs after surgery, inflammation, or radiotherapy [2].

Computed tomography, unlike US, provides excellent results in more robust patients, including those with abundant fat surrounding the organs. Multidetector CT (MDCT) technology, in addition to improving the spatial resolution and shortening the examination time, allows volumetric data acquisition and, accordingly, direct image reconstruction on any spatial plane, thus removing the previous limitation of single-detector scanners [2].

R. Pozzi Mucelli (✉)
Department of Radiology, "G.B. Rossi" University Hospital,
Verona, Italy

Magnetic resonance imaging offers good spatial and contrast resolution, the latter further increased by paramagnetic contrast media. Furthermore, with the availability of cholangio-Wirsung magnetic resonance (CWMR) sequences, an excellent view of the pancreatic ductal system and the adjacent biliary tree is obtained, reducing the diagnostic use of endoscopic retrograde cholangiopancreatography (ERCP) and avoiding potential complications (acute pancreatitis). Unfortunately, MRI is still strongly influenced by motion artifacts, nor can it be performed in patients with metal implants or suffering from claustrophobia. Moreover, it does not allow visualization of intraglandular and/or intraductal calcifications, both of which are clearly visible on US and CT [2].

While the correct use of the currently available imaging modalities reveals most pathologic conditions, a variety of anatomic entities, anatomic variants, and pathologies in and around the pancreas can simulate, at imaging, primary pancreatic tumors and vice versa, leading the radiologist to a misdiagnosis. In general, the potential causes of misdiagnosis may depend on operator experience or the adequacy of the diagnostic examination. Therefore, it is important that the radiologist be aware of the wide spectrum of anatomic variants and diseases that can mimic primary pancreatic neoplasia, in order to indicate the appropriate subsequent diagnostic and therapeutic procedures and avoid unnecessary or harmful choices [3].

13.2 Pitfalls

13.2.1 Anatomic Variants

Normal anatomic structures and anatomic anomalies may represent potential pitfalls in that they can mimic other diagnostic entities.

Pancreas divisum, i.e., lack of fusion of the ventral and dorsal embryonic buds, represents the most frequent anomaly of the pancreas. In these patients, the duct of Wirsung is very thin and short, draining only the lower part of the pancreatic head, whereas the duct of Santorini is long, dominant in size, and does not communicate with the duct of Wirsung. In incomplete forms, there is a communication between the two ducts, with the duct of Santorini still dominating. This anomaly can be associated with recurrent abdominal pain and recurrent pancreatitis because the minor papilla is not sufficiently large to support the flow of the pancreatic juices. In addition, this condition is often associated with the onset of ductal ectasia (Santorinicele) [4, 5] (Fig. 13.1).

In annular pancreas, the second most common pancreatic anomaly, a stenotic ring, formed by the gland, surrounds the second duodenal portion, resulting in occlusion. In half of the cases it presents as a duodenal occlusion at birth, often associated with other intestinal malformations. In the other half it may persist into adulthood, causing non-specific digestive disorders or acute or chronic pancreatitis (15–20%) [2] (Fig. 13.2).

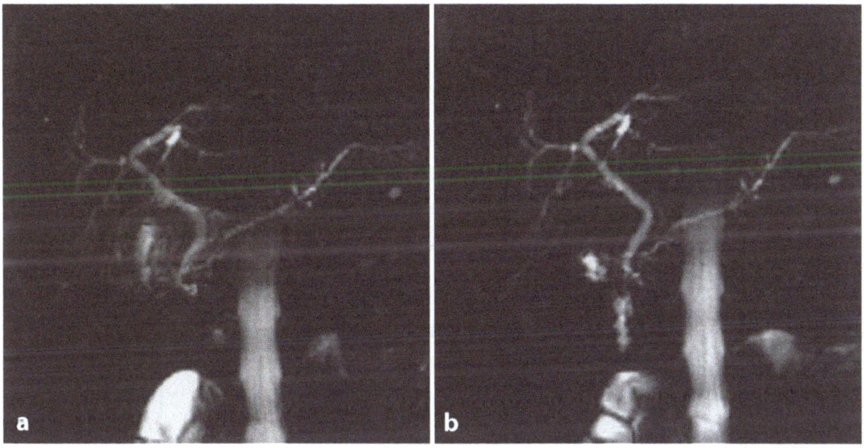

Fig. 13.1 a, b Anatomic variants. Example of pancreas divisum. MRCP without (**a**) and with (**b**) secretin stimulation shows the main pancreatic duct crossing the common bile duct and terminating in the papilla minor. The findings are better demonstrated with secretin stimulation

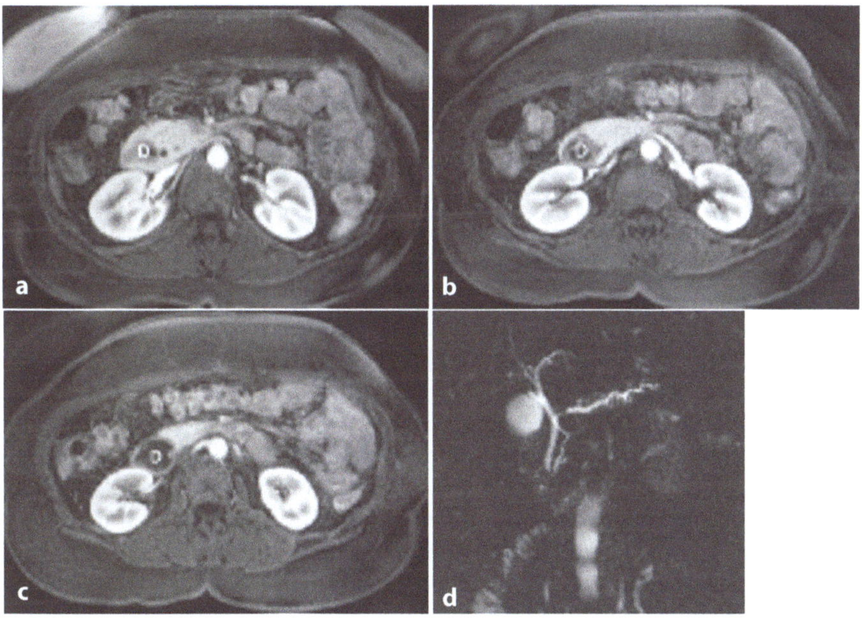

Fig. 13.2 a-d Anatomic variants. Example of annular pancreas. The duodenum (*D*) is included in the pancreatic head and is almost completely surrounded by the pancreatic parenchyma (**a-c**). Magnetic resonance cholangiopancreatography (MRCP) (**d**) shows irregularities, an increased diameter of the main pancreatic duct, and mild dilatation of several collateral branches, consistent with chronic pancreatitis

Ectopic pancreas is relatively common (0.6–14%), although it is often suspected by endoscopy or at surgery and then histologically confirmed. The extrapancreatic glandular islets can be localized within the wall of the stomach, duodenum, jejunum, ileum, or Meckel's diverticulum. More rarely, other sites, such as the colon, esophagus, gallbladder, biliary tract, liver, gut, and mesentery, are involved. An ectopic pancreas is usually small, localized in the submucosa, generally asymptomatic, and clinically evident because of its complications (stenosis, ulcers, bleeding, intussusception, etc.) [5, 6].

Duodenal duplications may also be misinterpreted as pancreatic masses at CT or MRI. While rare in the gastrointestinal tract, approximately 12% of duplications occur in the gastroduodenal region. The duplications are usually non-communicating and in most cases located on the mesenteric side of the second and third portions of the duodenum. These patients typically present with symptoms of obstruction but may also develop biliary obstruction and pancreatitis [2].

Splenic variants, such as accessory spleen or splenosis, can also mimic a pancreatic mass. An accessory spleen occurs in approximately 10% of the population, and intrapancreatic accessory spleens, located in the pancreatic tail, in roughly 16% of these patients [2].

13.2.2 Inflammatory and Infectious Diseases of the Pancreas

In the differential diagnosis of pancreatic tumors, inflammatory and infectious diseases of the pancreas may be difficult to rule out. In fact, they can often manifest with unusual clinical manifestations or, even when associated with clinical data, their imaging appearance may be very similar to that of a pancreatic neoplasm.

Chronic pancreatitis can manifest with a variety of pancreatic abnormalities, such as atrophy or enlargement of the organ and ductal dilatation. In particular, when enlargement due to inflammation is focal it may be essentially indistinguishable from adenocarcinoma on the basis of morphologic features or enhancement pattern at CT or MRI [7] (Fig. 13.3).

Acute focal pancreatitis, even when supported by clinical data, can likewise cause problems in the differential diagnosis of neoplastic lesions [8, 9]. Complications such as hemorrhage, pseudocysts, and peripancreatic fat necrosis can mimic a pancreatic tumor, or in other cases [3] hide an underlying neoplasm that has formed in the meantime (Fig. 13.4).

Groove pancreatitis, a rare segmental chronic type of pancreatitis localized to the groove between the head of the pancreas, the duodenum, and the common bile duct, may also be confused with a pancreatic carcinoma of the pancreatic head. This condition is well demonstrated by T1-weighted MRI as a hypointense mass between the pancreatic head and the duodenal wall, while at CT it appears as a poorly enhancing lesion, reflecting a fibrous mass [10] (Fig. 13.5).

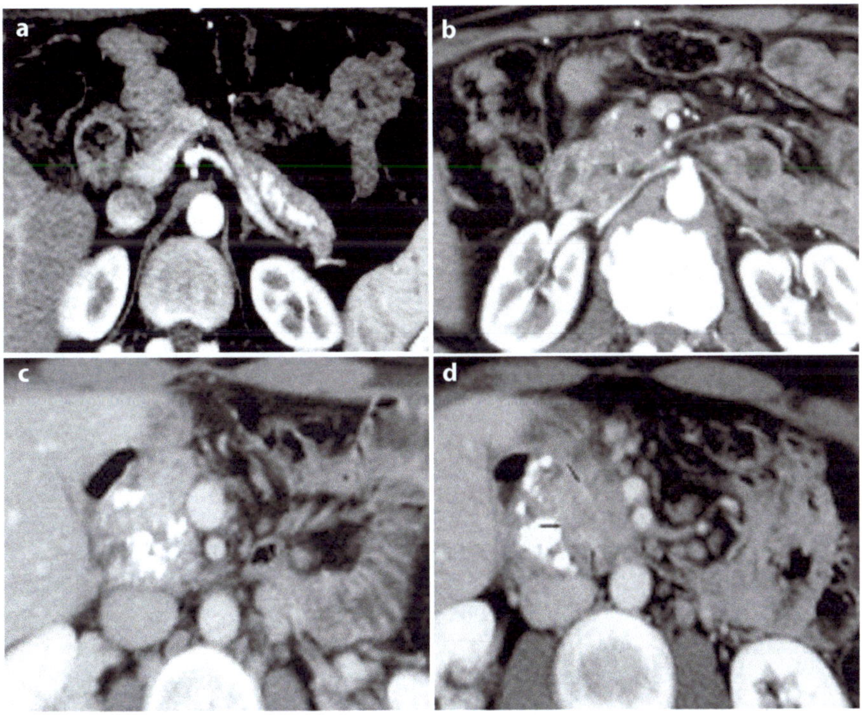

Fig. 13.3 a-d Differential diagnosis between adenocarcinoma and chronic pancreatitis. **a**, **b** False-negative: in this patient with chronic calcified pancreatitis a small mass (*asterisk*) in the pancreatic head was missed. This was a surgically proven adenocarcinoma. **c**, **d** False-positive: in this patient with chronic pancreatitis an apparent mass (*arrows*) in the pancreatic head was suspected to be a tumor; however, this was not proven at biopsy (chronic pancreatitis with diffuse calcifications)

Autoimmune pancreatitis, even if it typically manifests with diffuse pancreatic enlargement, may appear as a distinct mass in the pancreatic head and can be indistinguishable from a pancreatic carcinoma [11, 12] (Fig. 13.6).

13.2.3 Tumors

In the case of tumors, diagnostic problems include difficulties in the detection and characterization of these masses. There are also challenges and diagnostic problems in the staging of pancreatic carcinoma. This section focuses on detection and characterization.

Detection of Pancreatic Tumors

There are difficulties and potential pitfalls in the detection of pancreatic tumors, both with pancreatic adenocarcinoma and with tumors such as those of neuroendocrine origin. Pancreatic adenocarcinoma can be difficult to detect at imaging, whether US, CT, or MRI but for different reasons.

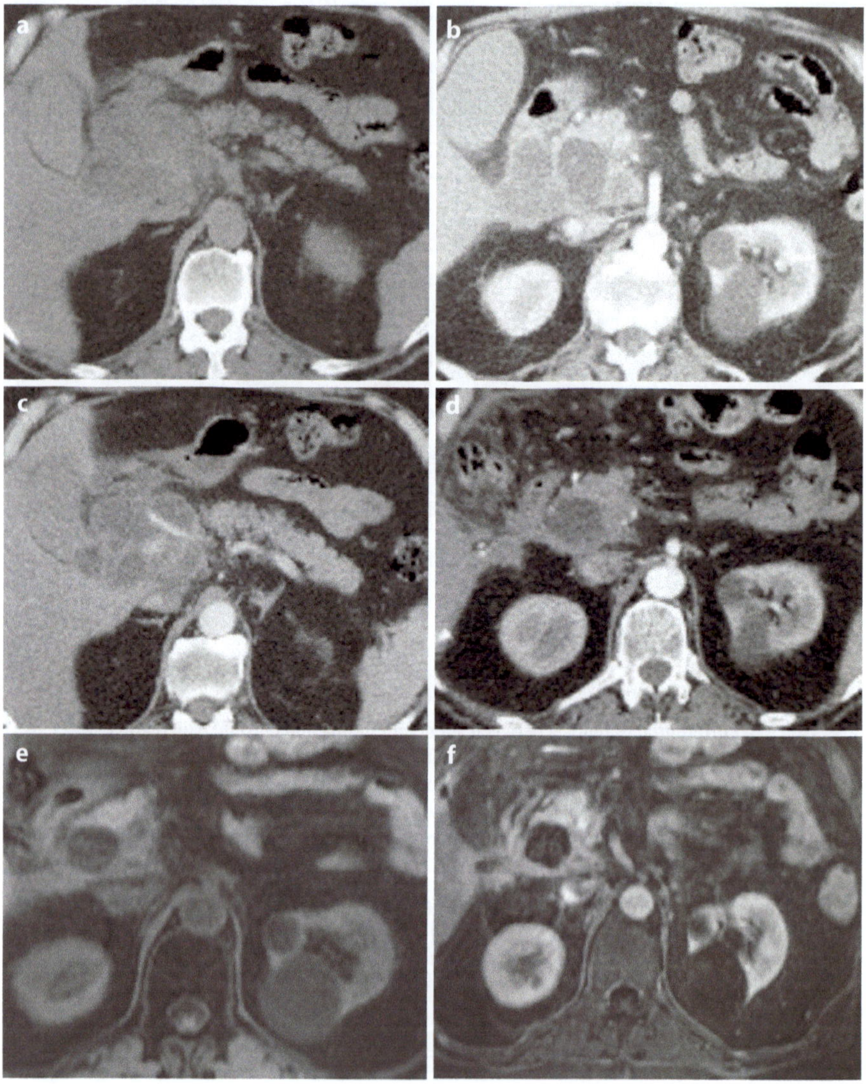

Fig. 13.4 a-f Infection mimicking a tumor mass. **a-c** Large mass of the pancreatic head, with extension into the hepatic hilum. The mass is heterogeneous, with fluid and solid components and irregular septations. The mass was considered to be a tumor with cystic components. The patient underwent surgery, which showed an inflammatory caseous mass (probably tubercular in origin, in spite of the absence of clinical symptoms of infection). **d-f** Residual cystic mass after surgery

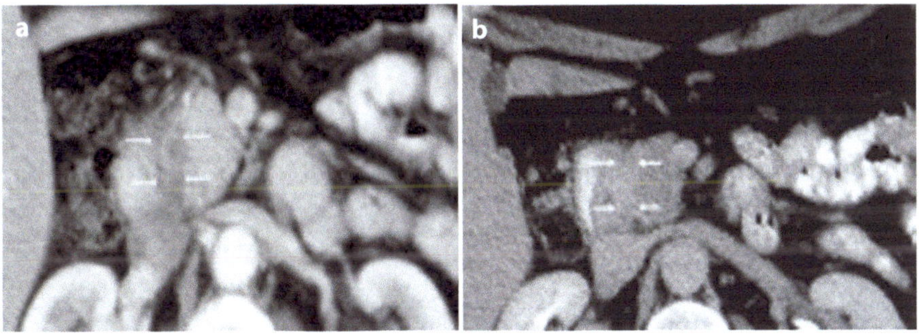

Fig. 13.5 a, b Groove pancreatitis. A low-density area (*arrows*) between the head of the pancreas and the duodenum is seen following contrast enhancement (**a**). In the delayed phase (**b**) a faint late enhancement is present in the same area (*arrows*) due to the fibrous component. This feature contributes to differentiating groove pancreatitis from a carcinoma of the head of the pancreas

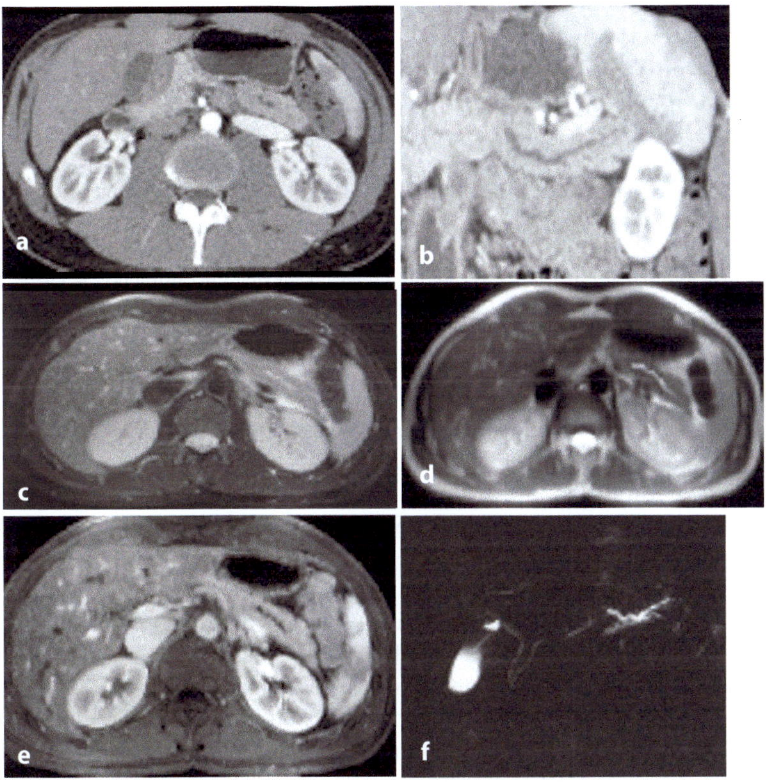

Fig. 13.6 a-f Autoimmune pancreatitis. **a, b** MDCT and **c, d** MRI T2-weighted images; **e** contrast-enhanced T1-weighted and **f** MRCP images. A mild dilatation of the common bile duct is seen in the tail of the pancreas, with a stenosis at the body-tail border. No lesion is visible on either MDCT or MRI at the level of the ductal stenosis. At surgery, a focal area of pancreatitis was found. Histology showed a lymphoplasmacellular infiltrate surrounding the main pancreatic duct, consistent with the diagnosis of autoimmune pancreatitis

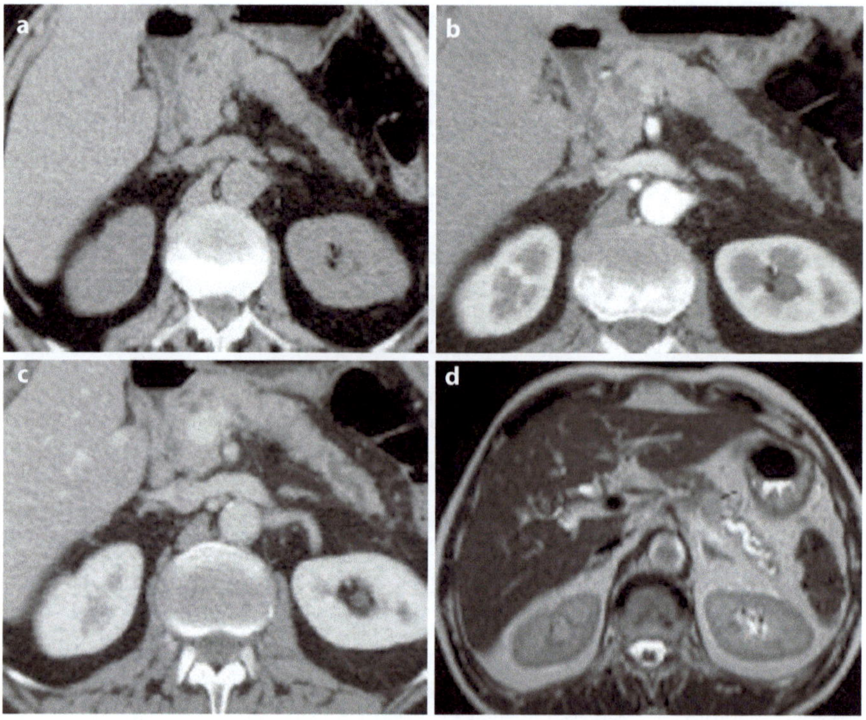

Fig. 13.7 a-d Small pancreatic adenocarcinoma undetected at CT. Non-contrast (**a**) and contrast-enhanced (**b**, **c**) CT. In the tail of the pancreas a dilatation of the main pancreatic duct is demonstrated together with mild atrophy of the gland, but no lesion causing the obstruction is visible. At MRI (**d**), due to the higher contrast resolution, an area of increased signal intensity (*arrow*) is seen together with dilatation of the main pancreatic duct

Difficulties in the US identification of pancreatic adenocarcinoma are related to the well known limiting factors that can obscure the pancreas, mainly bowel gas and obesity. The tail of the pancreas is more difficult to visualize with US and most undetected masses at US are located in this part of the gland. The other cause of a false-negative diagnosis for pancreatic tumor is the small size of the mass, as in small neuroendocrine tumors (NETs). These tumors, when hyperfunctioning and associated with typical symptoms (i.e., insulinomas, gastrinomas), are usually very small (1–2 cm or less) and may be very difficult to demonstrate. Improvements in US techniques, such as contrast-enhanced ultrasonography (CEUS) or endoscopic ultrasound, can reduce the number of false-negative diagnoses, although in many of these cases further imaging with CT and/or MRI is required to detect a small tumor or to confirm its presence.

At CT, the main causes of the undetectability of pancreatic tumors are the small size of these lesions and their isodensity with the surrounding parenchyma (Fig. 13.7). This is true for both pancreatic carcinoma and NETs. In the non-contrast examination, pancreatic adenocarcinoma is usually isodense or mildly hypodense compared to the normal pancreatic parenchyma, while following contrast enhancement it is invariably hypodense. However, these differences in CT densities may be slight or absent, and the tumor, although suspected, for instance, of causing the obstruction or dilatation of the common bile duct and/or the main pancreatic duct, is simply not visible.

Neuroendocrine tumors of the pancreas may be functioning or non-functioning but typically only functioning tumors cause diagnostic difficulties since they can be small or very small in size (Fig. 13.8). Non-functioning NETs of the pancreas are usually large and therefore more easily detected. The sensitivity of CT in the detection of functioning NETs is quite variable although nowadays this has improved with the wider availability of MDCT [13].

Nonetheless, in spite of technological improvements, a number of lesions go undetected due to their small size and/or isodensity in all phases of the contrast-enhanced examination. The sensitivity of MRI is similar to that of CT, although the availability of multiple sequences and parameters affecting signal intensity may favor the MRI-based detection of difficult tumors (Fig. 13.8).

Characterization of Pancreatic Tumors

There are difficulties and potential pitfalls in the characterization of pancreatic tumors, too; for example, in the differential diagnosis between pancreatic adenocarcinoma and other tumors of the pancreas. There may also be confusion with tumors surrounding the pancreas and with non-neoplastic diseases of the pancreas.

Differential Diagnosis Between Pancreatic Adenocarcinoma and Other Tumors of the Pancreas

Pancreatic adenocarcinoma is the most common tumor of the pancreas. In spite of improvements in diagnosis and treatment, the prognosis of these patients has remained poor with respect to 5-year survival. The differentiation of pancreatic adenocarcinoma from other pancreatic tumors is important because non-adenocarcinomatous pancreatic tumors can, in general, be more successfully treated, resulting in a longer survival of these patients. Once again, the most common differential diagnosis to be considered is with NETs, but in this case with the non-functioning variety.

There are a number of imaging characteristics that, if associated with clinical findings, simplify the differential diagnosis [14]. Comparisons of pancreatic adenocarcinoma and non-functioning NETs reveal differences as far as the type of growth, size, boundaries, structure, and vascular pattern are concerned. The type of growth is infiltrative for pancreatic adenocarcinoma, but expansive for non-functioning NETs. Adenocarcinomas tend to be small mainly because symptoms develop quite early, whereas non-functioning NETs, at detection, are larger since due to their lack of endocrine function they long remain asymptomatic. The infiltrative nature of pancreatic adenocarcinoma results in irregular boundaries whereas the expansive growth of most NETs produces

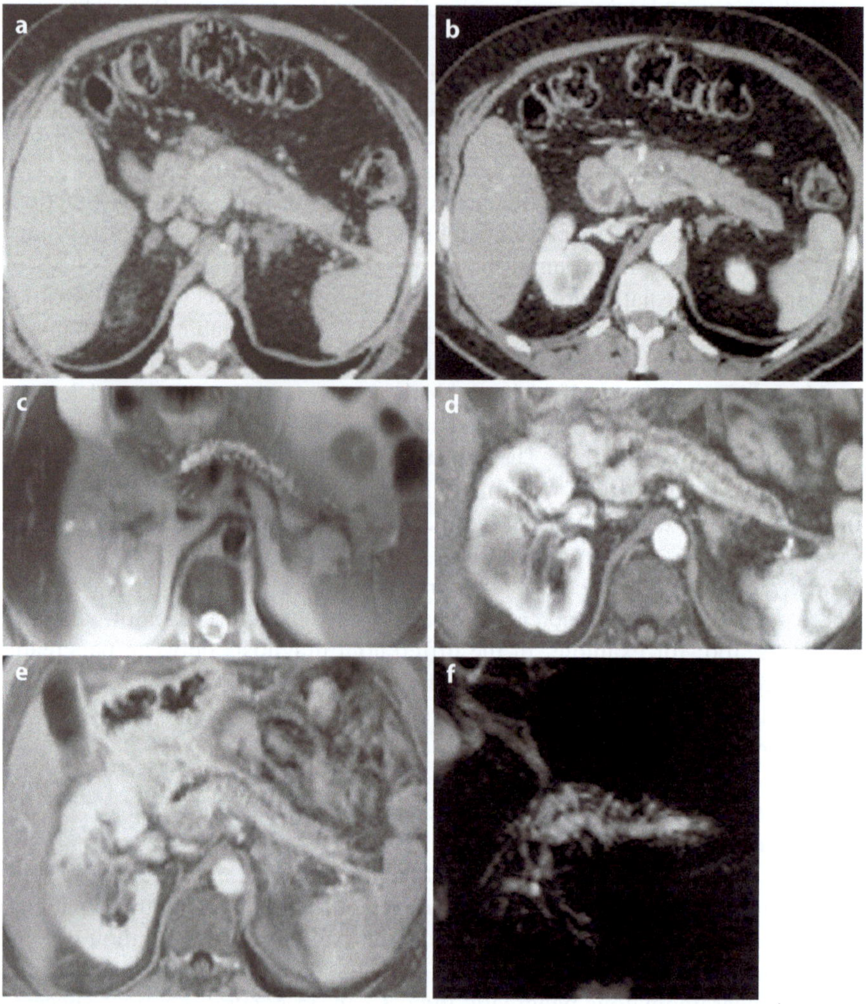

Fig. 13.8 a-f Small NET undetected at MDCT and MRI. MDCT without (**a**) and with contrast enhancement (**b**) demonstrates dilatation of the main pancreatic duct. No definite lesion is visible in the pancreatic head. **c** T2-weighted and **d**, **e** T1-weighted contrast-enhanced MRI in arterial and venous phases as well as **f** MRCP confirm dilatation of the main pancreatic duct without showing any lesion. At surgery, a small (< 1 cm) NET in the head of the pancreas and obstructing the main pancreatic duct was demonstrated

boundaries that are regular or relatively so. The internal structure is non-homogeneous in pancreatic adenocarcinoma, but predominantly homogeneous in NETs, with exceptions for large or very large tumor masses, in which internal areas of non-homogeneous density can be seen.

The vasculature is probably the characteristic on which the differential diagnosis between these two different tumors is mainly based: pancreatic

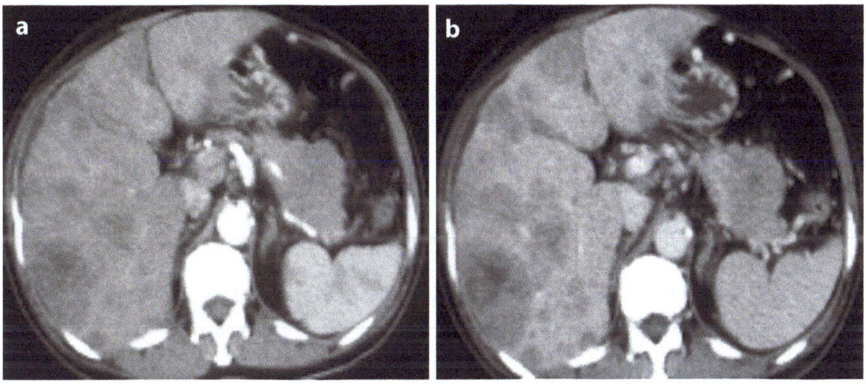

Fig. 13.9 a, b Hypovascular NET indistinguishable from pancreatic adenocarcinoma. MDCT in the arterial (**a**) and venous (**b**) phases shows a large hypodense, hypovascular mass in the tail of the pancreas. Multiple liver hypovascular metastases are also present

adenocarcinoma is hypovascualar in the arterial phase of contrast enhancement while NETs are hypervascular. Thus, in daily practice, the occurrence of a hypervascular tumor mass of the pancreas (especially if associated with the above-mentioned characteristics) should raise suspicion of a non-functioning NET. However, exceptions have been demonstrated in the 20–30% of patients whose NETs are hypovascular and therefore hypodense on contrast-enhanced CT and hypointense on contrast-enhanced MRI. Biopsy under imaging guidance is required in these cases to establish the correct diagnosis (Fig. 13.9).

Tumors other than non-functioning NETs may be included in “difficult” differential diagnoses but they are extremely rare, i.e., acinar cell carcinoma and anaplastic adenocarcinoma. Also, metastases can occur in the kidney but the multiplicity of these lesions and the clinical history usually excludes this possibility from the differential diagnosis.

A different group of lesions that sometimes need to be differentiated from pancreatic adenocarcinoma and, more generally, from solid pancreatic tumors are cystic tumors of the pancreas. The varieties of cystic neoplasm are quite numerous but the most common are the intraductal papillary mucinous tumors (IPMT), i.e., mucinous cystoadenoma (and cystoadenocarcinoma) and serous cystoadenoma. The IPMT can be further divided into central or peripheral depending upon the involvement of the main pancreatic duct or the collateral ducts. Since central IPMT present with ductal dilatation, other causes of ductal dilatation, such as an infiltrating pancreatic adenocarcinoma, should be ruled out. In a few instances, a serous cystoadenoma with numerous enhancing septae within the mass may have a solid or pseudo-solid appearance at CT or MRI, making the differential diagnosis with other pancreatic tumors problematic [15].

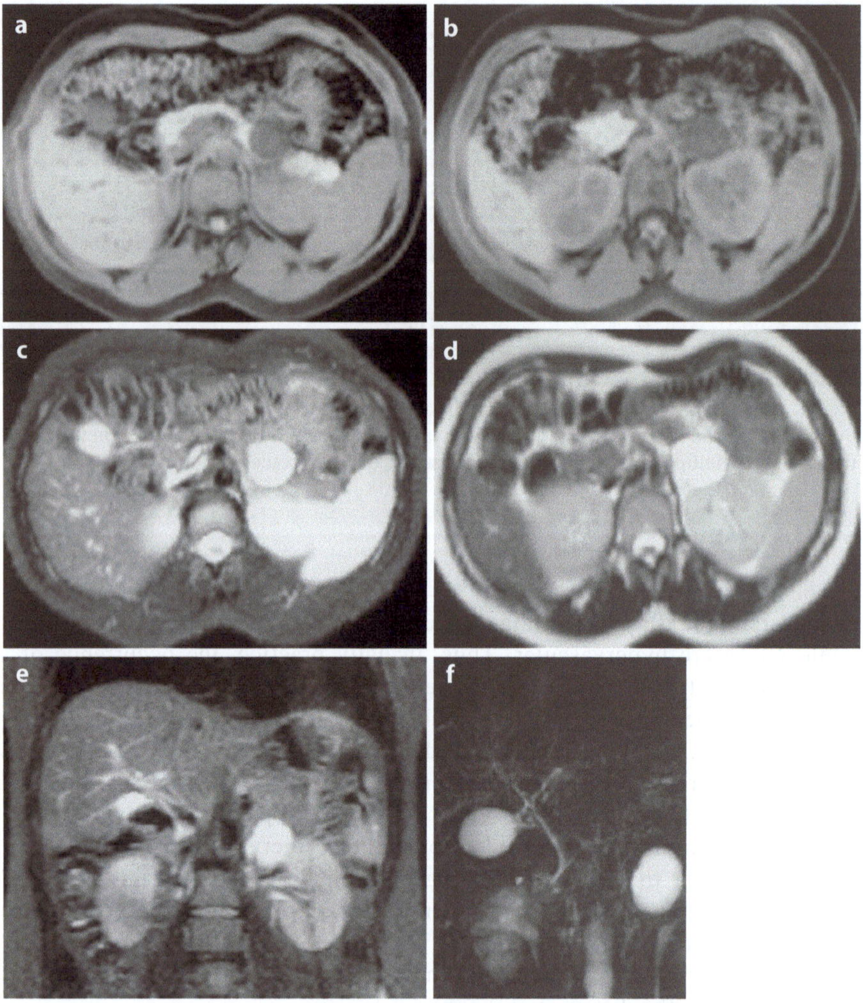

Fig. 13.10 a-f Adrenal mass mimicking a pancreatic cystic mass. **a**, **b** T1-weighted images; **c-e** T2-weighted images; **f** MRCP. There is a cystic mass in the tail of the pancreas (**a**, **c**); however, the mass is also contiguous with the left adrenal, as seen on axial (**b**, **d**) and coronal (**e**) images. MRCP (**f**) shows a normal common bile duct above the cystic mass

Differential Diagnosis with Tumors Surrounding the Pancreas

There is a long list of organs and tumors that potentially simulate pancreatic disease. Lawler et al. [16] and To'o et al. [3] listed a number of pseudo-lesions mimicking primary pancreatic neoplasms, dividing them according to the site (head, body, tail). Among these are anatomical variants, inflammatory conditions, tumors originating in the stomach, duodenum, or proximal jejunum but

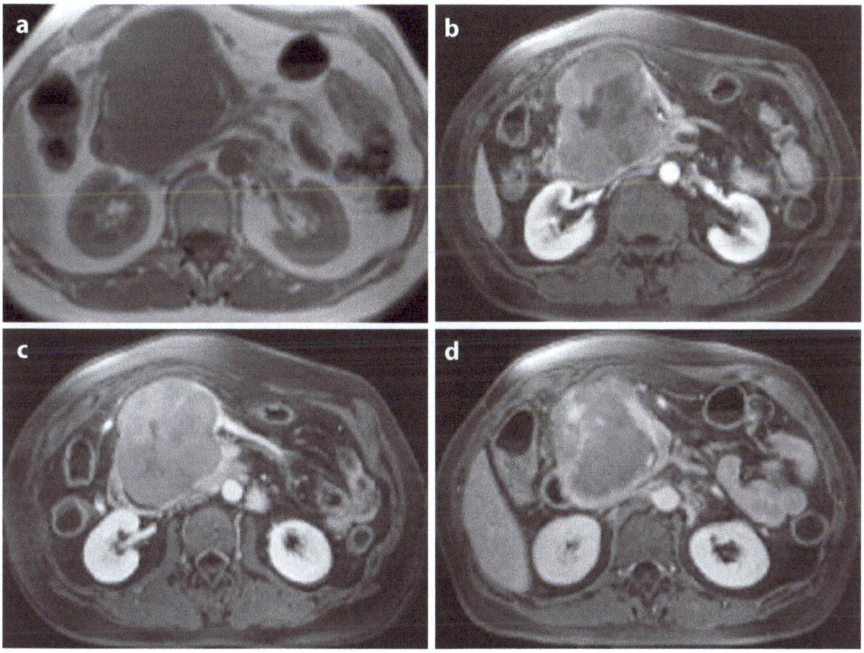

Fig. 13.11 a-d Lymphoma in the pancreatic region, indistinguishable from a pancreatic mass. **a** T1-weighted and **b-d** contrast-enhanced T1-weighted MRI in the arterial and venous phases. There is a large mass, with heterogeneous enhancement and occupying the pancreatic region; due to the large size of the mass, its origin could not be defined. US-guided biopsy demonstrated a lymphoproliferative disease (B-cell lymphoma)

also those from the adrenal glands and kidney. The most common tumor that can be mistaken for a pancreatic tumor is a tumor of the papilla of Vater. Although many of these tumors are malignant, the differential diagnosis between a pancreatic adenocarcinoma and a papillary tumor is important because patients with the latter have a better prognosis. Differentiation is based on a careful evaluation of the site of the lesion, which is more peripheral in papillary tumors. The evaluation of CT and MRI strategies should consider coronal reformations in order to obtain a more ideal view of the region of the papilla of Vater.

Other tumors that must be considered in the peripancreatic region include gastrointestinal stromal tumors (GIST) (mainly from the stomach) and, on the left side, adrenal (Fig. 13.10) and sometimes renal tumors. Lymphoadenopathies, when large and confluent, are a further cause of diagnostic difficulties. They can be observed in lymphomas, both Hodgkin and non-Hodgkin, and consist of multiple lymph nodes that can be separated or confluent. When confluent, they can present as large masses such that the differential diagnosis with a mass originating from the pancreas can be very difficult (Fig. 13.11).

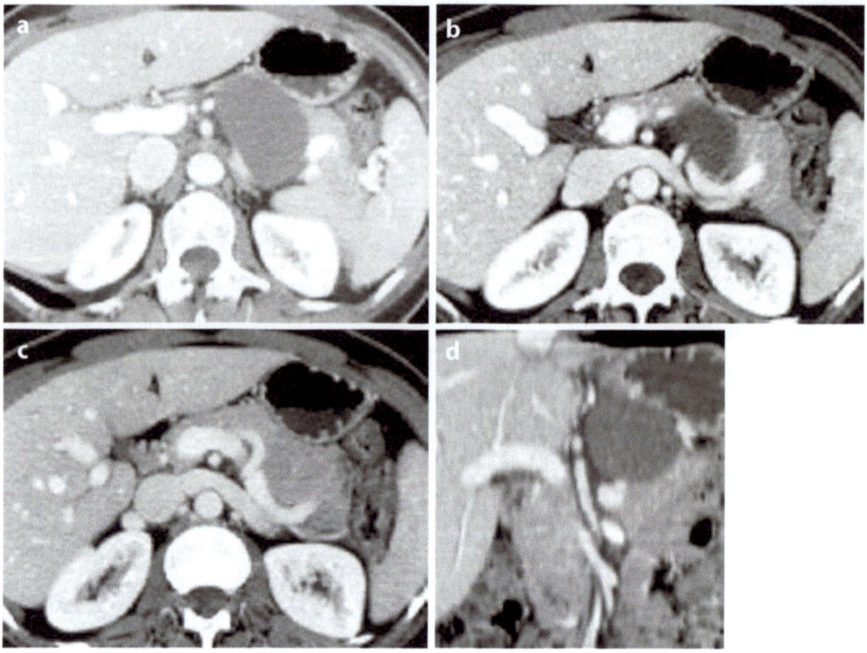

Fig. 13.12 a-d Retroperitoneal lymphangioma. A large cystic homogeneous mass in proximity to the pancreas. The differential diagnosis between a pancreatic cystic tumor and a retroperitoneal cystic mass can be difficult based on axial scans alone. Coronal reformations help in establishing the extrapancreatic origin of the mass

In some cases, also cystic masses originating in the proximity of the pancreas can be confused with cystic pancreatic masses (such as pseudo-cysts and cystic pancreatic tumors). Typical examples of these cystic masses are lymphangiomas and lymphoepithelial cysts originating in the retroperitoneum. A careful evaluation of thin contiguous CT sections and the use of coronal and sagittal reformations aid in the differential diagnosis of the origin of these masses (Fig. 13.12).

Differential Diagnosis with Non-neoplastic Diseases of the Pancreas

Diagnostic difficulties occur also with non-neoplastic diseases, which in some instances can simulate a pancreatic tumor. The main cause of misdiagnosis is represented by chronic pancreatitis, when it presents as a focal mass. The differential diagnosis is based not only on imaging findings but also on the clinical history and previous imaging examinations, if available.

Autoimmune pancreatitis, a particular form of chronic pancreatitis, is frequently misdiagnosed as a pancreatic adenocarcinoma and the differential diagnosis can be very difficult. This disease presents with two main imaging

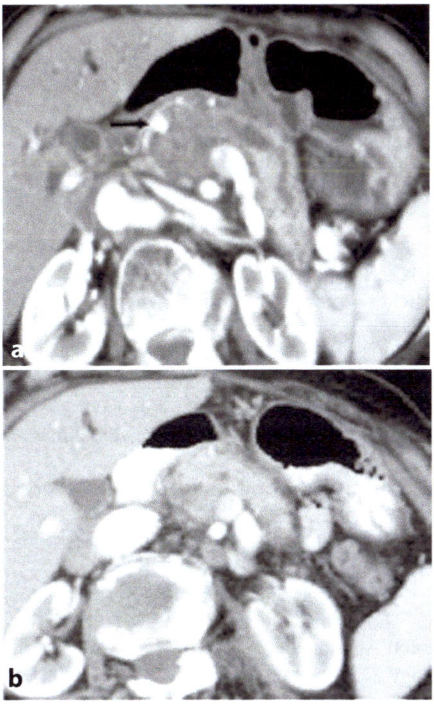

Fig. 13.13 a, b Autoimmune pancreatitis: focal form. **a** Initial MDCT showing a hypodense mass in the head of the pancreas and causing dilatation of the main pancreatic duct. A biliary prosthesis (*arrow*) is also seen since the patient presented with obstructive jaundice. **b** Follow-up CT after one month of steroid therapy shows regression of the pancreatic mass and the normal size of the main pancreatic duct

features: diffuse or focal. While the diffuse form has some characteristic imaging findings, the focal form can present as a focal mass that is hypodense and/or hypointense, respectively, on contrast-enhanced CT and MRI, thus indistinguishable from a pancreatic adenocarcinoma (Fig. 13.13). The differential diagnosis should consider other imaging findings, such as progressive enhancement of the focal mass in the venous and delayed phases, a positive response to steroid treatment at follow-up (favoring a diagnosis of autoimmune pancreatitis), the clinical history (previous autoimmune diseases), and elevated IgG4 levels in the blood [16, 17].

References

1. Matos C, Pezzullo M, Triantopoulou C (2011) Pearls and pitfalls of pancreatic imaging. In: Gourtsoyiannis NC (ed) Clinical MRI of the abdomen: why, how, when. Springer, Berlin Heidelberg, pp 255-277
2. D'Onofrio M (2012) Ultrasonography of the pancreas. Springer-Verlag Italia
3. Katherine J. To'o, Steven S. Raman et al (2005) Pancreatic and peripancreatic diseases mimicking primary pancreatic neoplasia. RadioGraphics 25:949-965
4. Manfredi R, Costamagna G, Brizi MG et al (2000) Pancreas divisum and "santorinicele": diagnosis with dynamic MR cholangiopancreatography with secretin stimulation. Radiology 217:403-408

5. Mortelé KJ, Rocha TC, Streeter JL, Taylor AJ (2006) Multimodality imaging of pancreatic and biliary congenital anomalies. Radiographics 26:715-731
6. Jovanovic I, Knezevic S, Micev M, Krstic M (2004) EUS mini probes in diagnosis of cystic dystrophy of duodenal wall in heterotopic pancreas: a case report. World J Gastroenterol 10:2609-2612
7. Johnson PT, Outwater EK (1999) Pancreatic carcinoma versus chronic pancreatitis: dynamic MR imaging. Radiology 212:213-218
8. Lore n I, Lasson A, Fork T et al (1999) New sonographic imaging observations in focal pancreatitis. Eur Radiol 9:862-867
9. D'Onofrio M, Zamboni G, Malagò R et al (2005) Pancreatic pathology. In: Quaia E (ed) Contrast media in ultrasonography. Springer-Verlag: Berlin, pp 335–347
10. Irie H, Honda H, Kuroiwa T et al (1998) MRI of groove pancreatitis. J Comput Assist Tomogr 22:651-655
11. Wakabayashi T, Kawaura Y, Satomura Y et al (2003) Clinical and imaging features of autoimmune pancreatitis with focal pancreatic swelling or mass formation: comparison with so-called tumor-forming pancreatitis and pancreatic carcinoma. Am J Gastroenterol 98:2679-2687
12. Taniguchi T, Seko S, Azuma K et al (2000) Autoimmune pancreatitis detected as a mass in the tail of the pancreas. J Gastroenterol Hepatol 15:461-464
13. Graziani R, Brandalise A, Bellotti M et al (2010) Imaging of neuroendocrine gastroenteropancreatic tumors. Radiol Med 115:1047-1064
14. Procacci C, Carbognin G, Accordini S et al (2001) Nonfunctioning endocrine tumors of the pancreas: possibilities of spiral CT characterization. Eur Radiol 11:1175-1183
15. Megibow AJ, Lombardo FP, Guarise A et al (2001) Cystic pancreatic masses: cross-sectional imaging observations and serial follow-up. Abdom Imaging 26:640-647
16. Manfredi R, Graziani R, Cicero C et al (2008) Autoimmune pancreatitis: CT patterns and their changes after steroid treatment. Radiology 247:435-443
17. Carbognin G, Girardi V, Biasiutti C et al (2009) Autoimmune pancreatitis: imaging findings on contrast-enhanced MR, MRCP and dynamic secretin-enhanced MRCP. Radiol Med 114:1214-1231

Errors in the Interpretation of the Non-traumatic Acute Abdomen

14

Antonella Filippone, Roberta Cianci, and Antonio R. Cotroneo

14.1 Introduction

The term "acute abdomen" defines a clinical syndrome characterized by the sudden onset of severe abdominal pain requiring emergency medical or surgical treatment [1]. In a review of approximately 30,000 patients with acute abdomen, de Bombal [2] observed that the most common causes of acute abdominal pain were represented by appendicitis, acute cholecystitis, and small-bowel obstruction whereas in one third of patients no cause could be determined. Since many of these conditions may have similar early clinical presentations, diagnostic imaging tools including abdominal plain film (APF), ultrasound (US), and multidetector computed tomography (MDCT) play a pivotal role in the management of patients presenting to the emergency department with acute non-traumatic abdominal pain.

In this chapter, we discuss the technical, perceptual, and interpretative errors in the diagnostic work-up of patients presenting with acute abdominal pain due to the frequently encountered urgent diagnoses such as appendicitis, diverticulitis, cholecystitis, and bowel obstruction.

14.2 Technical Errors

14.2.1 General Concepts

The most commonly initial imaging examination performed in the diagnostic work-up of patients with acute abdominal pain is APF. In evaluations of the

A. Filippone (✉)
Department of Neurosciences and Imaging, Section of Radiological Imaging,
"G. d'Annunzio" University,
Chieti, Italy

gallbladder in all patients and in assessment of the appendix in children and women of reproductive age, US has developed a niche. However, CT has evolved as the premier technique for triaging most patients. The diffusion of multidetector technology is such that a significant number of CT protocols have been developed for a multitude of pathologies. Accordingly, technical errors in imaging of acute abdominal pain usually reflect the erroneous choice of CT scanning protocols and scanning parameters.

The use of intravenous (I.V.) contrast agent is advocated, with the exception of patients with a history of contrast media allergy. One of the most common error is to perform abdominal CT without I.V. contrast agent. The use of contrast material in most cases ensures a high level of accuracy and diagnostic confidence, especially in rendering diagnoses in thin patients, in whom fat interfaces may be almost absent.

Morover, the lack of enteral contrast material does not seem to hamper the accurate reading of CT images obtained in patients with acute abdominal pain. In fact, positive oral contrast medium may obscure the diagnosis of bowel hemorrhage or ischemia as well as limit the detection of ureteral stones, appendicoliths, bile duct stones, and bowel wall contrast-enhanced pattern. There are also practical difficulties that include the inability of sick patients to consume and retain sufficient quantities of oral contrast material.

Recently, tailored limited CT protocols have been advocated to increase the sensitivity and specificity of CT over conventional radiography [3-6]. Limited CT scan tailored to confirm or exclude a specific suspected cause of acute abdomen may reduce the examination time, the cost, and the need for I.V contrast material, while improving accuracy for a specific diagnosis. However, there is a risk of prematurely narrowing the diagnostic focus in the clinical setting. Indeed, diagnostic errors will occur if the anatomic coverage is dictated solely by the vagaries of clinical diagnosis. In our experience it is best to obtain a general survey examination that includes the entire abdomen and pelvis.

14.2.2 Appendicitis

In the mid 1980s, graded compression sonography emerged as a promising imaging technique for the evaluation of suspected appendicitis, especially in children [7]. Unfortunately, sonography is highly operator-dependent, requires a high level of skill and expertise, and may be difficult in some situations (severe pain, overlying gas, large and overweight adults). Anecdotally, our personal experience with sonography in the diagnosis of appendicitis has been disappointing. Moreover, one of the cause of delayed diagnosis is a false-negative or inconclusive sonography result. In these situations we recommend proceeding with MDCT, to avoid a missed diagnosis.

The optimal CT technique for appendicitis remains controversial, and a variety of methods have been advocated. Some centers suggest examination

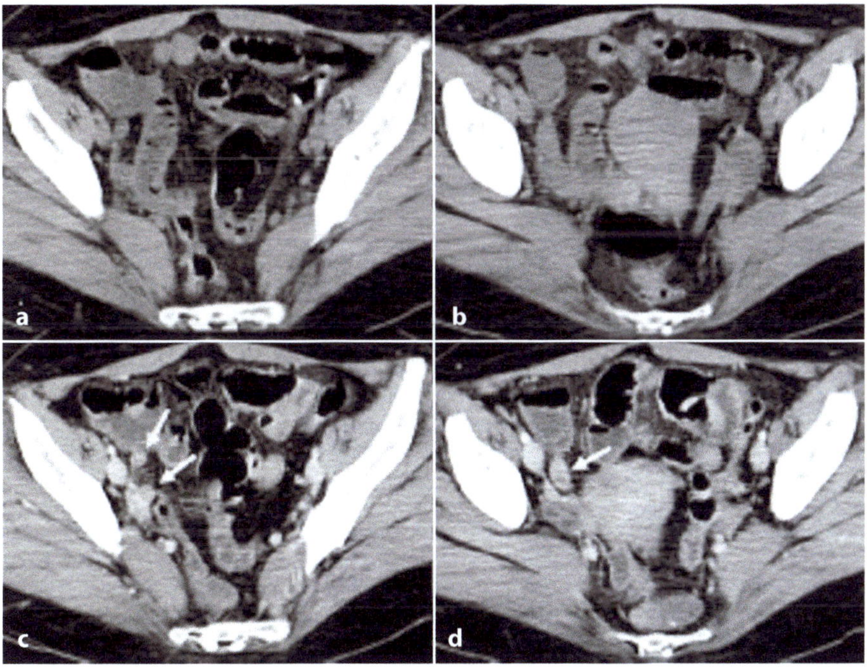

Fig. 14.1 Axial CT images from a 46-year-old woman suspected of having appendicitis. At non-enhanced CT (**a**, **b**), the appendix was not confidently visualized and the pericecal fat was not involved. These features were not considered to be indicative of acute appendicitis. Two days later, as her symptoms had not resolved, a CT scan was performed after I.V. contrast administration, revealing a thickened inflamed appendix with mural enhancement and minimal peri-appendiceal fat stranding (*arrows* in **c**, **d**). Surgery was performed, with a final diagnosis of catarrhal acute appendicitis, consistent with the diagnosis based on the enhanced CT study

without I.V. contrast agent [5, 8]. A lack of I.V. contrast agent may be a cause of error in patients with a paucity of intrabdominal fat or in patients with early signs of inflammation. In the former category, a non-enhanced scan may be inconclusive, because the inflamed appendix is not confidently visualized. Similarly, enhanced scans avoid a false-negative diagnosis in patients with early acute appendicitis (mild wall thickening and mural hyper-enhancement with minimal or no fat stranding) (Fig. 14.1) [9].

Some authors advocate a focused CT examination from the right renal lower pole through the entire pelvis. However, the focused CT technique may be a cause of missing other diseases that mimic appendicitis clinically. In one study of 100 patients presenting to the emergency department with right lower quadrant pain, Kamel et al. [10] showed that if the only CT exam that had been performed was focused CT, then 7% of patients with abnormalities outside the pelvis (4% of whom required surgery) would have been undiagnosed.

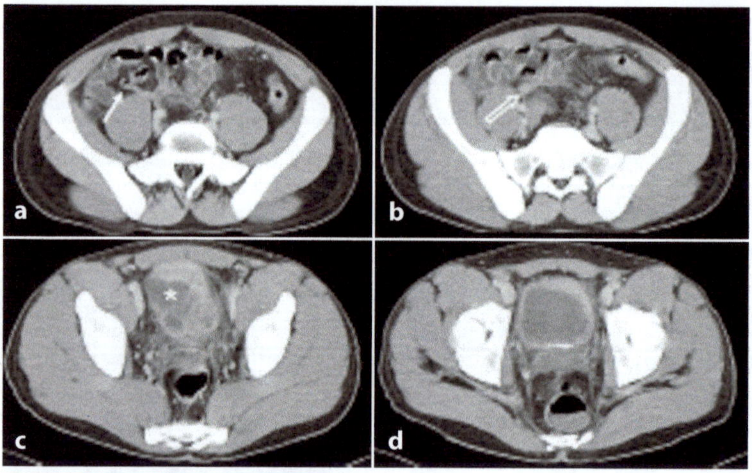

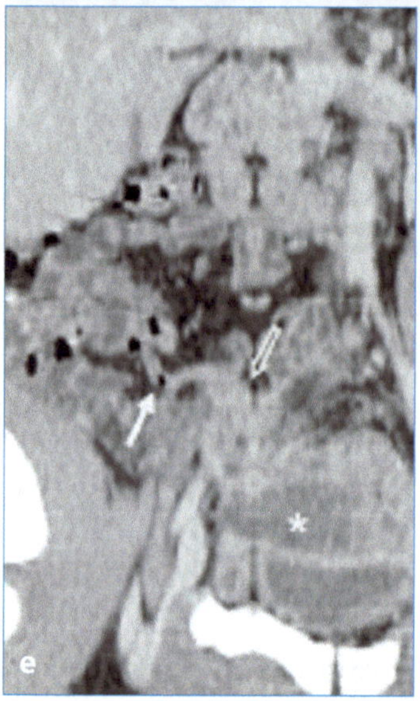

Fig. 14.2 MDCT examination in a 26-year-old man with acute right lower quadrant pain and sepsis due to complicated tip appendicitis. Axial CT images (**a-b**) show the presence of an abscess (*asterisk in* **c**) with extensive fat inflammatory changes in the pelvis above the urinary bladder. Surgery proved that the abscess was due to a complicated tip appendicitis. On review, the appendix appears normal and gas-filled in its proximal course (*white arrow in* **a**), whereas it shows inflammation of its tip (*open arrow in* **b**). Coronal reformation (**e**) clearly shows the entire length of the appendix (*white arrow in* **e**), with a better visualization of the distal portion (*open arrow in* **e**) and its contiguity with the abscess (*asterisk in* **e**) located above the urinary bladder

When considering scanning parameters. section thicknesses ≥ 5 mm may be a cause of a missed diagnosis. As a matter of fact, the use of thin-section (< 5 mm) images has been shown to improve visualization of abnormal appendiceal inflammation. The use of thin sections also results in multiplanar reformations (MPRs) with a spatial resolution similar to that of the axial plane. Several studies have shown that coronal MPRs improve physician confidence in both the diagnosis and the exclusion of appendicitis [11, 12]. The entire length of the appendix is often easier to delineate on coronal images and may reduce the risk of missing tip appendicitis (Fig. 14.2). Coronal views may be particularly helpful in patients with a paucity of abdominal fat, in whom periappendiceal fat stranding can be difficult to visualize.

14.2.3 Intestinal Bowel Obstruction

More than 80% of cases of intestinal obstruction are secondary to adhesion, hernias, or malignancies. The radiologist's role is to identify the presence of bowel obstruction, define the site and the cause of obstruction, and determine possible strangulation.

The first radiologic examination in patients with suspected intestinal obstruction is APF. However, the diffusion of MDCT has dramatically improved the management of patients with suspected obstruction. A lack of I.V. contrast agent may delay the diagnosis of strangulation, which is a main cause of morbidity and mortality. Intravenous contrast agent highlights the abdominal viscera and lesions of the bowel or around the bowel; moreover, it allows an analysis of bowel wall enhancement, which is helpful when looking for strangulation.

In terms of scanning parameters, section thicknesses ≥ 5 mm may result in the transition zone being overlooked. Unlike the degree of dilatation, which is not a reliable criterion for differentiating bowel obstruction from a dynamic ileus, identification of the transition zone is a key point in the diagnosis of mechanical obstruction.

When the CT scans are equivocal the post-processing technique of MPR is especially beneficial, considerably increasing the radiologist's level of confidence in the diagnosis [13]. In some cases, in order to avoid overlooking the transition zone, reformatting views can be included. In small bowel obstruction (SBO) due to adhesion, it may not be possible to visualize the exact point of obstruction; rather, the diagnosis is based on the detection of dilated and collapsed bowel loops, with the cause of the obstruction remaining unclear. The actual adhesion cannot be seen on reformatting views but it may be highlighted as a beak-like narrowing at the obstruction site, without a focal intestinal or adjacent lesion at this point (Fig. 14.3).

14.3 Perceptual Errors

14.3.1 CT Window Settings

Regular soft-tissue windows apply a window width of 350 HU and window level 50 HU. The use of additional windows settings, particularly in evaluating the intra-abdominal fat, is very helpful. In patients with acute abdominal pain, the observation of intra-abdominal fat stranding is a helpful CT sign. According to some authors [14], it suggests that the pathologic process is centered in the mesentery, thus narrowing the differential diagnosis of gastrointestinal disorders to four main entities: diverticulitis, epiploic appendagitis, omental infarction, and appendicitis. The characteristic CT findings of each of these entities often allow a final diagnosis (Fig. 14.4).

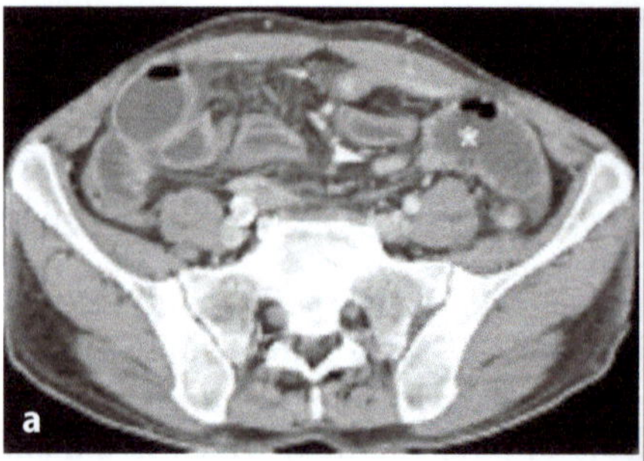

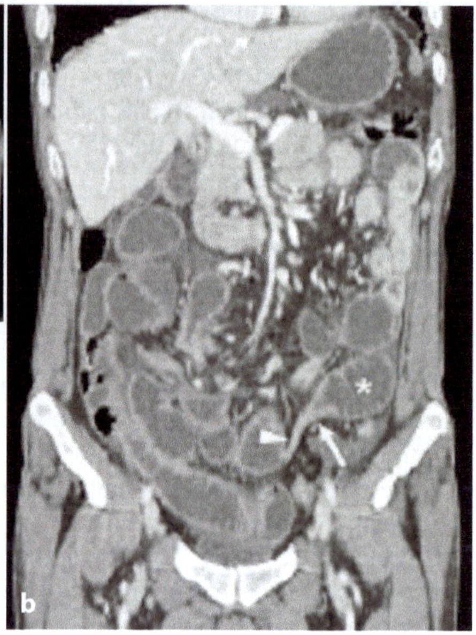

Fig. 14.3 Small bowel obstruction due to adhesion. On axial CT scan (**a**) the transition between dilated (*asterisk*) and collapsed (*arrowhead*) bowel loops is not clearly appreciable. Coronal reformation (**b**) accurately shows bowel loop tapering with a beak sign, indicating the transition site (*arrow*); this finding further supports a diagnosis of mechanical obstruction

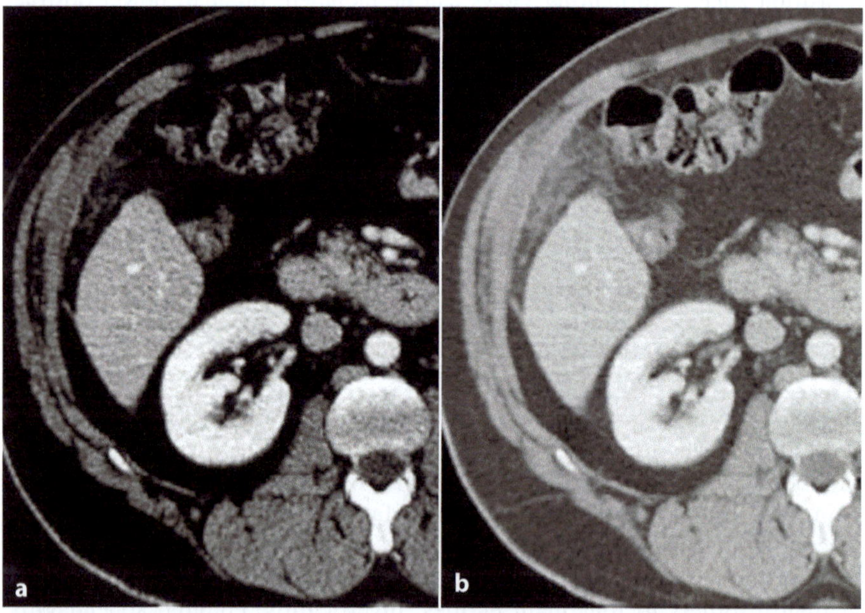

Fig. 14.4 a Acute right flank pain in a 46-year-old man. The heterogeneous fatty mass in the greater omentum and the peritoneal thickening are better appreciated by applying a wider window for image interpretation (**b**). The finding of extensive fat stranding without significant changes of the adjacent colon allows omental infarction to be diagnosed with confidence

14.3.2 Picture Archiving and Communication System

Image review is facilitated on workstations equipped with a picture archiving and communication system (PACS). The possibilities of continuous scrolling through the bowel loops enables extra-luminal fluid collections to be visually separated from adjacent bowel lumen, although these different entities quite often have the same density features.

14.4 Interpretative Errors

14.4.1 Appendicitis

Radiologists generally rely on a typical constellation of CT findings to diagnose appendicitis (distension of the appendix, inflammatory changes in the peri-appendiceal fat, focal cecal wall thickening, and an appendicolith). Causes of errors are represented by variants of appendiceal disease, including distal and stump appendicitis.

In case of distal or tip appendicitis, the proximal portion of the appendix is normal, whereas the distal portion is focally inflamed; stranding of the adjacent fat may be present or absent. By carefully following the appendix from its origin to its tip, the radiologist can avoid overlooking inflammation.

Stump appendicitis in patients with right lower abdominal pain after appendectomy can delay diagnosis and treatment. As the CT findings may not be specific, an awareness of the possibility of stump appendicitis, combined with a high index of suspicion, are needed to make the diagnosis. CT findings in the handful of cases described in the literature include pericecal inflammatory changes, abscess formation, fluid in the right paracolic gutter, cecal wall thickening, and an ileocecal mass [15] (Fig. 14.5).

Appendicitis, with its secondary inflammatory changes in the right lower quadrant, may cause reactive dilatation of the small bowel [16] that may be significant enough to mimic SBO. This, in turn, can result in a missed diagnosis of the underlying problem, i.e., the inflamed appendix, that is causing the small bowel dilatation. In these cases, especially in patients with an apparent SBO who have no prior history of surgery and no cause for obstruction, the diagnosis of appendicitis should be actively excluded (Fig. 14.6).

14.4.2 Acute Cholecystitis

Sonographic signs of acute cholecystitis include gallbladder distension, wall edema, stones, pericholecystic fluid, air in the wall, sloughed mucosa, and the Murphy sign. Of these, wall edema is a key feature in the diagnosis of acute cholecystitis, although this finding may lead to overdiagnosis. It should be kept in mind that gallbladder wall edema, which appears as a thin or striated

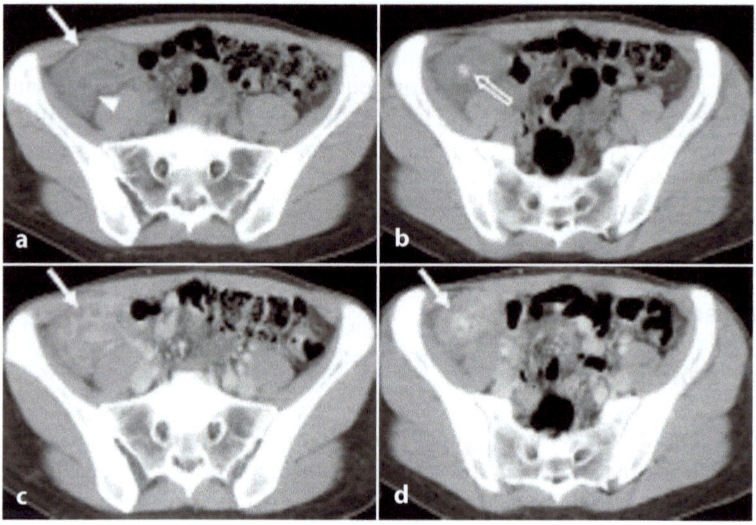

Fig. 14.5 This 38-year-old woman presented with right lower quadrant pain and a history of prior appendectomy. CT report was inconclusive. Two days later, due to unremitting abdominal pain, the patient underwent laparoscopic exploration, which showed an inflamed short appendiceal stump. On review, cecal wall thickening (*arrows in* **a**, **c**, **d**), inflammatory changes in the pericecal fat (*arrowhead in* **a**), and an appendicolith (*open arrow in* **b**) are appreciable on the CT images. The diagnosis is suggested by a combination of the CT features and the awareness that stump appendicitis can occur, even in the absence of a distended appendiceal stump

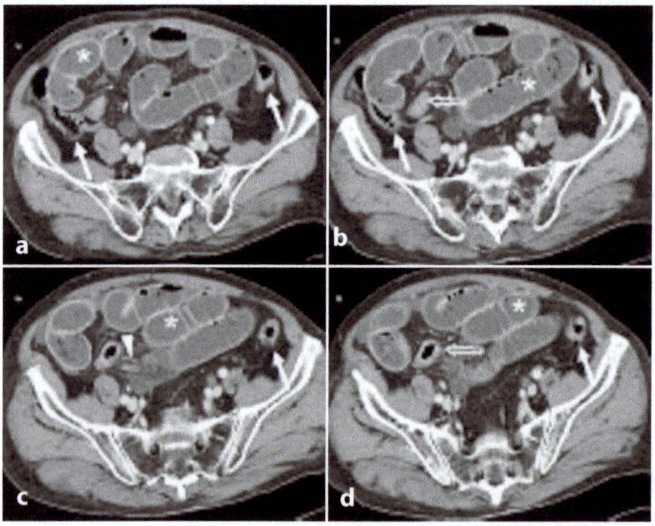

Fig. 14.6 Tip appendicitis and involvement of the distal ileus in a 57-year-old man. CT images show dilated small bowel loops (*asterisks in* **a**-**d**), with collapse of colon (*white arrows in* **a**-**d**) and distal ileus (*open arrow in* **b**). The scan was interpreted as showing distal small-bowel obstruction, but at surgery tip appendicitis was found with involvement of distal ileus. On review, the distal portion of the appendix (*arrowhead in* **c**) appears to be inflamed, with adjacent fat stranding and inflammatory involvement of the distal ileus (*open arrow in* **d**)

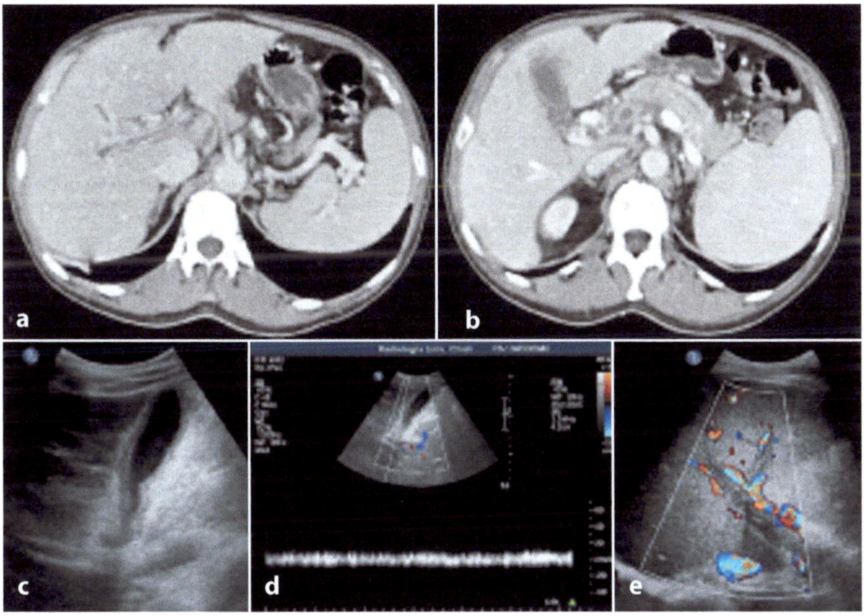

Fig. 14.7 Chronic hepatitis and epigastric pain in a 65-year-old man. The CT scan (**a**, **b**) revealed portal vein thrombosis; the gallbladder showed diffuse wall thickening, erroneously interpreted as wall edema due to acute inflammation. Since this diagnosis did not convince the clinicians, Doppler US was performed, which confirmed the portal vein thrombosis (**e**) and the gallbladder wall thickening, with an intraparietal venous signal (**c**, **d**). This finding, combined with the lack of gallbladder distension, was considered indicative of edema caused by venous congestion due to increased hepatic sinusoid pressure. The diagnosis of acute cholecystitis could therefore be excluded

focal, circumferential, or discontinuous sonolucent band, may also occur in other pathologies, such as hypoproteinemia, acute hepatitis, liver disease with portal hypertension, congestive heart failure, and renal failure. In this setting, careful evaluation of additional imaging findings is needed to distinguish these entities from acute cholecystitis. The lack of a distended gallbladder lumen makes acute cholecystitis unlikely and a search for other causes of edema should be undertaken (Fig. 14.7).

Conversely, the diagnosis of acute cholecystitis cannot be based on gallbladder distension alone, as the latter also occurs as a consequence of diminished gallbladder emptying due to prolonged fasting and parenteral nutrition, or the administration of cholestatic drugs, particularly narcotics.

On CT, the most important early predictor of acute cholecystitis is pericholecystic increased liver enhancement on arterial phase. However, this sign can be misinterpreted as focal fatty sparing around the gallbladder. One there-

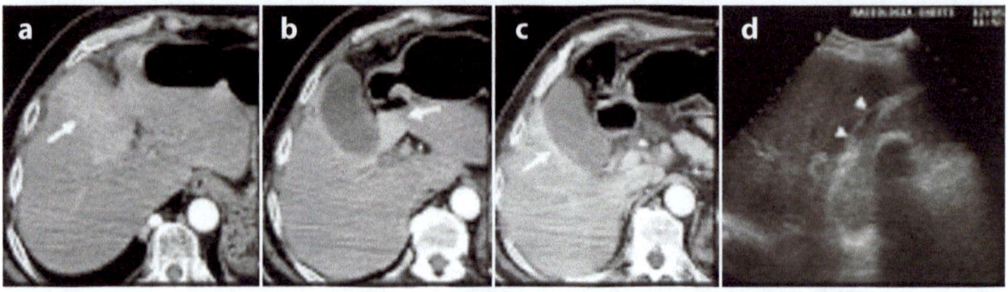

Fig. 14.8 Acute epigastric pain due to surgically proved acute cholecystitis in a 67-year-old woman. CT images (a-c) show the mildly distended gallbladder with a high-density rim in the surrounding liver (*arrows*), representing arterial hyperenhancement. This finding was interpreted as focal fatty sparing around gallbladder. On review, the liver did not show fatty infiltration on unenhanced images. The next day, due to unremitting abdominal pain, the patient underwent an US exam (d), which showed gallbladder distension and wall thickening (*arrowheads*) indicative of inflammatory edema

fore has to be familiar with the signs of acute cholecystitis on CT, and a routine examination of the gallbladder for any abnormality is essential, especially in patients with a non-specific clinical presentation (Fig. 14.8).

14.4.3 Intestinal Bowel Obstruction

Severe obstruction may cause the bowel loops to completely fill and become distended by intestinal fluid, such that on APF the main radiographic feature is the total absence of intestinal gas. It is important not to confuse this condition with "spastic ileus," i.e., the hypertonic-spastic condition of the small bowel loops, which could represent the early appearance of an acute abdomen [17]. In patients with spastic ileus, parietal-visceral findings are prominent, such as contours of the psoas and margins of the abdominal parenchymal organs [17], which otherwise are less well visualized in the presence of SBO. In this clinical setting, US or CT could be very helpful in visualizing fluid-filled bowel loops and in not overlooking a diagnosis of SBO, thus delaying adequate treatment (Fig. 14.9).

In patients with severe large bowel obstruction, CT will reveal the presence of gas within the bowel wall due to a severe distension of the colonic lumen with mechanical disruption of the mucosa [18]. The use of I.V. contrast agent will allow visualization of normal colonic wall enhancement and thereby avoid misinterpretation of bowel wall pneumatosis, indicative of intestinal infarction (Fig. 14.10).

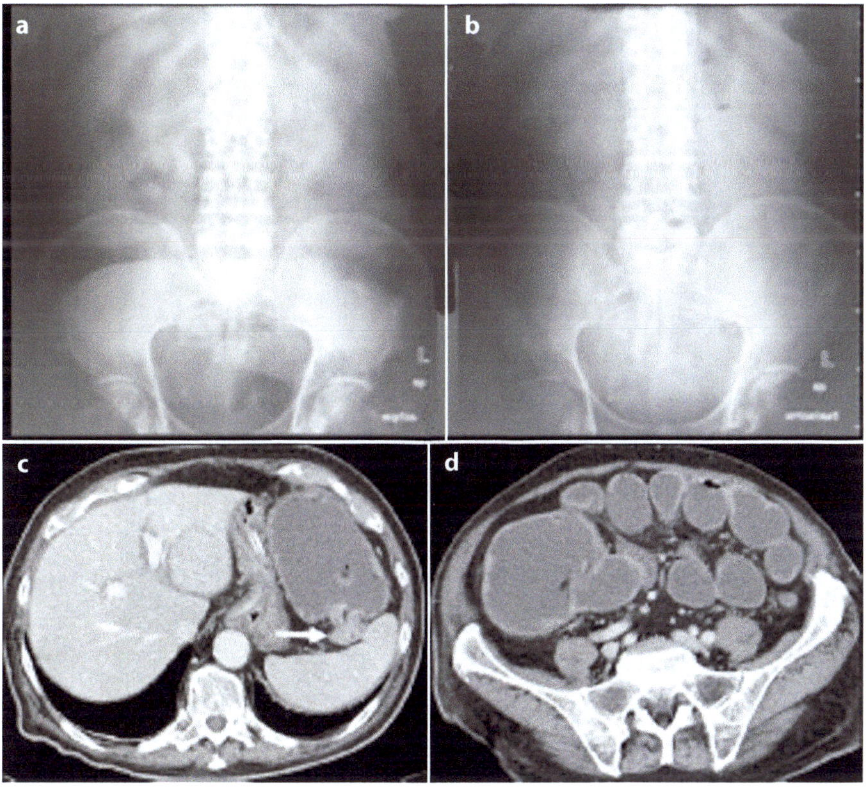

Fig. 14.9 Severe intestinal obstruction due to colonic neoplasm in a 76-year-old man. The APF (**a**, **b**) was erroneously interpreted as "spastic ileus." The day after, due to a worsening of symptoms, the patient underwent a CT scan (**c**, **d**), which showed a severe mechanical obstruction with completely fluid-filled tenual and colonic loops until the left colic flexure. A neoplastic thickening of the left colic flexure was the cause of the obstruction (*arrow in* **c**)

14.4.4 Diverticulitis

The most common CT finding of acute diverticulitis is paracolic fat stranding associated with the presence of ill-defined or blurry diverticula and mild colonic wall thickening (usually < 5 mm) [16]. In some instances, small localized collections of gas and/or fluid are identified adjacent to the colonic wall. All these additional findings represent a key diagnostic feature to avoid mistaking diverticulitis for epiploic appendagitis. In acute epiploic appendagitis, the involved colonic segment is short (Fig. 14.11) whereas in acute diverticulitis a lengthy segment of thickened colonic wall is a typical CT feature [19].

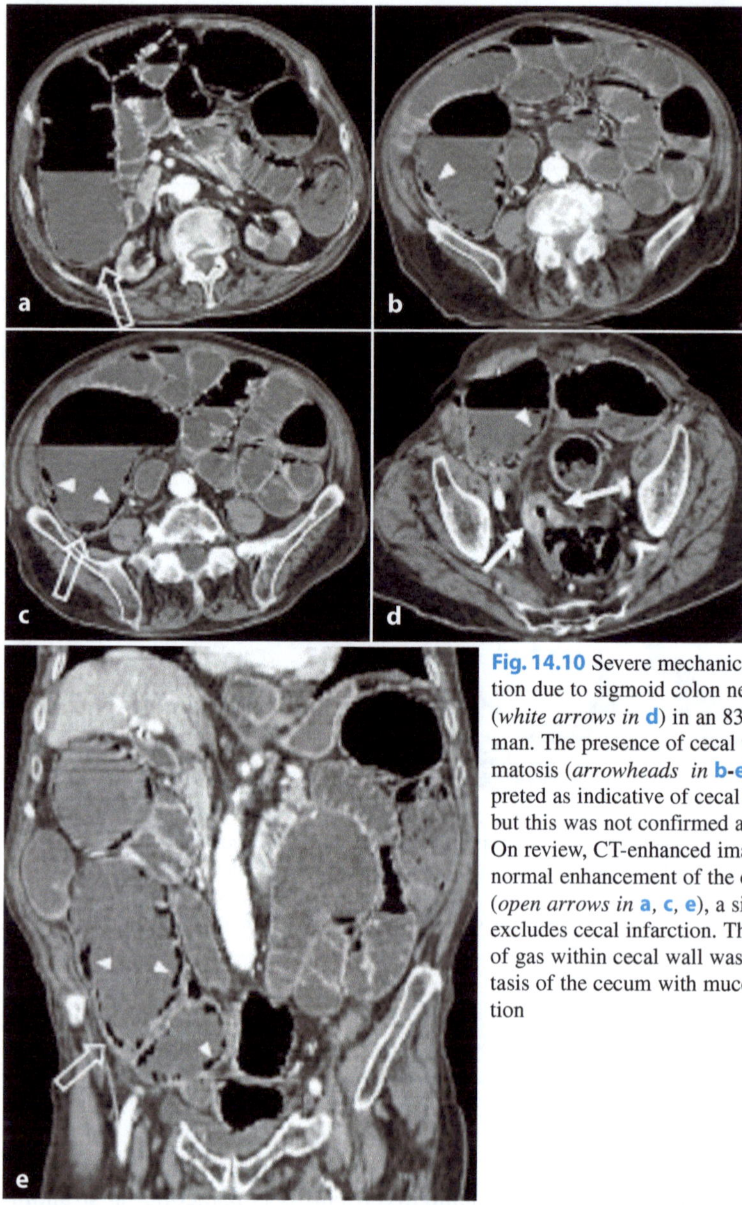

Fig. 14.10 Severe mechanical obstruction due to sigmoid colon neoplasm (*white arrows in* **d**) in an 83-year-old man. The presence of cecal wall pneumatosis (*arrowheads in* **b-e**) was interpreted as indicative of cecal infarction, but this was not confirmed at surgery. On review, CT-enhanced images showed normal enhancement of the cecal wall (*open arrows in* **a**, **c**, **e**), a sign that excludes cecal infarction. The presence of gas within cecal wall was due to diastasis of the cecum with mucosal disruption

Sometimes on non-enhanced CT images not only bowel wall pneumatosis due to mucosa disruption but also the presence of gas within the mesenteric and/or portal vessels is observed. The finding of normal bowel wall enhancement on enhanced CT prevents a mistaken diagnosis of bowel infarction (Fig. 14.12).

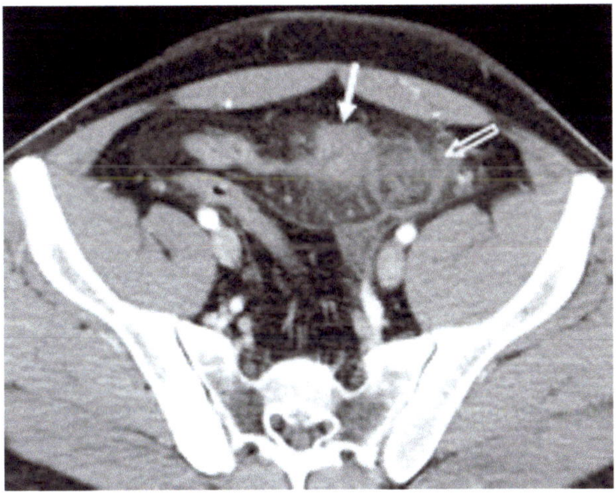

Fig. 14.11 Primary epiploic appendagitis in a 23-year-old man with clinical diagnosis of presumed colonic diverticulitis. Axial contrast-enhanced CT scan shows perisigmoid fatty lesion surrounded by hyperattenuating ring (*open arrow*) associated with very mild and short thickening of sigmoid colon (*white arrow*), without evidence of any diverticulum. All these findings are indicative of epiploic appendagitis

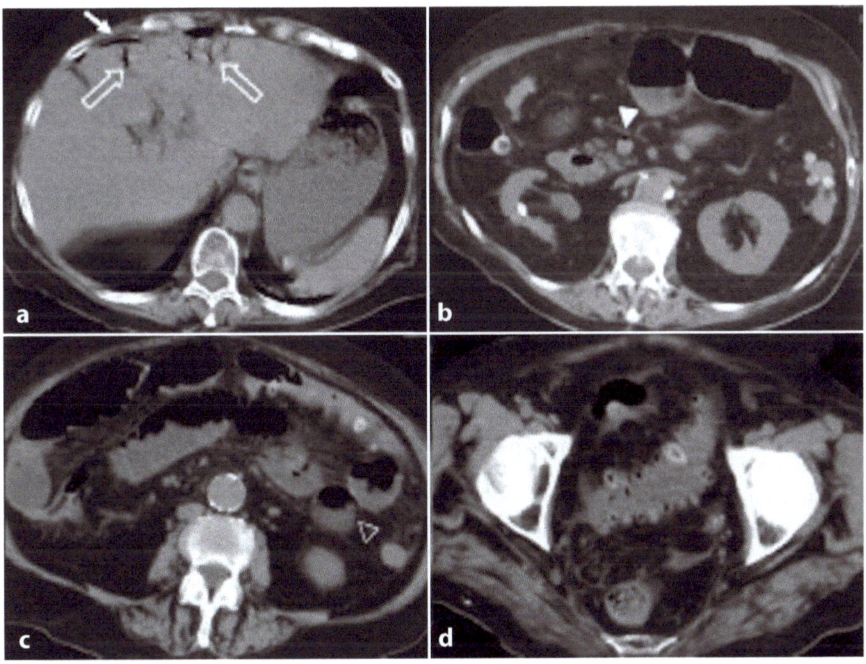

Fig. 14.12 Diffuse abdominal pain and bloody feces in a 66-year-old woman. Non-enhanced CT scans demonstrated the presence of free intraperitoneal air (*white arrow in* **a**) together with gas within the intrahepatic portal veins (*open arrows in* **a**), superior mesenteric vein (*arrowhead in* **b**), and bowel wall (*open arrowhead in* **c**).These findings were interpreted as bowel infarction, for which I.V. contrast medium was judged to be not useful for diagnosis. At surgery, no sign of bowel ischemia was found, but there was an evidence of acute diverticulitis

14.5 Conclusions

Awareness of the spectrum of factors that contribute to the misinterpretation of the information provided by the various diagnostic tools may improve the radiologist's performance, which ultimately translates into improved patient care.

References

1. Silen W (1996) Cope's early diagnosis of the acute abdomen, 19th ed. Oxford University Press, New York
2. de Bombal FT (1991) Introduction. In: de Bombal FT (ed) Diagnosis of acute abdominal pain, 2nd ed. Churchill Livingstone, Edinburgh, pp 1-10
3. Mindelzun RE, Jeffrey RB Jr (1997) Unenhanced helical CT for evaluating acute abdominal pain: a little more cost, a lot more information. Radiology 205:43-47
4. Malone AJ Jr, Wolf CR, Malmed AS, Melliere BF (1993) Diagnosis of acute appendicitis: value of unenhanced CT. Am J Roentgenol 160:763-766
5. Lane MJ, Katz DS, Ross BA et al (1997) Unenhanced helical CT for suspected acute appendicitis. Am J Roentgenol 168:405-409
6. Rao PM, Rhea JT, Novelline RA et al (1997) Helical CT technique for the diagnosis of appendicitis: prospective evaluation of a focused appendix CT examination. Radiology 202:139-144
7. Puylaert JB, Rutgers PH, Lalisang RI et al(1987) A prospective study of ultrasonography in the diagnosis of appendicitis. N Engl J Med 317:666-669
8. Lane MJ, Liu DM, Huynh MD et al (1999) Suspected acute appendicitis: non-enhanced helical CT in 300 consecutive patients. Radiology 213:341-346
9. Miki T, Ogata S, Uto M et al (2005) Enhanced multidetector-row computed tomography (MD-CT) in the diagnosis of acute appendicitis and its severity. Radiat Med 23:242-255
10. Kamel IR, Goldberg SN, Keogan MT et al (2000) Right lower quadrant pain and suspected appendicitis: non focused appendiceal CT-review of 100 cases. Radiology 217:159-163
11. Paulson EK, Harris JP, Jaffe TA et al (2005) Acute appendicitis: added diagnostic value of coronal reformations from isotropic voxels at multidetector row CT. Radiology 235:879-885
12. Zangos S, Steenburg SD, Phillips KD et al (2007) Added diagnostic value of coronal reformations with 64-slice multidetector row computed tomography. Acta Radiol 14:19-27
13. Aufort S, Charra L, Lesnik A et al (2005) Multidetector CT of bowel obstruction: value of post-processing. Eur Radiol 15:2323-2329
14. Pereira JM, Sirlin CB, Pinto PS et al (2004) Disproportionate fat stranding: a helpful CT sign in patients with acute abdominal pain. RadioGraphics 24:703-715
15. Shin LK, Halpern D, Weston SR et al (2005) Prospective CT diagnosis of stump appendicitis. Am J Roentgenol 184:62-64
16. Levine CD, Aizenstein O, Lehavi O, Blachar A (2005) Why we miss the diagnosis of appendicitis on abdominal CT: evaluation of imaging features of appendicitis incorrectly diagnosed on CT. Am J Roentgenol 184:855-859
17. Grassi R, Di Mizio R, Pinto A et al (2004) Serial plain abdominal film findings in the assessment of acute abdomen: spastic ileus, hypotonic ileus, mechanical ileus and paralytic ileus. Radiol Med 108:56-70
18. Felzko PJ, Mezwa DG, Farah MC, White BD (1992) Clinical significance of pneumatosis of the bowel wall. RadioGraphics 12:1068-1078
19. Ahneida AT, Melão L, Viamonte B et al (2009) Epiploic appendagitis: an entity frequentely unknown to clinicians-diagnostc imaging, pitfalls, and look-alikes. Am J Roentgenol 193:1243-1251

Errors in the MDCT Diagnosis of Intestinal Ischemia and Infarction

15

Stefania Romano, Gianluca Ponticiello, and Giovanna Russo

15.1 Introduction

The diagnosis of vascular intestinal disorders continues to pose a crucial challenge in the evaluation of computed tomography (CT) scans in patients with acute abdominal syndrome. The ability to distinguish between and correctly interpret the related findings of ischemia (a potentially reversible event) and infarction (a non-reversible event, with inevitable death of the involved bowel segment) is the first step in a correct diagnostic workup and image analysis. In fact, ischemia and infarction indicate different stages of an injury caused by interruption of the blood supply to the tissue [1, 2]. Three main conditions underlie an intestinal ischemic event: (1) a deficiency in the arterial blood supply, mainly related to embolism or thrombosis (splanchnic); (2) impaired venous drainage (post-splanchnic); (3) decreased mesenteric blood flow (the "low-flow" state) due, for example, to cardiac failure, myocardial infarction, bleeding, hypovolemia (pre-splanchnic) [2-4].

The added value of a multidetector CT (MDCT) exam in a patient with an acute abdomen related to mesenteric ischemia has been well established. Indeed, MDCT has become the preferred imaging technique for patients with suspected acute intestinal ischemia [2, 5] as it allows efficient evaluation of the mesenteric vasculature, intestinal wall, and other abdominal hollow and solid structures [2]. Major problems hindering an effective diagnosis are related to the radiologist's lack of knowledge of ischemic disease progression and the accompanying pathologic changes that occur in the intestinal wall, which offer a virtual staging of the disease [2].

S. Romano (✉)
Department of Diagnostic Radiological Imaging, "A. Cardarelli" Hospital, Naples, Italy

L. Romano, A. Pinto (eds.), *Errors in Radiology*,

15.2 Errors in the CT Diagnosis of Intestinal Ischemia

The basic steps in an efficient evaluation of the MDCT findings in a patient with acute intestinal disease due to vascular disorders begins with the recognized absence of any other acute condition that could justify the abdominal syndrome. The ability to differentiate between intestinal inflammatory changes due to infections and those related to ischemic disease is fundamental to understanding the important role of the radiologic report in the therapeutic work-up of the patient. Further steps in the interpretation process are related to efficiently distinguishing ischemic disease from infarction, as the latter is a point of no-return that requires resection of the "dead" intestinal segment.

The image evaluation process is supported by a correct examination that fully addresses the indications using a state-of-the-art protocol, thus allowing visualization of the anatomical structures of interest. It is therefore imperative that radiologists are able to evaluate the caliber and endoluminal opacification of the mesenteric arterial and venous districts, diagnose early-stage ischemic disease, correctly identify parietal damage due to reperfusion, suggest correct follow-up in terms of additional diagnostic imaging exams or interventional procedures, and note the signs of intestinal infarction. with a comprehensive assessment of the extent of the damage [2, 6].

The basis of the process applied to interpret the CT images of acute intestinal disease due to arterial supply deficiency or impaired venous drainage rests upon knowledge of the early morphologic changes of the intestine due to the acute injury and the type of evolution, in terms of parietal wall alterations, that might be evident [2, 6]. Alterations in the enhancement or appearance of the intestinal wall or in the mesenteric vasculature could be absent in the neurogenic response of a spastic reflex ileus (intestinal loops collapsed) and in the hypotonic state (the loops distended by gas) [2, 7], such that consideration of the clinical history and laboratory parameters are needed to suggest very early ischemic disease. From this early stage, in the absence of reperfusion, intestinal ischemia of arterial origin may progress to infarction.

Signs of reperfusion damage [8] are more often observed in exams performed at a reasonable time after the onset of symptoms. CT findings at this stage could be informative regarding bowel wall appearance, especially the presence of submucosal edema, possible moderate hyperdensity of the mucosa, as well as potential anomalies in the patency and caliber of the mesenteric vessels [2]. Differentiation between the normal enhancement of the bowel wall and abnormal hyperdensity from mural hemorrhage is essential at this stage as well. In fact, the CT findings can be correlated to the histopathologic changes that occur in the intestine after an ischemic event, ranging from epithelial damage to the inflammation, edema, and submucosal hemorrhage evidencing reperfusion injuries [7], as an ischemic enteritis (Fig. 15.1). The differential diagnosis of this stage and any other type of intestinal inflammatory condition affecting the intestine is a crucial diagnostic step (Figs. 15.2-15.4).

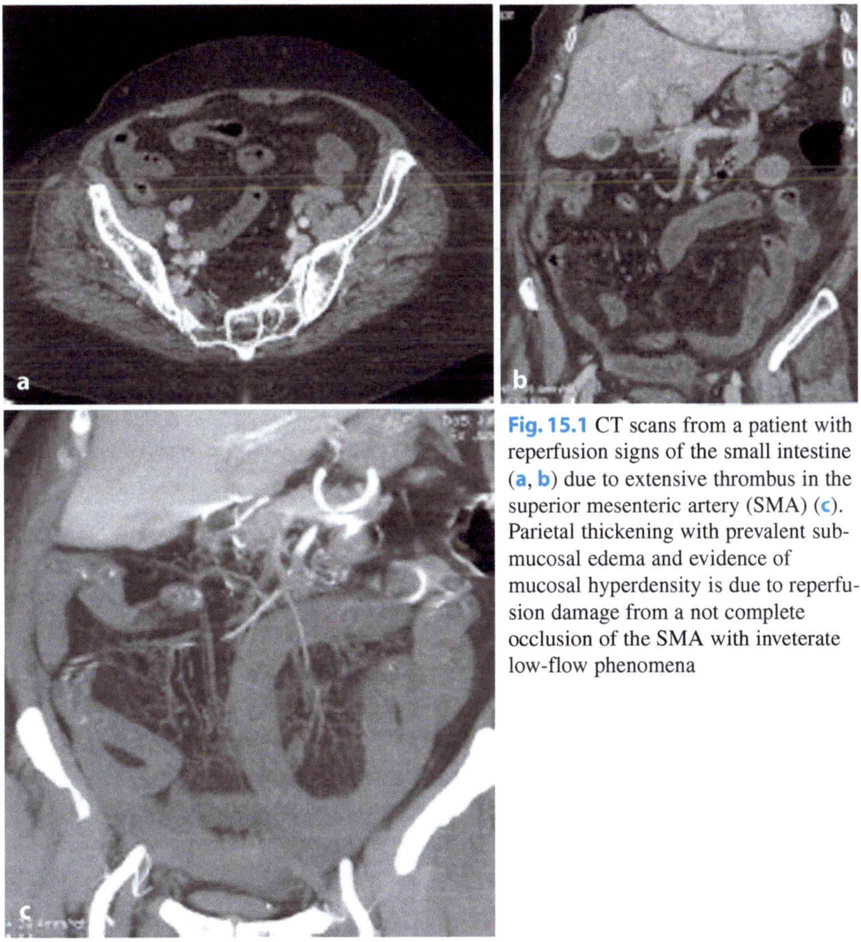

Fig. 15.1 CT scans from a patient with reperfusion signs of the small intestine (**a**, **b**) due to extensive thrombus in the superior mesenteric artery (SMA) (**c**). Parietal thickening with prevalent submucosal edema and evidence of mucosal hyperdensity is due to reperfusion damage from a not complete occlusion of the SMA with inveterate low-flow phenomena

Moreover, the CT findings related to late-stage intestinal vascular disease, in which there is intestinal infarction, death, and necrosis of the involved bowel can be effectively correlated with the absence of enhancement of the infarcted wall segment, the presence of pneumatosis (parietal, mesenteric, portal), and, if perforation of the bowel has occurred, free peritoneal air [2, 6, 7]. At this stage, correct interpretation of the signs of intestinal necrosis requires careful attention to the endoluminal opacification of the mesenteric vessels [2, 6], especially in case of "benign" pneumatosis, in which bubbles of air penetrate from the lumen into the wall through micro-fissurations in an overly distended bowel but not due to parietal necrosis.

Other important considerations are intestinal disorders related to medium- to advanced-stage injury reflecting impaired venous drainage, in which case the intestinal infarction is of venous origin. CT findings evidencing vascular

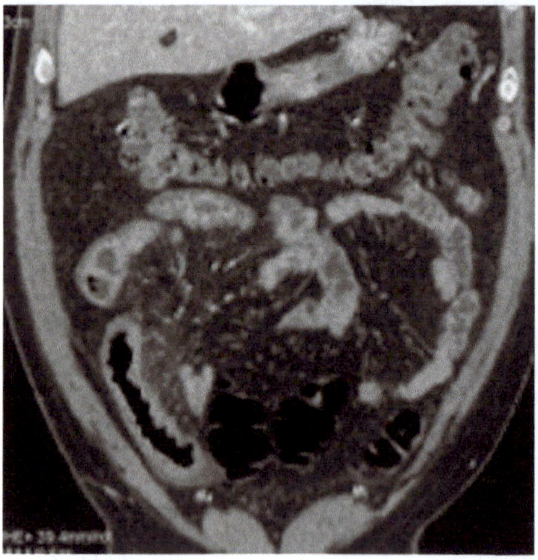

Fig. 15.2 CT coronal scan from a patient with proven early-stage Crohn's disease. Note the parietal edematous swelling of the affected small bowel loops, with more evident mucosal hyperdensity

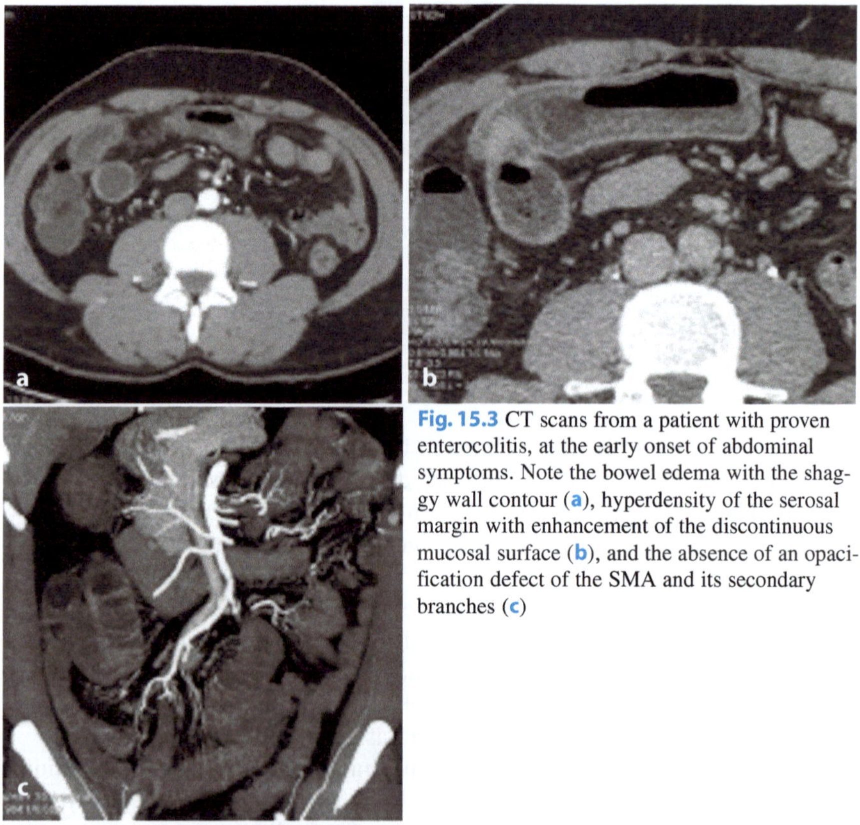

Fig. 15.3 CT scans from a patient with proven enterocolitis, at the early onset of abdominal symptoms. Note the bowel edema with the shaggy wall contour (a), hyperdensity of the serosal margin with enhancement of the discontinuous mucosal surface (b), and the absence of an opacification defect of the SMA and its secondary branches (c)

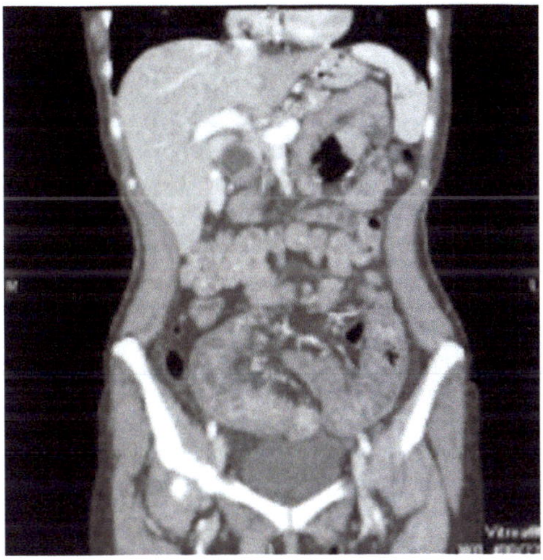

Fig. 15.4 CT coronal scan of patient with enteritis related to vasculitis. Note the marked thickening, submucosal edema, and greater enhancement of the mucosal surface of some small bowel loops

disorder due to impaired venous drainage from venous occlusions are those related to the pathologic changes in the bowel wall, varying from congestion and swelling with edema to hemorrhage, with blood flowing out from the bowel and mesentery into the peritoneal cavity. This sequence of events was already observed many years ago in animal experimental models [2, 9-11], in which the progression to infarction with bowel necrosis occurred in a few hours, By contrast, according to clinical observations, the entire process in humans is longer because of differences in the collateral circulation [11]. Thus, the CT appearance of the bowel wall altered by impaired venous drainage comprises evidence of mesenteric venous thrombosis, small-bowel thickening, greater enhancement due to intramural hemorrhage, evidence of submucosal edema, and alternating layers of different density, including a hypodense submucosa [2, 7]. It is important to note that an intestinal injury caused by impaired venous drainage has the potential to heal with correct medical therapy; however, persistence of the disease causes a chronic alteration in the intestinal wall that in rare cases progresses to intestinal infarction [2, 7]. The main findings of the latter are the absence of enhancement at the expected delay time as well as signs of parietal death with necrosis (Fig. 15.5).

In the colon, a potential diagnostic error related to CT findings of intestinal ischemic changes is a consequence of the fact that effective signs are not easy to detect, especially in the absence of alterations in the mesenteric vessels, since a swollen edematous submucosa and mucosal hyperemia are also seen in other pathologies acutely affecting the large intestine (Fig. 15.6). In addition, the low-flow state of the small intestine may be misinterpreted if the inexperienced radiologist, lacking the expert's "diagnostic eye," fails to recognize the lumen distension, the features of the bowel wall, and the different enhancement pattern.

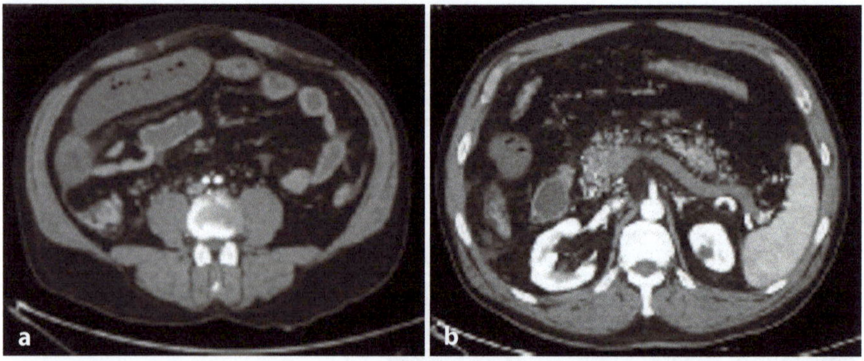

Fig. 15.5 CT scans of a jejunal infarction (**a**) due to extensive spleno-portal-mesenteric thrombosis (**b**). Note the appearance of the infarcted loop, with marked parietal thickening, the absence of enhancement, and the altered appearance of the remnant small intestine, in which injury is due to impaired venous drainage, not infarction

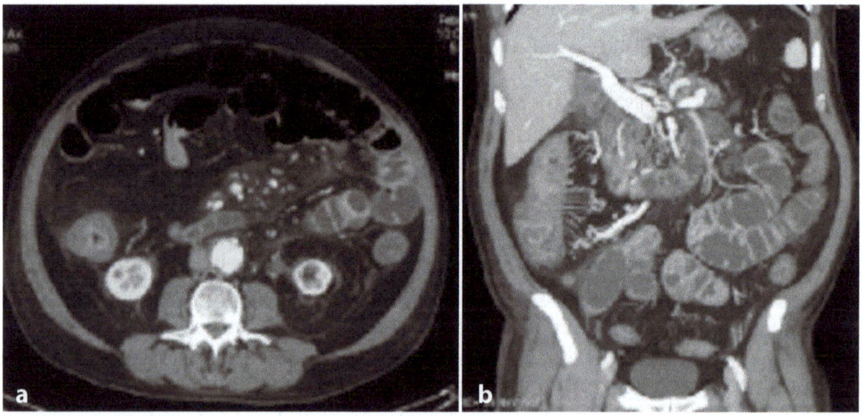

Fig. 15.6 CT axial scan from a patient with acute abdominal symptoms related to proven acute active Crohn's disease affecting also the large bowel. The parietal thickening and appearance of the colon (**a**) must be differentiated from ischemic colitis. A coronal reconstruction well shows the inflammatory changes of the large intestine, with its engorged vasa recta (**b**)

One of the major challenges in evaluating the intestinal tract under emergency conditions is the post-operative appearance of the bowel (even if the primary surgery was not pertinent to the intestines), in which reperfusion damage of different levels of severity can simulate other pathologies, especially inflammatory and infectious diseases, drug reactions, or other pathologic entities that alter both the normal enhancement of the wall layers and intestinal motility (Fig. 15.7).

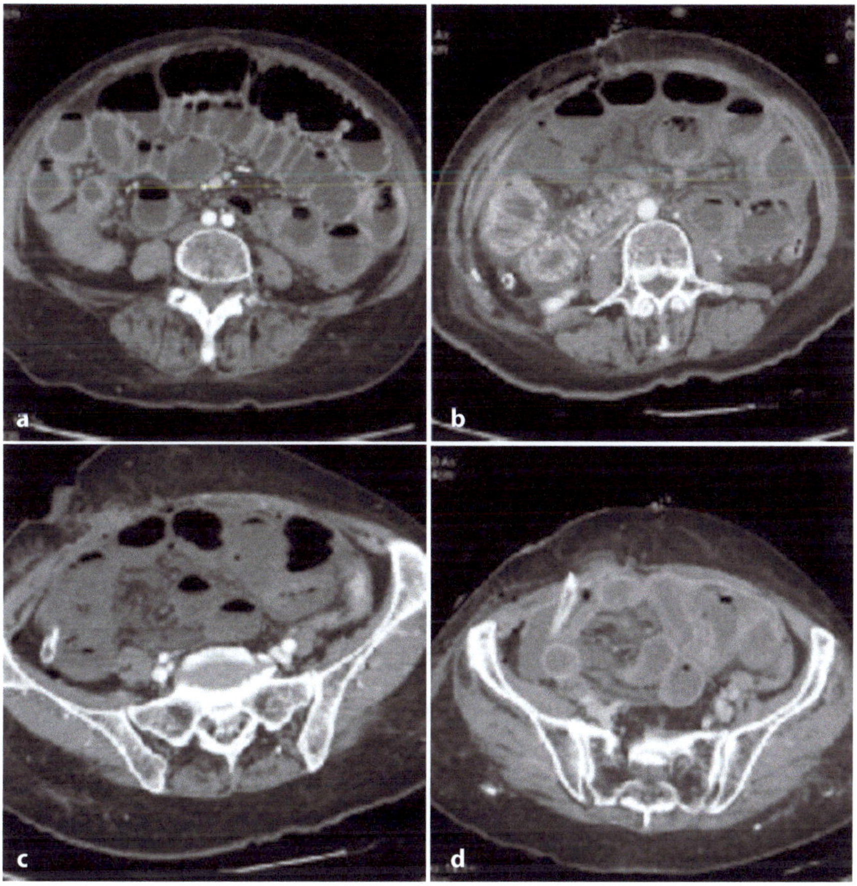

Fig. 15.7 CT scans from a patient who underwent surgery for cancer in the right colon (a). In the early post-operative days, the patient developed abdominal pain. While CT findings related to reperfusion damage were well evident (b, c), the diminished enhancement of some small bowel loops did not correspond to any altered laboratory parameters. No additional surgery was performed but a CT exam several days later evidenced the improved conditions resulting from reperfusion of the postoperative damage to the small intestine (d)

15.3 Conclusions

In the diagnosis of intestinal tract ischemia, the imaging findings may be confusing, such that a high index of suspicion is needed in order to correctly distinguish among the relatively non-specific presenting symptoms and signs [5]. Accordingly, the differential diagnosis of patients with abdominal pain should include bowel ischemia and infarction. An aggressive diagnostic and therapeutic approach should be followed, thereby improving the patient survival rate in this potentially lethal disorder [5]. To limit any potential errors in the presence of clinical suspicion of a vascular intestinal disorder, evaluation of the imaging findings related to the bowel wall and other abdominal structures must also consider the clinical history of the patient, the laboratory parameters, the type of abdominal pain, and the results of any recent diagnostic imaging exam performed [2]. Important and essential safeguards to reach a correct diagnosis are well defined knowledge of the definitions and criteria used to differentiate the CT findings of intestinal ischemia from those of infarction and the ability to make full use of imaging in evaluating the intestine, especially in intermediate-stage disease, with recognition of reperfusion injury and all conditions occurring in the interval from "early" to "late" disease.

References

1. Fenoglio-Preiser C.M, Noffsinger AE, Stemmermann GN et al (2008) The nonneoplastic Small Intestine. In: Fenoglio-Preiser CM, Noffsinger AE, Stemmermann GN et al (eds) Gastrointestinal pathology. An atlas and text, 3rd edn. Wolters Kluwer – Lippincott Williams & Wilkins, Philadelphia, PA USA, pp 326-339
2. Romano S, Romano L (2011) Acute mesenteric ischemia and ischemic colitis. In: Taourel P (ed) CT of the acute abdomen. Medical radiology. Diagnostic imaging. Springer-Verlag, Berlin Heidelberg, pp 183-197
3. Paterno F, Longo WE (2008) The etiology and pathogenesis of vascular disorders of the intestine. Radiol Clin North Am 46: 877-885
4. Klatte EC, Becker GJ, Yune HY et al (1982) Angiographic studies of the upper gastrointestinal tract. In: Scott HW, Sawyers JL (eds) Surgery of the stomach, duodenum and small intestine. Blackwell Scientific, Cambridge MA, USA, pp 194-197
5. Gore RM, Yaghmai V, Thakar KH et al (2008) Imaging in intestinal ischemic disorders. Radiol Clin North Am 46: 845-875
6. Romano S, Niola R, Maglione F et al (2008) Small bowel vascular disorders from arterial etiology and impaired venous drainage. Radiol Clin North Am 46: 891-908
7. Romano S, Lassandro F, Scaglione M et al (2006) Ischemia and infarction of the small bowel and colon: spectrum of imaging findings. Abdom Imag 31: 277-292
8. Chou CK, Mak CW, Tzeng WS et al (2004) CT of small bowel ischemia. Abdom Imaging 29:18-22
9. Noer RJ (1943) The blood vessels of the jejunum and ileum: a comparative study of man and certain laboratory animals. Am J Anat 73: 293-334
10. Polk HC Jr (1966) Experimental mesenteric venous occlusion III. Diagnosis and treatment of induced mesenteric venous thrombosis. Ann Surg163:432-444
11. Laureano BA, Wade TP (1998). Mesenteric venous disease. In: Longo WE, Peterson GJ, Jacobs DL (eds) Intestinal ischemia disorders. Quality Medical, St. Louis MO, USA, pp 207-219

Crohn's Disease: Errors of Interpretation in Emergency MDCT Evaluation

16

Luigia Romano, Maria Giuseppina Scuderi, and Stefania Daniele

16.1 Introduction

Computed tomography (CT) is increasingly being used as a screening modality for patients with symptoms of acute abdomen. As such, it has become the preferred small bowel imaging approach for assessing intestinal disorders. However, errors in the interpretation of the intestinal radiological CT findings are a common occurrence in acute conditions, given the large spectrum of pathologies, including inflammatory, infectious, vascular, and neoplastic diseases. In fact the differential diagnosis is often challenging, as intestinal emergency findings are similar, such that pitfalls are common.

Crohn's disease—a chronic, transmural, granulomatous inflammatory pathology of unknown etiology—is the major inflammatory small bowel disorder. Its early symptoms are often non-specific, leading to frequent emergency presentations, such as small bowel obstruction, intestinal hemorrhage, septic status, and acute abdominal pain. Histologically, it typically affects the entire bowel wall, in contrast to ulcerative colitis, which is restricted to the mucosal intestinal layer. Due to these particular spreading features, patients develop major complications during the disease course, such as obstruction (Fig. 16.1), hemorrhage, fistulas, and abscesses.

Although other methods, such as magnetic resonance imaging (MRI) and CT enterography, are preferred for assessing small bowel chronic inflammatory diseases, patients with abdominal pain who have an acute presentation of the disorder typically undergo contrast-enhanced emergency CT of the abdomen. Moreover, for acutely ill patients, CT is often the only study required, as it provides crucial information allowing the accurate diagnosis of Crohn's disease and its associated complications [1].

L. Romano (✉)
Department of Diagnostic Radiological Imaging, "A. Cardarelli" Hospital, Naples, Italy

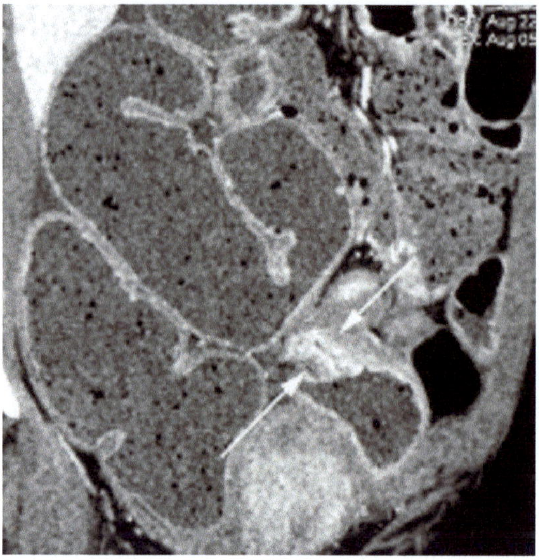

Fig. 16.1 Coronal CT reformatted image obtained with intravenous contrast medium (CM) shows a circumferential thickening of a segmental small bowel loop, obstructing the lumen. The wall has a homogeneous and hyperattenuating pattern (*white arrows*). The other loops have thin walls; their lumen is enlarged and filled by fluid and air bubbles. CT findings suggest small bowel Crohn's disease with obstruction. Surgery and biopsy confirmed the diagnosis

16.2 MDCT Protocol Design Considerations

The MDCT protocol is for a 64-row scanner: images acquired at a 0.625 mm collimation, a reconstruction axial slice thickness of 2.5 mm, a pitch of 0.984, and a gantry rotation time of 0.5 s. The abdominal volumetric scan begins at the level of the diaphragmatic dome and ends at the pubic symphysis.

Since bowel wall alterations may be very subtle, the use of a thin section, high-volume, rapid-bolus scanning technique with state-of-the-art CT technology is important in differentiating intestinal abnormalities. Indeed, intravenous administration of contrast medium (CM) is mandatory for discovering intestinal wall abnormalities. In selected cases, the oral administration of CM could be useful. A preliminary unenhanced abdominal CT scan is obtained to detect pre-existing hyperattenuating material in the bowel wall and lumen, such as suture materials, foreign bodies, drugs, blood (Fig. 16.2), clots, or retained CM.

Intravenous injection of 100–120 ml of iodinated CM is generally necessary to evaluate enhancement alteration of the bowel wall and mesenteric folds. Even better visualization of enhancement alterations is achieved with contrast agents containing higher concentrations of iodine (400 mg/ml) and high injection rates (at least 4 ml/s), followed by a 30- to 50-ml saline chaser injected at a rate of 4 ml/s.

After the abdominal pre-contrast scan, automated bolus tracking is used to time the beginning of CM acquisition during the arterial phase. Bolus tracking requires precise placement of the region-of-interest (ROI) cursor in the lumen of the abdominal aorta. Image acquisition is triggered at an attenuation threshold of

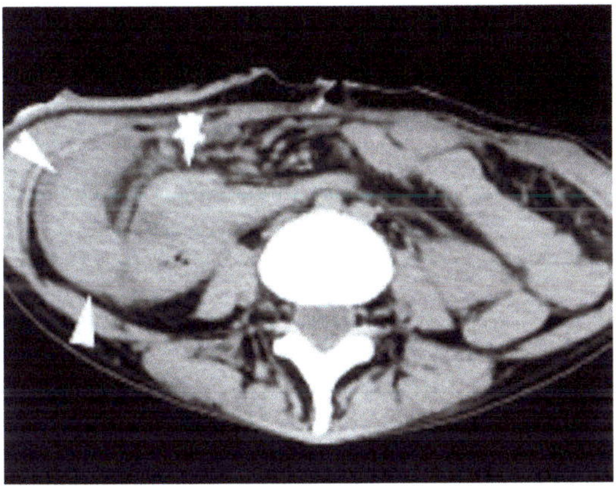

Fig. 16.2 Axial pre-contrast CT scan shows hyperdense fluid, representing blood, in the lumen of the small intestine (*white arrowheads*). Without intravenous CM, further information is not possible

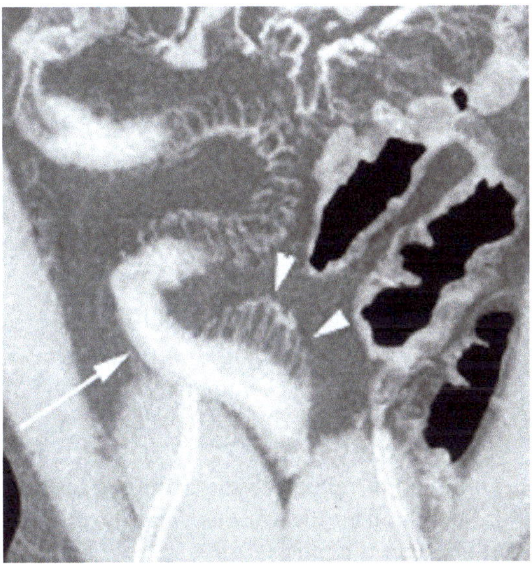

Fig. 16.3 Coronal CT reformatted image obtained with intravenous CM shows hypervascularity of the mesentery with vessel dilatation, tortuosity and prominence of the vasa recta, producing the comb sign (*white arrow heads*). There is a transmural inflammation near a thickened bowel wall that appears homogeneously hyperdense

150 HU. The CM arterial phase is mandatory to detect arterial anomalies associated with intestinal findings, such as the mesenteric comb sign (Fig. 16.3).

The scan delay until the following portal-venous phase is 70 s. Acquisition in this phase provides for maximum bowel wall attenuation, useful in evaluating intestinal enhancement alterations, wall thickness, and the venous mesenteric drainage.

Sagittal and coronal MIP reformatted images aid in localizing the pathological segment of bowel within the abdomen (Fig. 16.4) and in evaluating the mesenteric vessels and their peripheral branches.

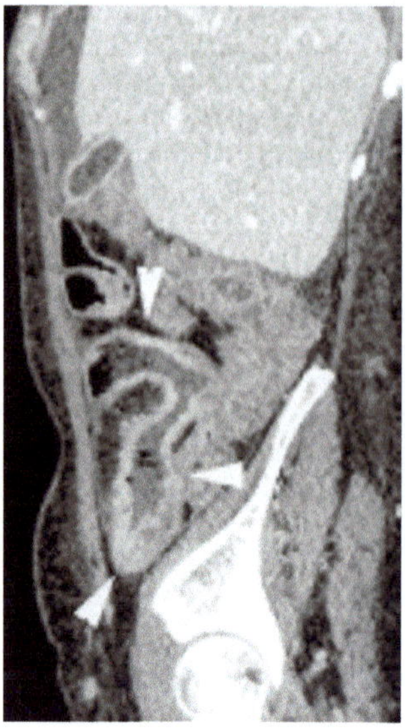

Fig. 16.4 Sagittal reformatted image obtained with intravenous CM demonstrates the entire pathological intestinal segment, with hyperattenuated wall thickening (*white arrowheads*)

16.3 Scanning Technique Pitfalls

Residual fluid within the lumen and covering the mucosa of the bowel wall may be seen as a thickened layer of the wall without enhancement. In these cases, a disease process may be difficult to exclude.

It should be emphasized that idiopathic inflammatory bowel disease can present many different attenuation patterns, corresponding to different phases of the disease process and their physiologic status. The attenuation pattern is also dependent on the volume of CM, the speed of its intravenous delivery, and the timing of the scan.

The pitfalls of the scanning technique are related to the different patterns of bowel wall enhancement that are common in the various small bowel diseases, which in turn can lead to an incorrect diagnosis.

16.4 CT Findings of Crohn's Disease and Related Pitfalls

The inflammatory process of Crohn's disease results in full-thickness intestinal alterations that can lead to significant complications caused by microperforation of the wall, such as the development of fistulas, abscesses and mesenteric phlegmons (Fig. 16.5).

The severity of the intestinal inflammatory process depends on several pathological components: nodular transformation of the mucosal layer, superficial and deep ulcers, stenosis or obstruction of the intestinal lumen, mesenteric fold thickening, mesenteric lymph nodes, fibrofatty proliferation of the

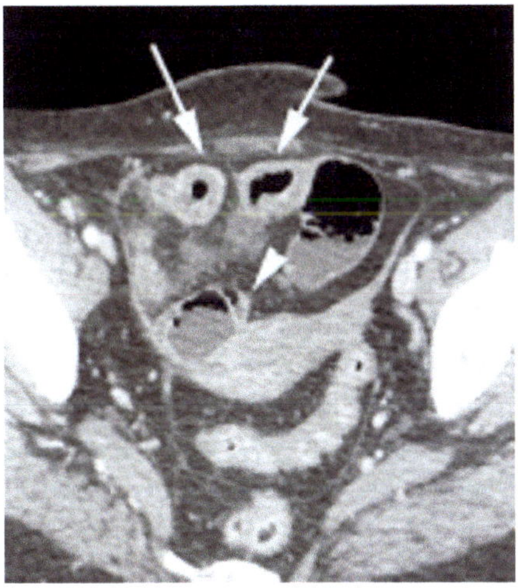

Fig. 16.5 Axial post-contrast CT pelvic scan shows small bowel wall edema (*white arrows*) with stranding of adjacent fat and an abscess involving the right broad ligament (*white arrowhead*)

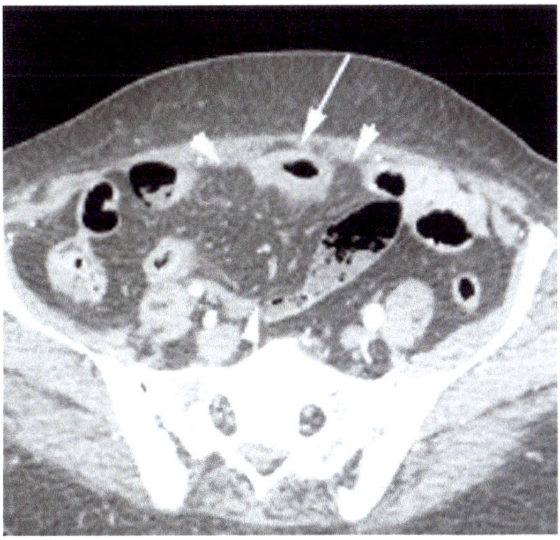

Fig. 16.6 Axial post-contrast CT pelvic scan demonstrates fibrofatty mesenteric proliferation (*white arrowheads*) with displacement of small bowel loops (*white arrow*)

mesentery (Fig. 16.6), fistulas, mesenterial hypervascularity (comb sign), phlegmon, abscesses, and the discontinuity of the multi-segmental inflammatory process [2].

The CT findings of Crohn's disease include:

- Intestinal wall thickness;
- Segmental mural hyperenhancement;
- A prominent peri-enteric vasculature (comb sign);
- Length of the intestinal involvement;
- Associated abnormalities (stenosis of the lumen, enlarged local lymph nodes) and local mesenteric alterations.

16.4.1 Intestinal Wall Thickness

The normal small bowel wall is thin, but its exact thickness depends on the degree of luminal distension. Typically, it measures 1–2 mm when the lumen is well distended and 2–3 mm if the lumen is collapsed or partially collapsed. Importantly, the wall of the normal small bowel is of symmetric thickness.

A precise assessment of the intestinal wall thickness contributes significantly to establishing the correct differential diagnosis. The CT findings that need to be analyzed when assessing the thickened bowel wall include degree of thickening, symmetric versus asymmetric thickening, focal, segmental or diffuse involvement, attenuation pattern, and associated peri-enteric abnormalities. Any perceptible thickening generally indicate disorders including inflammatory conditions, infectious conditions, and neoplastic diseases [3].

Pitfalls

Bowel wall thickening may be related to a number of entities, including normal variants, inflammatory conditions, and neoplastic diseases.

Potential pitfalls exists when the normal small bowel is filled with water or enteric fluid, because its wall may then appear thicker. The wall should measure < 3 mm, but it is often imperceptible [4].

Bowel wall thickening is not specific for Crohn's disease [5].

Entities that cause mild (5–10 mm) or severe (10–20 mm) bowel thickening often overlap and include inflammatory diseases (Crohn's disease and ulcerative colitis), infectious conditions, neoplasm, radiation enteritis, graft versus host disease, and ischemic bowel disorders.

Since in patients with ulcerative colitis the inflammatory process is limited to the mucosal layer whereas in Crohn's disease it is often transmural, bowel

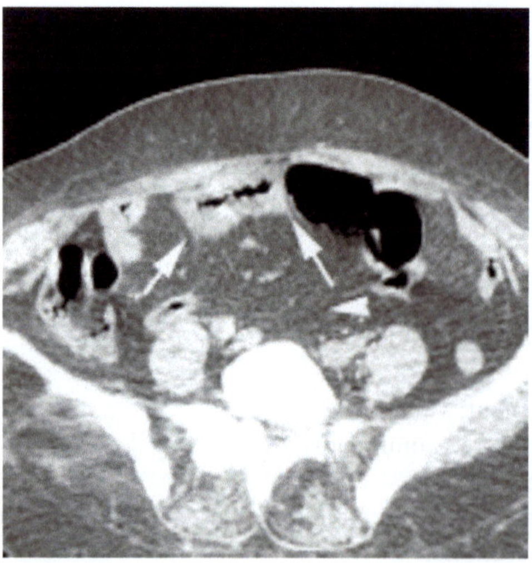

Fig. 16.7 Contrast-enhanced axial CT image shows mild small bowel wall thickening (*white arrows*) associated with lumen narrowing and fibrofatty mesenteric proliferation (*white arrowhead*) in a patient with abdominal pain. No lymphadenopathy was present. The CT findings were erroneously interpreted as chronic small bowel Crohn's disease. Surgery revealed intestinal adenocarcinoma

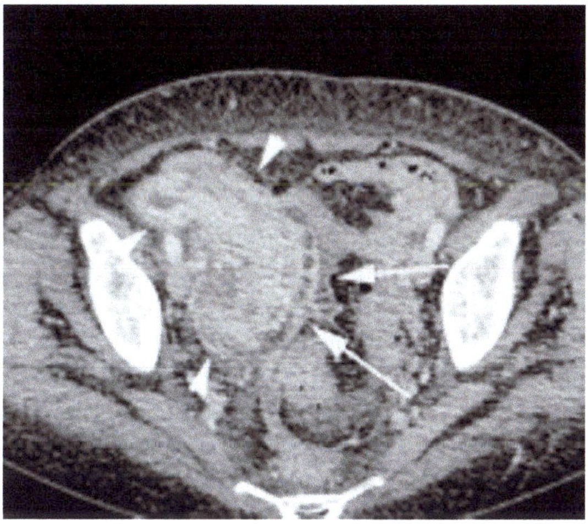

Fig. 16.8 Axial post-contrast CT pelvic scan from a patient with acute right-sided abdominal pain demonstrates severe hyperenhanced thickening of the terminal ileum (*white arrowheads*) with fluid and stranding in the adjacent mesenteric fold (*white arrows*). The CT findings were erroneously interpreted as acute terminal ileum Crohn's disease. Retrograde endoscopy revealed intestinal lymphoma

wall thickening is usually greater in Crohn's disease. Primary intestinal neoplasms often consist of shorter segments of bowel wall thickening (Fig. 16.7).

Another feature used to evaluate the inflammatory involvement of intestinal wall thickening is whether the involved segments are symmetrically or asymmetrically thickened. Symmetric thickening is present when the involved abnormal segment shows the same degree of thickening throughout its circumference. Symmetric thickening is seen in the acute phase of Crohn's disease, intestinal inflammatory conditions, infections, bowel edema and ischemia, and submucosal hemorrhage. Asymmetric thickening relates to different degrees of eccentric thickening around the circumference of the involved segment and is often seen in intestinal lymphoma (Fig. 16.8) and cancer.

16.4.2 Segmental Mural Hyperenhancement

The attenuation pattern of a thickened segment of bowel wall is an important criterion for establishing a differential diagnosis.

The bowel wall normally enhances after an adequate bolus of intravenous CM; the enhancement is usually greater on the mucosal aspect of the bowel wall and should not be mistaken for a disease process. Recognizing that the wall is not thickened and peri-enteric inflammation is not present differentiates normal enhancement from a disease process. Attenuation changes in the intestinal wall are frequently correlated with the thickened bowel wall.

Segmental mural hyperenhancement is defined as a post-CM attenuation of the wall of a segmental intestinal loop that is greater than the attenuation in adjacent small bowel loops. Common diagnoses with this pattern include idiopathic inflammatory bowel disorders, such as Crohn's disease, and vascular small bowel alterations.

After intravenous CM administration, there are two distinct patterns of bowel wall attenuation: homogeneous and non-homogeneous.

Homogeneous (White) Attenuation Pattern
The white homogeneous attenuation pattern represents high CM enhancement that can uniformly affect the majority of the thickened bowel wall. This finding can depend on a vasodilatation or an intramural vessel plexus injury with interstitial leakage. The increased wall enhancement associated with idiopathic inflammatory bowel disease reflects the hyperemic and hypervascular state seen classically in the acute phase of inflammation (Fig. 16.9).

If the bowel wall is enhanced to a degree equal to or greater than that of venous lumen opacification in the same CT scan, it should be classified as a white attenuation pattern (Fig. 16.9). However, it must be taken into account that this finding is dependent on the concentration, volume, rapidity of intravenous CM delivery, and timing of the CT scan [6, 7].

Pitfalls. The identification of bowel enhancement classified as a white attenuation is almost subjective and depends on technical factors, CM injection, and the patient's circulatory dynamics. The standard method used to quantify the white attenuation pattern is the enhancement of the venous system in the same axial scan images (Fig. 16.9).

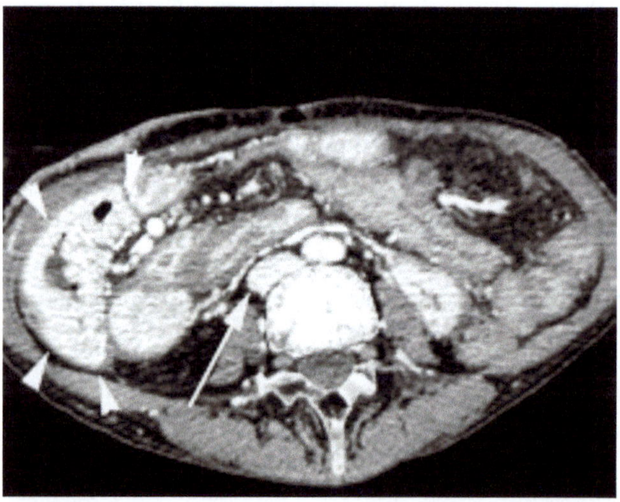

Fig. 16.9 Axial post-contrast CT scan shows evidence of the white attenuation pattern in a small bowel loop (*white arrowheads*) due to hyperemia and hypervascularity and associated with wall thickening. The attenuation of the affected loops is the same as the lumen of the vena cava (*white arrow*). These CT findings classically seen during the acute phase of inflammation were interpreted as an acute presentation of Crohn's disease. After only a week of antibiotic and anti-inflammatory therapy, the clinical and CT findings completely disappeared. The final diagnosis was an acute inflammatory intestinal disorder of indeterminate origin

Segmental mural enhancement is not a specific finding of Crohn's disease, as it is present in other inflammatory or infectious diseases (Fig. 16.10), in cancer, and in vascular intestinal disorders. In fact, the homogeneous attenuation pattern of a thickened bowel wall is also a feature of chronic Crohn's disease, radiation-therapy-induced submucosal hemorrhage, ischemic bowel loops, small bowel lymphoma, and cancer [8, 9].There is a considerable overlap in the findings of these different intestinal disorders, and other, associated morphological findings are necessary to make the correct diagnosis. A diagnosis based on this finding alone could be an erroneous one (Fig. 16.10). In particular, chronic Crohn's disease and chronic radiation enteritis may show the same homogeneous attenuation on contrast-enhanced CT.

In patients with long-standing Crohn's disease or radiation enteropathy, transmural fibrosis develops. During the chronic phase, the typical findings on intravenous contrast-enhanced CT of a target appearance are no longer present. Small bowel lymphoma (Fig. 16.8) is depicted on CT as a single segment or multiple segmental areas of circumferential thickening with homogeneous attenuation and enhancement [9].

The increased vascular permeability due to hypoperfusion of the intestinal wall in small bowel ischemia can lead to thickening and increased enhancement on CT scan, because of slowed perfusion and the interstitial leakage of CM molecules [10, 11].

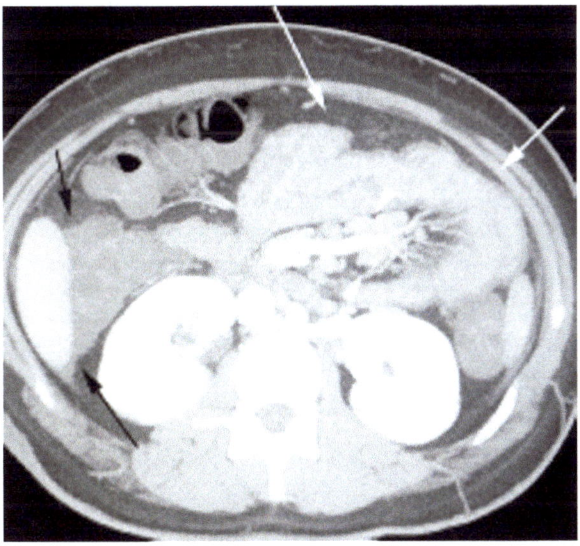

Fig. 16.10 Axial post-contrast CT scan shows the white attenuation pattern of a left-sided cluster of small bowel loops (*white arrows*) associated with multiple mesenteric lymph nodes (*white arrowheads*) and peritoneal free fluid (*black arrows*) in a patient with acute abdominal pain and diarrhea. These signs were initially interpreted as an acute presentation of Crohn's disease but the final diagnosis was viral enteritis

Heterogeneous (Stratified) Attenuation
Heterogeneous attenuation is the second pattern that may be depicted on a CT image of a thickened bowel wall segment. The mural stratification may be bilaminar, resulting in the *double-halo sign*, or trilaminar, producing a *target sign* (Fig. 16.11) [12]. Recognition of these stratified layers is based on the detection of either of these signs in the bowel wall

The double-halo sign is a generic term indicating stratification within a thickened bowel wall in which two continuous, symmetrically thickened layers are present. Specifically, there is an inner low-attenuation ring determined by edema (gray attenuation), surrounded by an outer higher-attenuation ring (white attenuation) that corresponds to the muscularis propria and indicates the presence of hyperemia [13]. Other conditions that can produce this sign include idiopathic inflammatory bowel diseases, vascular disorders, infectious diseases, and radiation damage [14].

In the target sign, inner and outer layers of high attenuation surround a central area of decreased attenuation. This finding is better visualized during the arterial phase. The "target" is composed of three rings: an outer strongly enhancing muscularis propria, a middle ring of gray attenuation that corresponds to submucosal edema, and an inner ring of high enhancement of the mucosal layer (Fig. 16.12) [15].

Pitfalls. The double halo and target signs are of similar significance and usually indicate an acute inflammatory or ischemic condition. The finding of stratified attenuation in a thickened intestinal segment, although non-specific, should be used only to exclude malignant conditions.

The two signs are present in many bowel pathological alterations, such as Crohn's disease, ulcerative colitis, acute-early inflammatory bowel disease, infectious disorders, radiation enteritis, vasculitis, lupus erythematous, cirrho-

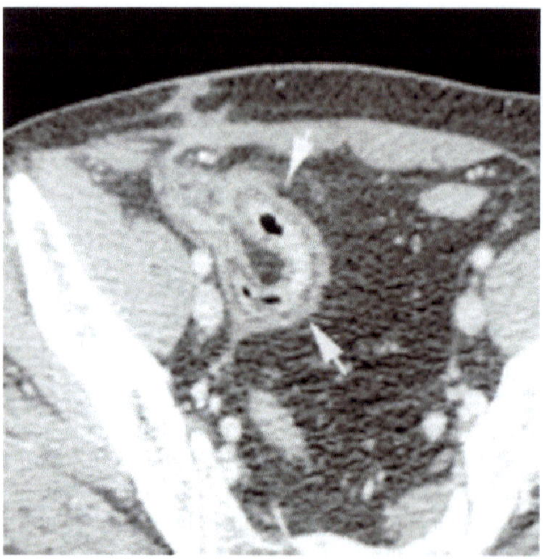

Fig. 16.11 Axial post-contrast CT scan demonstrates the classical mural trilaminar appearance of the terminal ileum wall (*white arrows*) in a patient with established Crohn's disease

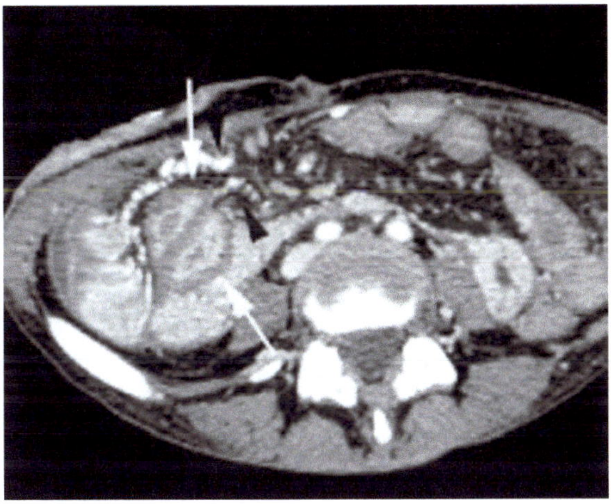

Fig. 16.12 Axial post-contrast CT scan demonstrates the target sign in the right-sided small bowel loops: the classical high enhancement of the outer muscularis propria layer, a middle ring of gray attenuation corresponding to edema of the submucosal layer, and a highly enhancing inner ring of the mucosal layer (*white arrows*). There is also a prominent peri-enteric vasculature (*black arrowheads*). These signs were initially interpreted as an acute presentation of Crohn's disease in a patient with abdominal pain and incomplete obstruction. The symptoms and findings resolved after medical treatment. The final diagnosis was an acute inflammatory intestinal disease of indeterminate origin

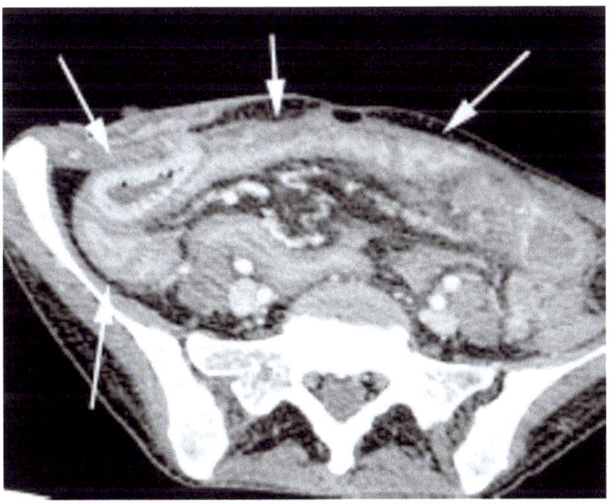

Fig. 16.13 Axial post-contrast CT scan demonstrates a double halo sign in the thickened small bowel loops (*white arrows*), misinterpreted in an emergency CT scan as idiopathic small bowel inflammation in patient with acute abdominal pain. Appropriate laboratory tests were negative; echocardiography revealed left atrial enlargement with peripheral thrombotic deposits. The final diagnosis was intestinal ischemia due to peripheral mesenteric arteriolar plexus microembolism

sis, ischemia, and vascular intestinal disorders (Fig. 16.13). In an emergency condition involving a patients without any previous history of inflammatory bowel disease, misinterpretation is common [6].

Heterogeneous attenuation and a thickened bowel are signs that are also indicative of ischemia, in addition to being seen in high-grade, poorly differentiated gastrointestinal neoplasms such as adenocarcinoma and stromal cell tumors. In these cases, the CT signs are related to rapid tumor growth, ischemia, and necrosis.

A potential pitfall may arise when residual fluid and oral CM fill the bowel lumen to mimic the target sign.

Fat Halo Sign

The fat halo sign refers to a three-layered target sign of thickened bowel in which the middle or submucosal layer shows fatty attenuation [16, 17] (Fig. 16.14). Common diagnoses referring to this finding include idiopathic inflammatory bowel and colon disease during the chronic phase. The fat halo is more frequently seen in ulcerative colitis than in Crohn's disease [6].

Pitfalls. The fat halo sign has also been described in patients who have undergone radiation therapy many years previously (Fig. 16.15). It has also been attributed to cytoreductive effects in the small bowel and colon following chemotherapy [17].

Intramural fat may be present in both the distal ileum and descending colon as a normal variant in patients without abdominal pain or gastrointestinal symptoms or in those with a history of intestinal disorders.

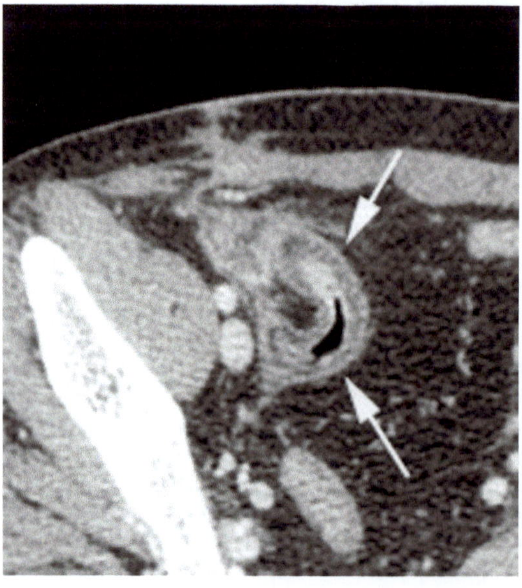

Fig. 16.14 Axial post-contrast CT scan demonstrates the classical fat halo sign (*white arrows*), i.e., a three-layered target sign of thickened ileal bowel loop in which the middle or submucosal layer has a fatty attenuation

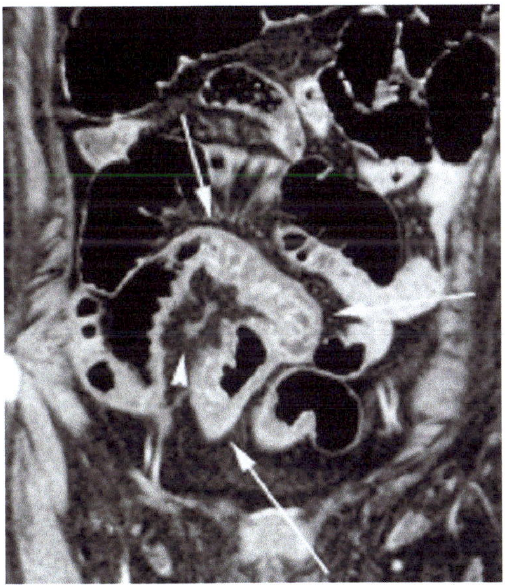

Fig. 16.15 Coronal CT reformatted image obtained from a patient with abdominal pain and intestinal obstruction symptoms. A scan with intravenous CM shows a fat halo sign in a thickened ileal bowel loop (*white arrows*) with mesenteric fold stranding and fluid (*white arrowhead*), misinterpreted in an emergency as Crohn's disease. The patient had undergone radiotherapy many years earlier for uterine cancer and the definitive diagnosis was postradiation chronic enteritis

In the small intestine, the normal intramural fat layer is generally very thin, usually thinner than the fat layer seen with idiopathic inflammatory bowel diseases. This finding is more often a feature of collapsed loops than of distended ones.

The fat halo sign in the normal terminal ileum is difficult to differentiate from the initial phase of Crohn's disease, especially in patients with abdominal pain and intestinal symptoms.

16.4.3 Prominent Peri-enteric Vasculature (Comb Sign)

The *comb sign* arises from the regional prominence and increased separation of the vasa recta in the ileum; it has also been called vascular jejunization of the ileum [18]. The engorged vasa recta, i.e., the extra-enteric portion of the vessels supplying the bowel, take on a parallel arrangement that resembles the teeth of a comb and is an expression of active disease (Fig. 16.3).

The tortuosity and dilatation of the vasa recta and their prominent comb-like arrangement in the small bowel mesentery is a finding of active Crohn's disease. The long, dilated, tortuous and widely spaced vasa recta of the ileum resemble the vasa recta of the jejunum. In fact, Crohn's disease causes a substantial increase in the arterial flow volume and a decrease in the resistance index at Doppler sonography [19].

Various factors have been proposed as the cause of hypervascularity in patients with Crohn's disease, including a granulomatous vasculitis in the muscularis propria.

Pitfalls

Hypervascularity of the mesentery with vascular dilatation, tortuosity, and prominence of the vasa recta, together producing the comb sign, should suggest that in this patient Crohn's disease is clinically active and advanced, but

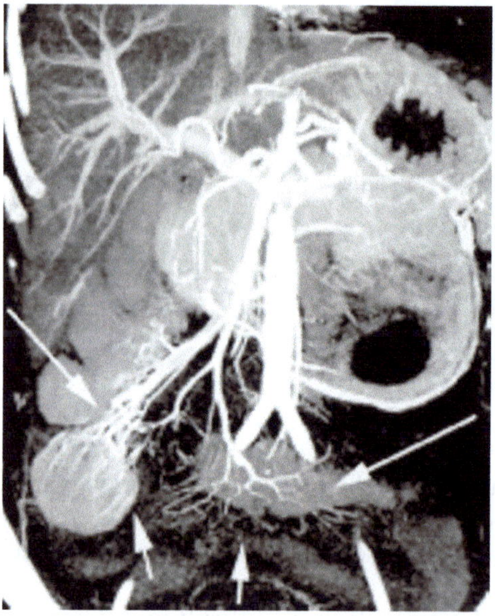

Fig. 16.16 Coronal MIP reformatted image obtained with intravenous CM during the arterial phase demonstrates segmental prominence, tortuosity, and the separation of peripheral mesenteric arteries (*white arrows*). This finding should suggest Crohn's disease but in this case a vasculitis due to lupus erythematosus was present

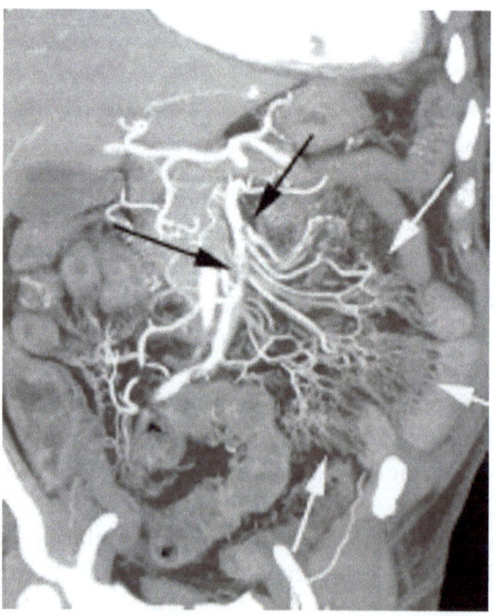

Fig. 16.17 Coronal MIP reformatted image obtained with intravenous CM during the arterial phase shows the comb sign (*white arrows*) due to an upper mesenteric artery embolism (*black arrows*)

these findings are not specific for the diagnosis [20]. In patients presenting with clinical symptoms for the first time, while this CT presentation should raise the possibility of Crohn's disease, it is not absolutely pathognomonic, as the comb sign has also been described in cases of lupus mesenteric vasculitis (Fig. 16.16) [21]. In fact, in systemic lupus erythematosus with abdominal pain, the comb sign is present in 87% of patients and it is frequently associated with CT findings of ischemic bowel disease, featuring segmental small bowel hyperattenuation. During emergency CT evaluation, these two findings could be misinterpreted as Crohn's disease.

Furthermore, there are several other disease processes in which engorgement of the mesenteric vessels has been reported, including other types of mesenteric vasculitis (polyarteritis nodosa, Henoch-Schönlein syndrome, microscopic polyangiitis, Behcet syndrome), mesenteric thromboembolism (Fig. 16.17), strangulated bowel obstruction, and ulcerative colitis: all of these intestinal disorders can mimic Crohn's disease during an emergency CT evaluation [8, 22].

16.4.4 Segment Length Involvement

It is important to determine whether the bowel wall thickening is focal (a few centimeters), segmental (10–30 cm), or diffuse (involving most of the small bowel).

Pitfalls

Inflammatory or neoplastic conditions may overlap with respect to segment length involvement. A segmental distribution is usually caused by Crohn's disease, infectious ileitis, radiation enteritis, intestinal ischemia, intestinal lymphoma, intramural hemorrhage, vasculitis, and lupus erythematosus [14, 21, 23].

16.4.5 Associated Abnormalities

Asymmetric mural enhancement and thickening are frequently seen along the mesenteric border. Since Crohn's disease is a transmural inflammatory process, changes may occur in the adjacent peri-enteric fat and small bowel mesentery. Increased density in the peri-enteric fat results from extension of the inflammatory process outside the bowel wall. Fibrofatty proliferation refers to an increased fatty proliferation along the mesenteric border of the bowel (Fig. 16.6) [24].

Penetrating disease refers to the presence of fistulas, phlegmons, and abscesses (Fig. 16.5) and occurs in up to 20% of Crohn's patients [25].

The associated features of Crohn's disease include mesenteric lymph nodes, mesenteric stranding, sinus tracts, fistulas, abscesses, the proliferation of mesenteric fat, and mesenteric vascular abnormalities.

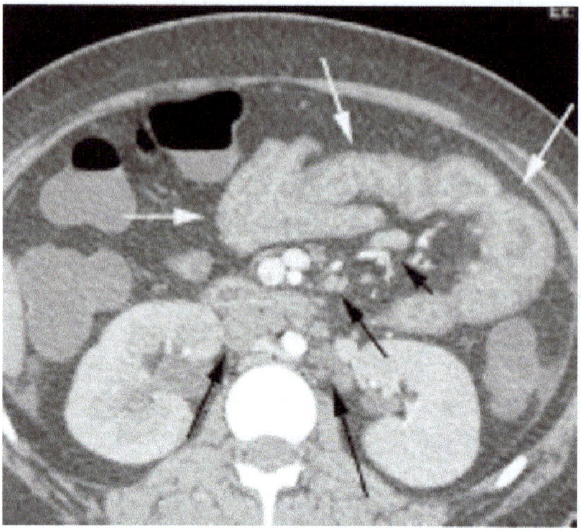

Fig. 16.18 Axial post-contrast CT scan demonstrates multiple peri-aortic and mesenteric lymph nodes (*black arrows*) associated with a cluster of small bowel loops in which the halo sign of the thickened wall can be seen. In an emergency setting, these signs were presumed to indicate Crohn's disease. However, alterations of the vasculature, the mesenteric border of the bowel loops, and the mesenteric fat were absent. Reassessment of the CT findings and clinical symptoms and an evaluation of the laboratory tests led to a final diagnosis of infectious enteritis

Pitfalls

Lymph nodes. The presence of lymph nodes in association with chronic inflammatory disease requires that the differential diagnosis include cancer, especially intestinal lymphoma, in addition to Crohn's disease (Fig. 16.18).

Mesenteric stranding. A frequent pitfall when interpreting CT findings of apparent bowel wall thickening is differentiating a disease process from residual fluid. When the peri-enteric fat adjacent to a thickened segment of bowel is normal, an acute inflammatory condition is less likely.

Abscesses, sinus tracts and fistulas. CT findings of mild, symmetric bowel wall thickening with or without a target sign in the distal ileum requires a differential diagnosis comprising infectious enteritis, Crohn's disease, vasculitis, and radiation enteritis. Secondary findings that help to establish the diagnosis of Crohn's disease include fistulas, sinus tracts, peri-enteric abscesses, and fibrofatty proliferation.

Fibrofatty proliferation. Intestinal tuberculosis is particularly difficult to distinguish from Crohn's disease [26].

16.5 Conclusions

Several alterations in the intestinal bowel loops characterize inflammatory Crohn's disease, such as wall enhancement pattern, the degree, symmetry, asymmetry and thickness of the altered wall, the mesenteric comb sign, and associated findings (stenosis of the lumen, fistulas, abscesses, mesenteric fibrofatty proliferation, mesenteric stranding), can indicate Crohn's disease and, in a differential diagnosis, when they appear together usually provide evidence for its confirmation.

Although none of the solitary CT signs is by itself specific, the accurate analysis of all small intestinal wall parameters and of the associated mesenteric alterations will allow most pitfalls to be avoided and either lead to a correct diagnosis or, at least, narrow the differential diagnosis of intestinal diseases with acute pain presentation.

References

1. Wills JS, Lobis IF, Denstman FJ et al (1997) Crohn disease: state of the art. Radiology 202:597-610
2. Gourtsoyiannis N, Papanikolau N, Grammatikakis J et al (2000) Magnetic resonance imaging of the small bowel using a true- FISP sequence after enteroclysis with water solution. Invest Radiol 12:2651-2658
3. Karahan OI, Dodd GD III, Chintapalli KN et al (2000) Gastrointestinal wall thickening in patients with cirrhosis: frequency and patterns on contrast enhanced CT. Radiology 215:103-107
4. Horton KM, Corl FM, Fishman EK et al (2000) CT evaluation of the colon: inflammatory disease. RadioGraphics 20:399-418
5. Phillpotts LE, Heiken JP, Westcott MA et al (1994) Colitis: use of CT findings in differential diagnosis. Radiology 190:445-449
6. Gore RM, Balthazar EJ, Ghahremani GG et al (1996) CT features of ulcerative colitis and Chron's disease. AJR 167:3-15
7. Tomei E, Discinti D, Marini M et al (1996) Computed Tomography of bowel wall in patients with Crohn's disease: relationship of inflammatory activity to biological indices. Ital J Gastroenterol 28:487-492
8. Rha SE, Ha HK, Lee SH et al (2000) CT and MR imaging features of bowel ischemia from various primary causes. RadioGraphics 20:29-42
9. Horton KM, Abrams RA, Fishman EK (2000) Spiral CT of colon cancer: imaging features and role in management. RadioGraphics 20:419-430
10. Sivit CJ, Taylor GA, Bulas DL et al (1992) Post traumatic shock in children: CT findings associated with hemodynamic instability. Radiology 182:723-726
11. Mirvis SE, Shanmuganathan K, Erb R (1994) Diffuse small-bowel ischemia in hypotensive adults after blunt trauma (shock bowel): CT findings and clinical significance. AJR 163:1375-1379
12. Gore RM, Marn CS, Kirby DF et al (1984) CT findings in ulcerative, granulomatous and indeterminate colitis. AJR 143:279-284
13. Baltazar EJ (1991) CT of the gastrointestinal tract: principles and interpretation. AJR 156:23-32
14. Horton KM, Corl FM, Fishman EK (2000) CT evaluation of the colon: inflammatory disease. RadioGraphics 20:399-418
15. Macari M, Balthazar EJ (2001) CT of bowel wall thickening: significance and pitfalls of interpretation. AJR 176:1105-116
16. Jones B, Fishmann EK, Hamilton SR et al (1986) Submucosal accumulation of fat in inflammatory bowel disease: CT pathologic correlation. J Comput Assist Tomogr 10:759-763
17. Muldowney SM, Baife DM, Hammermann A et al (1995) "Acute" fat deposition in bowel wall submucosa: CT appearance. J Comput Assist Tomogr 19:390-393

18. Meyers MA, McGuire PV (1995) Spiral CT demonstration of hypervascularity in Crohn disease: "vascular jejunization of the ileum" or "the comb sign". Abdom Imaging 20:327-332
19. Giovagnorio F, Discinti D, Vernis P (1998) Doppler sonography of the superior mesenteric artery in Crohn's disease. AJR 170:123-126
20. Lee SS, Ha HK, Yang SK et al (2002) CT of prominent pericolic or perienteric vasculature in patients with Crohn's disease: correlation with clinical disease activity and findings on barium studies. AJR 179:1029-1036
21. Byun JY, Ha HK, Yu SY et al (1999) CT features of systemic lupus erythematosus in patients with acute abdominal pain: emphasis on ischemic bowel disease. Radiology 211:203-209
22. Kim JK, Ha HK, Byun JY et al (2001) CT differentiation of mesenteric ischemia due to vasculitis and thromboembolic disease. J Comput Assist Tomogr 25:604-611
23. Blumeke DA, Fishman EK, Kuhlman JE et al (1991) Complications of radiation therapy: CT evaluation. RadioGraphics 11:581-600
24. Bodly KD, Fletcher JG, Solem CA et al (2006) Crohn disease mural attenuation and thickness at contrast-enhanced CT enterography-correlation with endoscopic and histologic findings of inflammation. Radiology 238:505-516
25. Bruining DH, Siddiki HA, Fletcher Jg et al (2008) Prevalence of penetrating disease and extraintestinal manifestations of Crohn's disease detected with CT enterography. Inflamm Bowel Dis 14:1701-1706
26. Podolsky DK (1991) Inflammatory bowel disease. N Engl J Med 325:928-937

Pitfalls of MRCP in the Evaluation of the Biliary Tract and Pancreatic Duct

17

Rosaria De Ritis, Isabella Iadevito, and Carlo Cavaliere

17.1 Introduction

Magnetic resonance cholangiopancreatography (MRCP) is a non-invasive imaging method that has proved to be valuable for the assessment of biliary and pancreatic disorders [1]. This technique basically exploits the long T2 relaxation times of slow-moving or stationary fluid to display bile and pancreatic juices with a high signal intensity on T2-weighted images.

Multiple studies have documented the accuracy of MRCP in the evaluation of choledocholithiasis, chronic pancreatitis, and anatomic variants of the biliary tract and pancreatic duct [2-5]. The sensitivity, specificity, and diagnostic accuracy of the MRCP/MRI assessment of the biliary tree and main pancreatic duct have been reported in numerous publications [6-9]. In fact, the diagnostic performance of MRCP is comparable to that of endoscopic retrograde cholangiopancreatography (ERCP) or percutaneous cholangiography, but without the risks associated with these procedures. Moreover, there is no use of ionizing radiation or iodinated contrast.

However, despite its established role in the diagnostic pathway of patient with pancreato-biliary disorders, MRCP has several limitations as well as pitfalls [10, 11] in which various pathologic conditions mask or simulate others. These pitfalls derive from both technical and interpretive limitations, such that MRCP results require a careful analysis in order to avoid diagnostic errors related to image misinterpretation.

In this chapter, we review the various pitfalls of MRCP, identifying the sources as well as the possible solutions.

R. De Ritis (✉)
Department of Diagnostic Radiological Imaging, MR Body Unit, "A. Cardarelli" Hospital, Naples, Italy

17.2 Technique

Two unique properties of bile that are exploited by nearly all MRCP sequences to aid in visualization are its relatively high water content and its stasis compared with blood flowing through adjacent vessels in the portal tracts [12]. Basically, MRCP uses heavily T2-weighted sequences to return a high signal from stationary or slow-moving fluid in the biliary and pancreatic ducts, which have long T2 relaxation times [13], and to suppress signal from background tissue and adjacent solid organs, such as the liver and pancreas, because of their shorter T2 relaxation times.

To date, a variety of MRCP techniques have been developed for a broad range of applications. For example, rapid T2-weighted acquisition with relaxation enhancement (RARE) sequences (single-shot fast spin echo sequences [14], or double-echo/multi-echo half-Fourier-acquisition single-shot turbo spin-echo sequence [15, 16]) is one of the more rapid pulse sequences used to obtain MRCP images and may well prove optimal for most analyses [17-21]. With this technique, individual slices are obtained during quiet breathing or in a breath-hold manner, reducing breathing and motion artifacts [21].

Technical considerations other than pulse sequences include two-dimensional versus three-dimensional acquisitions, respiratory triggering versus breath-hold scanning, and single-section versus multi-section acquisition [18, 20, 22-24]. The two most common two-dimensional MRCP techniques are the single-section and multi-section approaches. The latter (Fig. 17.1a) generates multiple thin slices (3–6 mm) best viewed sequentially in a cine-mode manner or post-processed for maximum intensity projection (MIP) to create a single overview image, In the single-slice approach [25] (Fig. 17.1b), a first thick slice (preferably around 3 cm [26]) is obtained during a breath-hold of a few seconds, with the process repeated with variable positions and orientations to encompass the entire pancreato-biliary system.

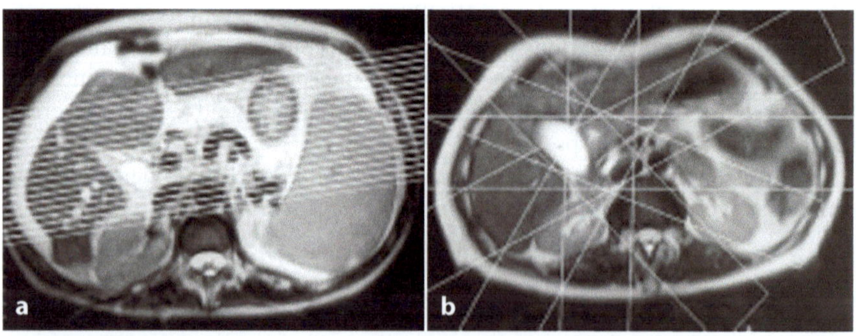

Fig. 17.1 Two-dimensional MRCP techniques. **a** Multi-section approach consisting of multiple thin slices (4 mm) that may be post-processed to create a single overview image. **b** Slice approach consisting of a single thick slice (3 cm) with variable positions and orientations to encompass the entire pancreato-biliary system

Although the many MRCP techniques can efficiently represent the pancreato-biliary system, at present, there is no clear consensus regarding the optimal MRCP protocol and optimal acquisition parameters, as all of the different approaches are susceptible to the technical pitfalls discussed in the following.

17.3 Technical Pitfalls

17.3.1 Incomplete Imaging

To accurately study the biliary tract and pancreatic duct, it is essential that all portions of the ductal system be visualized at MRCP, in particular the peripheral intrahepatic ducts (e.g., sclerosing cholangitis) and pancreatic ductal side branches (e.g., chronic pancreatitis) [27]. Especially in the two-dimensional single-slice MRCP technique (Fig. 17.1b), the relevant anatomy (generally, the distal tract of the common bile duct is used as a marker) must be identified by the imaging technician to allow correct slice positioning, as the different slices positions and orientations enable visualization of the entire pancreato-biliary system.

Accordingly, MRCP should always be performed in conjunction with cross-sectional imaging of the upper abdomen. This combined approach will improve the detection of subtle or more extensive parenchymal abnormalities without compromising ductal integrity, and better characterize putative non-specific ductal abnormalities.

17.3.2 Static Images

Unlike ERCP or percutaneous transhepatic cholangiography (PTC), MRCP yields only static images of the ducts, and in the physiologic, non-distended state, thereby decreasing the sensitivity of this technique to subtle ductal abnormalities [13], small or impacted biliary stones, short communications between cystic lesions and the pancreato-biliary system [28], and pancreato-biliary maljunction [29, 30].

This limitation is particularly evident in fasting and thin patients, in whom the secretion of bile and pancreatic juice is decreased such that the normal main pancreatic duct may be segmentally collapsed. It is also readily apparent on MIP reconstructions.

The physiological segmental collapse may be a source of misinterpretation in patients with, for example, ductal stenosis, as MRCP imaging may overestimate the length and degree of narrowing. It is also problematic in the early stages of chronic pancreatitis, in which, as seen on the MRCP images, the irregular outline of diseased side branches may be interpreted as the physiologic collapse of the ductal walls. Another potential pitfall related to the lack of ductal distention in MRCP imaging is the detection of small or impacted

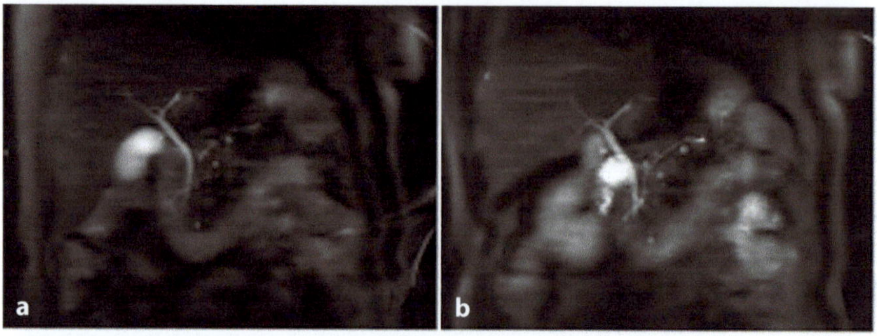

Fig. 17.2 Secretin-enhanced MRCP. **a** The pancreatic duct appears dilated by several cystic lesions in the pancreatic parenchyma. **b** Ten min after intravenous secretin injection (1 IU/kg), the pancreatic duct becomes more evident, revealing the communication between the cystic lesions and the second-order branches of the main pancreatic duct

biliary stones, which may be not appreciated due to the scarcity or absence of surrounding fluid.

Moreover, due to the absence of intraductal contrast material, used in ERCP and PTC procedures, it may be difficult to demonstrate a communication between a duct and surrounding fluid collections [11]. This may occur in attempts to determine the presence of a communication between a cystic lesion and the main pancreatic duct [28] (Fig. 17.2a), or, similarly, in patients with Caroli disease, in whom it may be difficult confirm that all cystic spaces represent dilated bile ducts and not simple hepatic cysts.

In such cases, investigators have proposed the use of secretin-enhanced MRCP to improve the delineation of the pancreatic duct architecture [31]. Secretin stimulates the exocrine pancreas to secrete fluid and bicarbonate, resulting in a transient increase in the diameter of the main pancreatic duct and therefore improvement in its depiction (Fig. 17.2b).

With dynamic secretin-enhanced MRCP, an initial acquisition is performed prior to the intravenous injection of secretin at a dose of 1 IU/kg body weight, followed by a series of acquisitions at 1-min intervals after the injection, with a total acquisition time of 10 min [32, 33].

Alternatively, intravenous morphine is also useful in improving distention of the biliary and pancreatic ducts as it reduces fluid outflow at the ampulla of Vater, which increases intraluminal pressure [34].

17.3.3 Acquisition and Reconstruction Artifacts

The optimization of acquisition parameters and post-processing algorithms is crucial for the correct interpretation of MRCP imaging findings. As far as acquisition parameters, the choice of an adequate slice thickness, echo time, and T2-weight (to optimize contrast resolution and differentiate ductal filling defects) are particularly important. Conversely, artifacts related to MIP and 3D volume-rendered reconstructions (e.g., lower spatial resolution, respiratory motion influence, and overestimation of ductal narrowing) are well known [35-37].

Slice thickness is also a critical parameter, especially in single-slice MRCP technique, as thicker slices allow the inclusion of more anatomy with a better signal-to-noise ratio; on the other hand, the contrast resolution in the image decreases, with significant volume averaging. Consequently, small filling defects may be obscured by partial volume effects, and pseudo-dilatations can occur if the cystic duct courses parallel to the common bile duct or if extraductal fluid-filled structures (e.g., intestine, pseudocysts, gallbladder) are volume averaged with it [35]. Generally, a thickness of about 3 cm represents a good compromise.

As far as the echo time and T2-weight setting, it should be considered that the signal intensity of the structures of interest depends on the chosen echo time (higher echo time corresponds to a higher signal intensity) and the T2 relaxation time of the fluid. Indeed, the pancreato-biliary system may disappear if very long echo times are used, and the presence of hemorrhage, sludge, and/or thick bile may have the same effects, thus influencing duct visualization [24, 38-40]. Moreover, pneumobilia may be misinterpreted as bile duct stones, although it is easily recognized on axial images: air will rise to a non-dependent position whereas true stones will layer dependently (Fig. 17.3) [37]. Finally, dense iodinated contrast material injected into the biliary tree for ERCP and PTC procedures has low signal intensity on heavily T2-weighted MRI; thus, when MRCP is performed immediately after these procedures, the pancreato-biliary system may not be visualized.

In terms of reconstruction techniques, given the low spatial resolution of MRCP and of MIP reconstruction, the diagnosis of a ductal stricture based on MRCP findings alone should be avoided since both the differentiation between

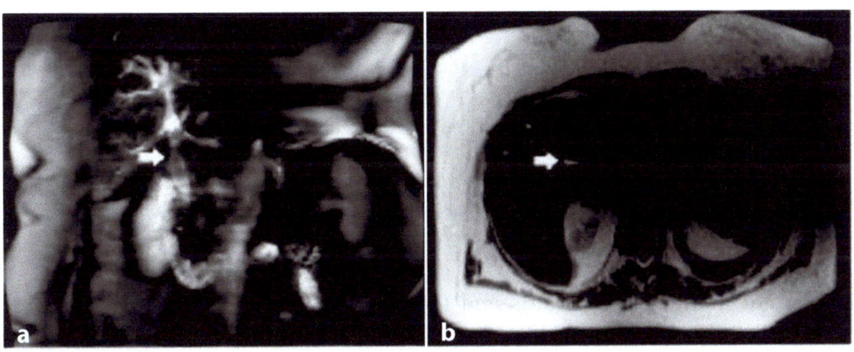

Fig. 17.3 Pneumobilia. **a** Air bubbles in the extrahepatic biliary duct (*arrow*) may be misinterpreted as bile duct stones. **b** Use of the non-dependent position in the axial T2-weighted image (*arrow*) resolves the doubt

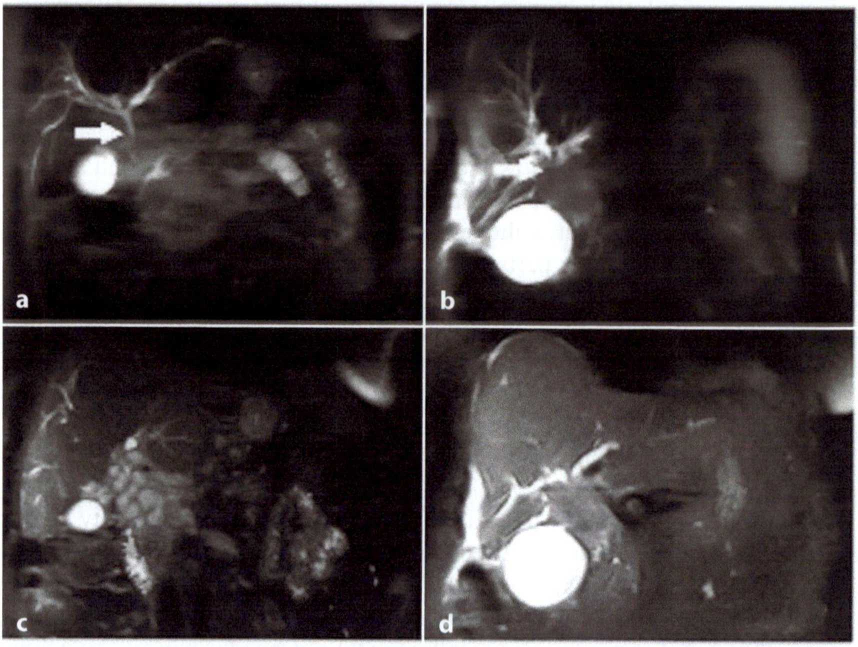

Fig. 17.4 MRCP alone fails to differentiate benign from malignant narrowing of biliary ducts. **a** A stenosis (*arrow*) caused by a portal cavernomatosis compresses the proximal tract of the common biliary duct. **b** A stenosis (*arrow*) caused by a heteroplastic lesion sited at segment I compresses and infiltrates the common bile duct at the confluence. **c, d** Coronal T2-weighted fat-saturated images demonstrate the different kind of lesions that determine biliary duct narrowing

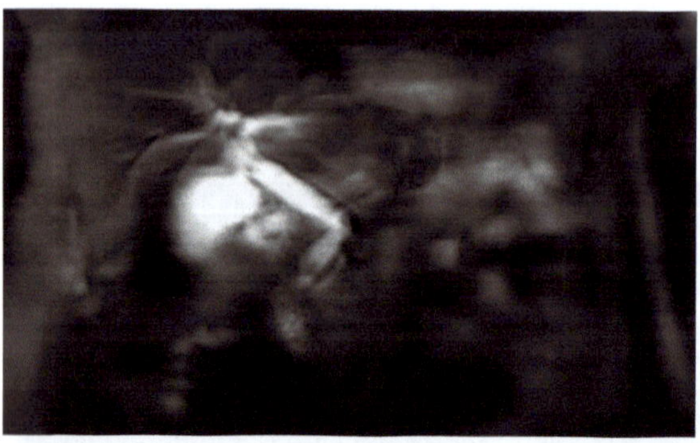

Fig. 17.5 Respiratory motion artifacts affect the visualization of the entire pancreato-biliary system, especially on maximum intensity projection reconstructions

benign and malignant strictures and the evaluation of pediatric patients [41] are difficult if not impossible. In fact, overestimation of ductal narrowing and pseudo-stricture results is inherent to MIP reconstruction and is a function of the technique's limited spatial resolution (Fig. 17.4) [37, 42], with corresponding effects.

Respiratory motion artifacts can present another problem in MIP reconstruction, If a patient does not perform an adequate breath hold [23], a misregistration of the common bile duct or main pancreatic duct will result [4, 37] (Fig. 17.5). Breathing artifacts are more common when the classic multiple thin-slice technique is used (typically with acquisition times > 10 s). To solve this problem, images may be obtained with respiratory gating by using the navigator echo approach. In addition, peristaltic motion is decreased in the fasted patient, whereas fat saturation and negative oral contrast agents can reduce artifacts from motion effects of the abdominal wall and bowel fluid, respectively.

In summary, both MIP and 3D volume-rendered images provide important information; however, the radiologist should always review the thin-section source images and not rely exclusively on post-processed images.

17.4 Interpretive Pitfalls

17.4.1 Pitfalls Related to Anatomic Variants

Ampullary and Papillar Region

The ampullary region represents a relative blind spot for MRI, due to the small size of the region, such that gastrointestinal images are often superimposed on the area of interest, and to the scarce/absent fluid, resulting in narrowing of the intramural segment of the bile duct. Consequently, an impacted stone near the ampulla is difficult to detect [37]. This condition should be suspected when dilatation of both the common bile duct and the pancreatic duct is evident, but this may also be detected with difficulty (Fig. 17.6). For example, the pancreatic duct may not be dilated, as in the case of pancreas divisum. Conversely, other conditions may induce concurrent dilatation of the common bile duct and pancreatic duct, as in focal pancreatitis or an ampullary carcinoma.

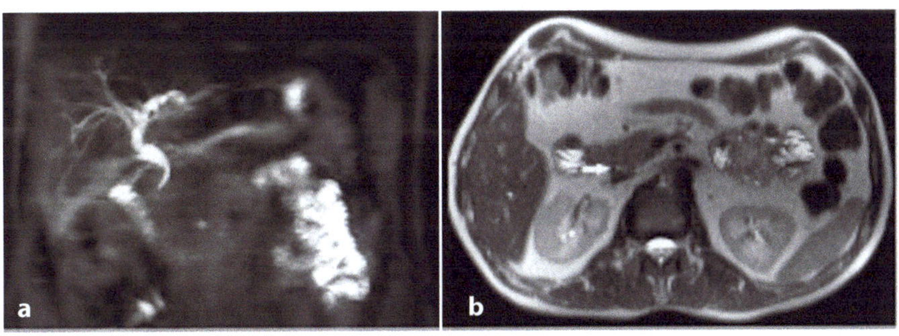

Fig. 17.6 Impacted stone in the ampullary region. **a** MRCP image shows a dilation of the distal common bile duct without identifiable causes. **b** The axial T2-weighted image shows a millimetric filling defect in the pre-ampullary tract of the duct (*arrow*) not previously identified

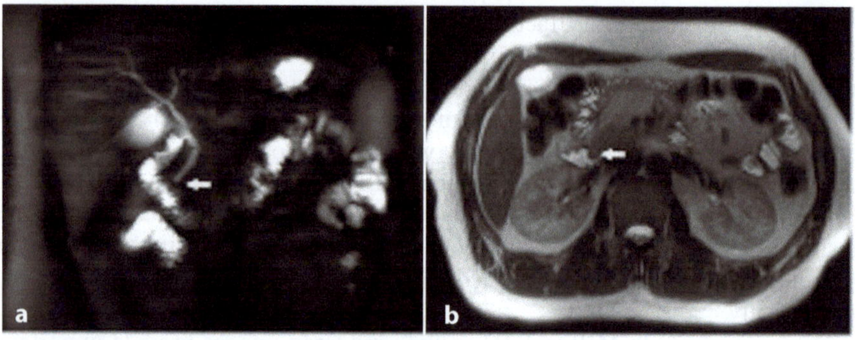

Fig. 17.7 Pseudocalculus sign. **a** The bulging appearance on MRCP of the sphincter of Oddi (*arrow*) mimics an obstructing stone. **b** Conventional MRI does not show stones or biliary sludge in this region, depicting the bulging profile of the papilla (*arrow*)

Nevertheless, when a filling defect or stricture is suspected in the peri-ampullary region, repeat MRCP and axial MRI should be performed.

On MRCP, the duodenal papilla can sometimes have a bulging appearance, which may be misinterpreted as the presence of an obstructing stone (Fig. 17.7). Moreover, extreme contraction of the sphincter of Oddi with retrograde "invagination" (also known as the pseudocalculus sign [43]) may mimic an impacted stone. A second MRCP and conventional MRI will clarify the precise local anatomy.

Cystic Duct Insertion and Morphology

The location of the insertion of the cystic duct with the common hepatic duct is variable. When the cystic duct runs parallel to the common hepatic duct for some distance, the two structures together may be mistaken for a dilated common bile duct. This pitfall is generally due to a MIP reconstruction artifact and can be avoided by reviewing source images. Moreover, occasionally, a signal void can be seen in the non-dependent central bile duct and misinterpreted as an intraductal filling defect (e.g., a stone). This flow artifact is uncommon but tends to appear in dilated ducts, when altered flow can occur, and at the insertion of a large cystic duct [44]. Flow-sensitive MRI (time-of- flight MR angiography) can demonstrate flow within the bile duct and resolve the problem.

Finally, when a dilated and tortuous cystic duct is detected, partial imaging of the redundant duct walls may mimic an intraductal filling defect, such as due to a stone. This pitfall can be avoided by changing the angle of image acquisition and by reviewing the axial images.

Pulsatile Vascular Compression: Hepatic Artery and Inferior Vena Cava

Vascular compression may induce a pseudo-obstruction of the biliary duct such that it may be difficult to differentiate between a signal void and a stone, hilar stenosis, or neoplasm on MIP images [45, 46]. The hepatic arteries and the gastroduodenal artery are often responsible for this artifact [10].

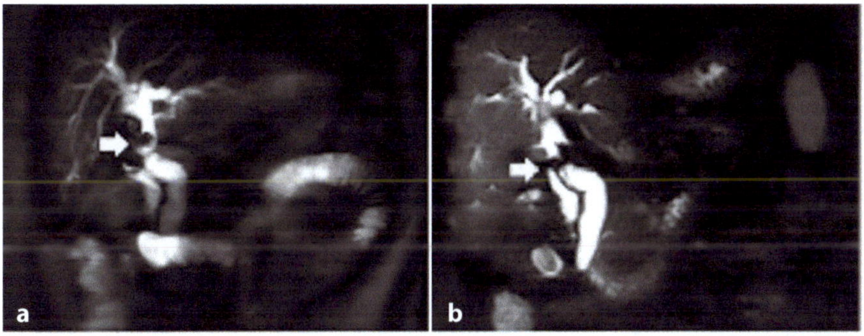

Fig. 17.8 Metallic clips simulate a filling defect in the biliary duct. **a** Metallic clips for a previous cholecystectomy determine a susceptibility artifact with loss of signal (*arrow*) in the proximal tract of the biliary duct. **b** This artifact is evident also in the coronal T2-weighted image

Specifically, as the right hepatic artery crosses posterior to the common hepatic duct below the bifurcation it can create an extrinsic impression on the duct that resembles an intraluminal filling defect. The same phenomenon can also be observed within the intrapancreatic portion of the common bile duct, where the many branches of the pancreatico-duodenal arcade may compress the biliary duct .

Similarly, pseudo-obstruction or motion artifacts of the extrahepatic bile duct may be produced by the back-and-forth motion of the anterior wall of the inferior vena cava (IVC) during the cardiac cycle [47-49].

Generally, the analysis of axial source images or a flow-sensitive sequence can be performed to identify the IVC.

17.4.2 Susceptibility Artifact

Infrequent causes of filling defects include susceptibility artifacts from adjacent clips, metallic bile duct stents, endovascular coils, gastrointestinal air, and calcifications (Fig. 17.8) [4, 42]. These different materials may produce adjacent signal loss and cause pseudo-obstruction [42], although MRCP is not as prone to this susceptibility artifact as other MRI sequences.

In particular, for gastrointestinal artifacts, the putative sources of this kind of pitfall include fluid located between gastric folds, the fluid/air contained in the gastric antrum, duodenal bulb, duodenal diverticulum or in an enteric duplication, or an overlapping hepatic cystic lesion. This artifact seems to be more prominent on fat-suppressed multi-section MRCP [50].

As in other pitfalls, the problem is often resolved by performing MRCP from a different angle of acquisition or with adjustments of section thickness. Alternatively, a negative oral contrast agent such as superparamagnetic iron oxide particles, gadolinium-meglumine compounds, or pineapple juice may be used [51-54].

Table 17.1 Pitfalls: summary

Pitfall	Description	Solution	References
Technical pitfall			
Incomplete imaging	It is essential that all portions of the ductal system be visualized at MRCP, in particular the intrahepatic peripheral bile ducts and branches of the pancreatic duct.	MRCP should be performed in conjunction with cross-sectional imaging of the upper abdomen.	[27]
Static images	MRCP yields only static images of the ducts, and in their physiologic, non-distended state, which decreases the sensitivity to subtle ductal abnormalities, small or impacted biliary stones, and thin communications between cystic lesions and the pancreato-biliary system.	Secretin or morphine administration may be useful.	[13, 28, 30, 31, 34]
Acquisition and reconstruction artifacts	The choice of an adequate slice thickness, echo time and T2-weight are crucial to avoid artifacts. Those related to MIP reconstruction (e.g., lower spatial resolution, respiratory motion influence, and overestimation of ductal narrowing) should be kept in mind.	Acquisition parameters should be optimized, e.g., by using respiratory gating, fasting, fat saturation and negative oral contrast agents to decrease motion artifacts. Thin-section source images should be analyzed.	[4, 35, 37]
Interpretative pitfalls			
Pitfalls related to anatomic variants	These are principally due to the lower spatial resolution of MRCP and MIP post-processing, and to flow artifacts in the biliary system, which determine intraductal filling defects.	Conventional MRI, or a flow-sensitive sequence may be useful.	[37, 43, 44, 46, 47]
Susceptibility artifacts	Adjacent clips, metallic bile duct stents, endovascular coils, gastrointestinal air, and calcifications may determine intraductal filling defects.	MRCP should be performed from a different angle of acquisition or with a different section thickness. Alternatively, a negative oral contrast agent may be used.	[4, 42, 54]

References

1. Fulcher AS, Turner MA, Capps GW (1999) MR cholangiography: technical advances and clinical applications. Radiographics 19:25-41
2. Fulcher AS, Turner MA, Capps GW et al (1998) Half-Fourier RARE MRCP in 300 subjects. Radiology 207:21-32
3. Chan Y, Chan ACW, Lam WWM et al (1996) Choledocholitiasis: comparison of MR cholangiography and endoscopic retrograde cholangiocgraphy. Radiology 200:85-89
4. Soto JA, Barish MA, Yucel EK et al (1995) Pancreatic duct: MR Cholangiopancreatography with three-dimensional fast spin-echo technique. Radiology 196:459-464
5. Taourel P, Bret PM, Reinhold C et al (1996) Anatomic variants of the biliary tree: diagnosis with MR cholangiopancreatography. Radiology 199:521-527
6. Kim JY, Lee JM, Han JK et al (2007) Contrast-enhanced MRI combined with MR cholangiopancreatography for the evaluation of patients with biliary strictures: differentiation of malignant from benign bile duct strictures. J Magn Reson Imaging 26:304-312
7. Kaltenthaler EC, Walters SJ, Chilcott J et al (2006) MRCP compared to diagnostic ERCP for diagnosis when biliary obstruction is suspected: a systematic review. BMC Med Imaging 6:9
8. Shanmugam V, Beattie GC, Yule SR et al (2005) Is magnetic resonance cholangiopancreatography the new gold standard in biliary imaging? Br J Radiol 78:888-893
9. Nguyen R, Pokorny CS (2003) Bile on the rocks: a guide to gallstones. Medicine Today 4:16-23
10. Irie H, Honda H, Kuroiwa T et al (2001) Pitfalls in MR cholangiopancreatographic interpretation. Radiographics 21:23-37
11. Van Hoe L, Mermuys K, Vanhoenacker P (2004) MRCP pitfalls. Abdom Imaging 29:360-387
12. Berry M, Chowdhary V, Mukhopadhyay S et al (eds.) (2006) Diagnostic radiology: gastrointestinal and hepatobiliary imaging. New Delhi, India. In Vashisht S, Thulkar S (2006) Imaging of obstructive biliopathy. 2nd edn. Jaypee Brothers Medical Publishers, New Delhi, pp 288-313
13. Vitellas KM, Keogan MT, Spritzer CE et al (2000) MR Cholangiopancreatography of bile and pancreatic duct abnormalities with emphasis on the single-shot fast spin-echo technique. Radiographics 20:939-957
14. Irie H, Honda H, Tajima T et al (1998) Optimal MR cholangiopancreaticographic sequence and its clinical application. Radiology 206:379-387
15. Van Hoe L, Vanbeckevoort D, Van Steenbergen W (2001) Atlas of cross-sectional and projective magnetic resonance cholangio-pancreaticography. A teaching file. Springer-Verlag, New York
16. Bosmans H, Van Hoe L, Gryspeerdt S et al (1997) Single-shot T2-weighted MR imaging of the upper abdomen: preliminary experience with double-echo HASTE technique. AJR 169:1291-1293
17. Fulcher AS, Turner MA (1997) HASTE MR cholangiography in the evaluation of hilar cholangiocarcinoma. AJR 167:1501-1505
18. Reuther G, Kiefer B, Tuchmann A (1996) Cholangiography before biliary surgery: single-shot MR cholangiography versus intravenous cholangiography. Radiology 198:561-566
19. Mizutani Y (1995) Short breath-hold MR Cholangiopancreatography with single slice method using HASTE sequence. Jpn J Magn Reson Med 15:187-195
20. Ichikawa T, Nitatori T, Hachiya J et al (1996) Breath-held MR cholangiopancreatography with half-averaged single shot hybrid rapid acquisition with relaxation enhancement sequence: comparison of fast GRE and SE sequences. J Comput Assist Tomogr 20:798-802
21. Miyazaki T, Yamashita Y, Tsuchigame T et al (1996) MR Cholangiopancreatography using HASTE (half-Fourier acquisition single-shot turbo spin-echo) sequences. AJR Am J Roentgenol 166:1297-1303
22. Reinhold C, Guibaud L, Genin G et al (1995) MR Cholangiopancreatography: comparison between two-dimensional fast spin-echo and three-dimensional gradient-echo pulse sequences. JMRI 4:379-384

23. Soto JA, Barish MA, Yucel EK et al (1995) MR cholangiopancreatography: Findings on 3D fast spin-echo imaging. AJR 165:1397-1401
24. Barish MA, Soto JA (1997) MR cholangiopancreatography: techniques and clinical applications. AJR 169:1295-1303
25. Ly JN, Miller FH (2002) MR imaging of the pancreas: a practical approach. Radiol Clin North Am 40:1289-1306
26. Topal B, Van de MM, Fieuws S et al (2003) The value of magnetic resonance cholangiopancreatography in predicting common bile duct stones in patients with gallstone disease. Br J Surg 90:42-47
27. Fulcher AS, Turner MA (1998) Pitfalls of MR Cholangiopancreatography (MRCP). J Comput Assist Tomogr 22:845-850
28. Irie H, Honda H, Aibe H et al (2000) MR cholangiopancreatographic differentiation of benign and malignant intraductal mucin-producing tumors of the pancreas. AJR Am J Roentgenol 174:1403-1408
29. Sugiyama M, Baba M, Atomi Y et al (1998) Diagnosis of anomalous pancreaticobiliary junction: value of magnetic resonance cholangiopancreatography. Surgery 123:391-397
30. Kamisawa T, Okamoto T (2004). Pitfalls of MRCP in the diagnosis of pancreatobiliary maljunction. JOP 5:488-490
31. Heverhagen JT, Burbelko M, Schenck zu Schweinsberg T et al (2007) Secretin-enhanced magnetic resonance cholangiopancreaticography: value for the diagnosis of chronic pancreatitis. Fortschr Rontgenstr 179:790-795
32. Fukukura Y, Fujiyoshi F, Sasaki M et al (2002) Pancreatic duct: morphologic evaluation with MR Cholangiopancreatography after secretin stimulation. Radiology 222:674-680
33. Matos C, Metens T. Deviere J et al (1997) Pancreatic duct: morphologic and functional evaluation with dynamic MR pancreatography after secretin stimulation. Radiology 203:435-441
34. Silva AC, Friese JL, Hara AK et al (2004) MR cholangiopancreatography: improved ductal distention with intravenous morphine administration. Radiographics 24:677-687
35. Yamashita Y, Abe Y, Tang Y et al (1997) In vitro and clinical studies of image acquisition in breath-hold MR cholangiopancreatography: single-shot projection technique versus multislice technique. AJR Am J Roentgenol 168:1449-1454
36. Anderson CM, Saloner D, Tsuruda JS et al (1990) Artifacts in maximum-intensity-projection display of MR angiograms. AJR 154:623-629
37. David V, Reinhold C, Hochman M et al (1998) Pitfalls in the interpretation of MR cholangiopancreatography. AJR Am J Roentgenol 170:1055-1059
38. Outwater EK, Gordon SJ (1994) Imaging the pancreatic and biliary ducts with MR. Radiology 192:19-21
39. McDermott VG, Nelson RC (1995) MR cholangiopancreatography: efficacy of three-dimensional turbo spin-echo technique. AJR 165:301-302
40. Kelekis NL, Semelka RC (1996) MR imaging of the gallbladder. Top Magn Reson Imaging 8:312-320
41. Irie H, Honda H, Jimi M et al (1998) Value of MR cholangiopancreatography in evaluating choledochal cysts. AJR Am J Roentgenol 171:1381-1385
42. Reinhold C, Bret PM (1996) Current status of MR cholangiopancreatography. AJR 166:1285-1295
43. Beneventano TC, Schein CJ (1969) The pseudocalculus sign in cholangiographic interpretation. Arch Surg 98:731-733
44. Hintze RE, Adler A, Veltzke W et al (1997) Clinical significance of magnetic resonance Cholangiopancreatography (MRCP) compared to endoscopic retrograde cholangiopancreatography (ERCP). Endoscopy 29:182-187
45. Watanabe Y, Dohke M, Ishimori T et al (2000) Pseudo-obstruction of the extrahepatic bile duct due to artifact from arterial pulsatile compression: a diagnostic pitfall of MR cholangiopancreatography. Radiology 214:856-860
46. Mortelé KJ, Rocha TC, Streeter JL et al (2006) Multimodality imaging of pancreatic and biliary congenital anomalies. RadioGraphics 26:715-731

47. Morita S, Saito N, Suzuki K et al (2007) Common bile duct pulsation synchronized with inferior vena cava anterior wall motion observed by cine-segmented true fast imaging with steady-state precession magnetic resonance imaging. Eur Radiol 17 Suppl 1:332.
48. Gullace G, Savoia MT (1984) Echocardiographic assessment of the inferior vena cava wall motion for studies of right heart dynamics and function. Clin Cardiol 7:393-404
49. Mintz GS, Kotler MN, Parry WR et al (1981) Real-time inferior vena cava ultrasonography: normal and abnormal findings and its use in assessing right-heart function. Circulation 64:1018-1025
50. Watanabe Y, Dohke M, Ishimori T et al (1999) Diagnostic pitfalls of MR cholangiopancreatography in the evaluation of the biliary tract and gallbladder. RadioGraphics 19:415-429
51. Takahara T, Yoshikawa T, Saeki M et al (1995) High concentration ferric ammonium citrate (FAC) solution as a negative bowel contrast agent. Nippon Igaku Hoshasen Gakkai Zasshi 55:425-426
52. Kato J, Kawamura Y, Watanabe T et al (2001) Examination of intra-gastrointestinal tract signal elimination in MRCP: combined use of T(1)-shortening positive contrast agent and single-shot fast inversion recovery. J Magn Reson Imaging 13:738-743
53. Papanikolaou N, Karantanas A, Maris T et al (2000) MR Cholangiopancreatography before and after oral blueberry juice administration. J Comput Assist Tomogr 24:229-234
54. Riordan RD, Khonsari M, Jeffries J et al (2004) Pineapple juice as a negative oral contrast agent in magnetic resonance cholangiopancreatography: a preliminary evaluation. Br J Radiol 77:991-999

18 Errors in Musculoskeletal MRI

Carlo Masciocchi, Laura Conti, Federico D'Orazio,
Armando Conchiglia, Giuseppe Lanni, and Antonio Barile

18.1 Introduction

The correct execution of magnetic resonance imaging (MRI) examinations under standardized and improved conditions can significantly increase their iconographic quality and facilitate their diagnostic interpretation. In MRI, errors may be technical, methodological, or interpretive in their origin.

18.2 Technical and Methodological Errors

Among the most common and frequent technical errors are movement artifacts, which are often due to the inability of the patient to maintain a correct position during the MRI examination. To avoid these artifacts, it is important to keep the examined anatomical region immobilized, to find the correct position inside the coil and, last but not least, to obtain maximum patient cooperation. The presence of ferromagnetic artifacts, often caused by clips, prostheses, or post-surgical outcomes can greatly impair image quality. These materials, in fact, can produce distortions or homogeneity alterations in the magnetic field, especially on STIR or gradient echo sequences.

Partial-volume effects are produced when different anatomical structures having different internal compositions are present within the same voxel, thereby influencing the MRI signal intensity. The thicker the slice, the higher the risk of partial-volume effects. A small field of view (FOV) of the anatomical area under examination increases the risk of wrap-around, aliasing, and backfolding artifacts.

A. Barile (✉)
Department of Radiology, University of L'Aquila, "S. Salvatore" Hospital,
L'Aquila, Italy

The term "magic angle" refers to the artifacts produced when the increase in the MRI signal is due to collagen fibers inclined at 55° with respect to the static magnetic field. The risk of producing these artifacts is much higher when short time of echo sequences are used. Menisci and tendons contain longitudinally oriented collagen fibers and the imaging of these structures is therefore likely to result in these artifacts (Fig. 18.1).

Methodological errors include those cases in which MRI examinations are improperly performed. The risk increases when a differential diagnosis algorithm is not followed or when incorrect scan planes or sequences are used, especially if, during the examination, the already acquired images are not taken into consideration in the planning of subsequent phases or are considered sufficient by themselves to allow a clear and supportable diagnosis. Obviously, the level of risk will be proportional to the operator's technical accuracy in executing the MRI examination [1, 2].

The term "pitfalls" includes all interpretative errors based on unapparent sources of misinterpretation for a non-expert radiologist; such errors cannot be attributed to a wrongly performed MRI examination alone.

18.3 Interpretation Errors

18.3.1 Bone

To correctly report musculoskeletal MRI examinations, it is essential to be aware of the MRI signal produced by bone marrow, because it is represented in every

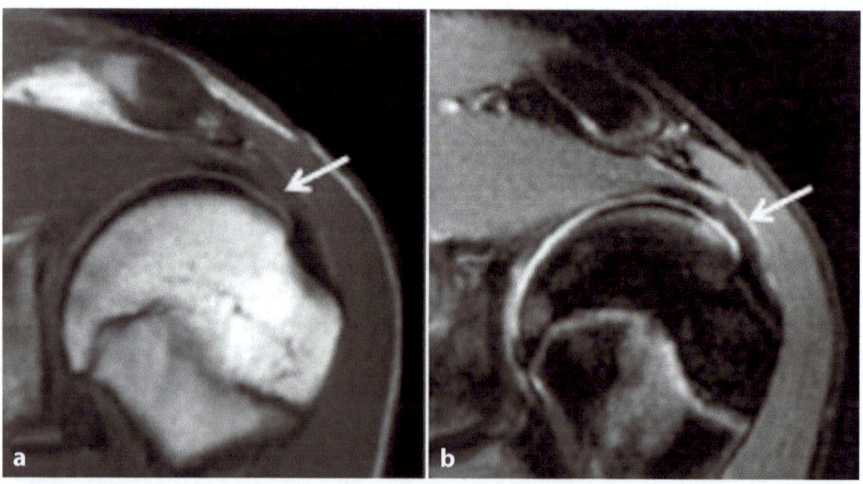

Fig. 18.1 During MRI, the "magic angle" artifact (*arrow*), evident here in the supraspinatus tendon of the shoulder, is present on the oblique-coronal short-TE image (**a**) and disappears on the long-TE oblique-coronal image (**b**)

anatomic region and must always be evaluated, analogous to other organs. The MRI signal of pathologic bone marrow is a sensitive but not sufficiently specific criterion of analysis. Firstly, T1-weighted sequences need to be used to evaluate cellular marrow content; STIR and T2-weighted sequences with fat saturation are also helpful. As is well known, fatty and hematopoietic elements are represented in different and variable proportions during developmental phases. Depending on their locations and representations, these bone marrow elements will generate different and opposite MRI signals, and thus vary in their appearance. Accordingly, problems will be encountered when studying the skeletal segments of a young patient with a recent history of trauma. During body growth, marrow conversion begins in the distal appendicular segments and reaches, after a period of months/years, the proximal segments. Within the long bones, conversion from red (hematopoietic) to yellow (fatty) marrow is initiated in the epiphyses and apophyses, then proceeds to the diaphysis, and finally to the metaphysis. In each of these regions, the conversion process starts centrally and then continues peripherally towards sub-cortical regions of the bone.

In the MRI examination of a young adult, red marrow with a "geographical" distribution is frequently found in the metaphysis, such that the bone has a typical "patchy" appearance (Fig. 18.2). The only diagnostic advantage for the radiologist in these cases is the frequently symmetrical distribution of red marrow; therefore, a comparison with the contralateral limb is a fundamental diagnostic aid [3].

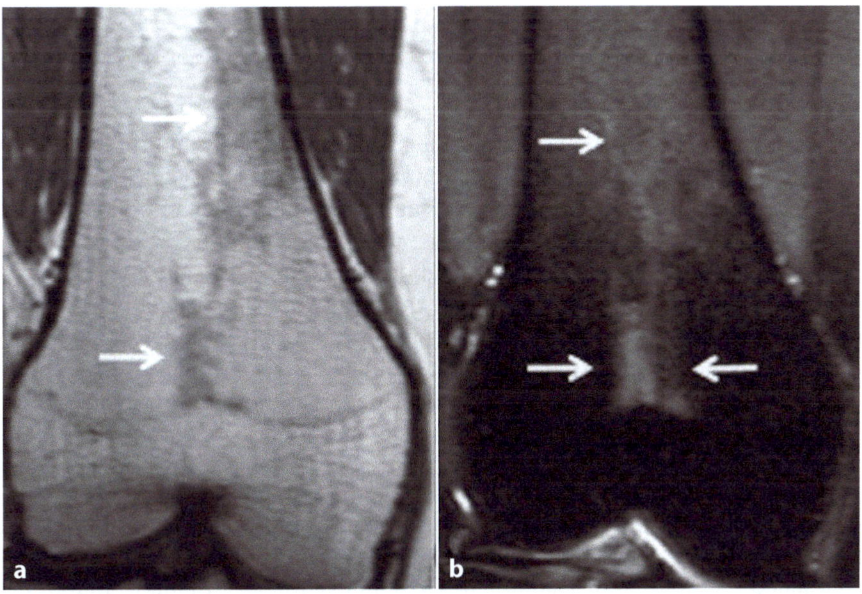

Fig. 18.2 MRI well documents the presence of "red" bone marrow (*arrows*) as an area of low signal intensity on the coronal T1-weighted image (**a**) and as an area of high signal intensity on the coronal STIR image (**b**)

Among the numerous pathologic conditions (traumatic and/or neoplastic) that comprise the differential diagnosis of benign alterations of the marrow signal are stress fractures and osteoid osteoma. In both cases, the distribution and signal intensity of intraspongious edema are similar to what is seen in residual red marrow. Thus, it is necessary to combine MRI and computed tomography (CT) to demonstrate the presence of a "nidus" or cortical extension of an overload fracture. Stress fractures are among the most frequent causes of non-neoplastic bone edema; their diagnosis is facilitated by accurate anamnesis of the patient and by the radiologist's familiarity with the most typical locations of these fractures.

In diagnostic practice, a reduction of normal hematopoietic cells and their replacement by fatty elements is a common finding in patients undergoing radiotherapy or chemotherapy. These marrow alterations are seen as focal aspects during or after radiotherapy but are more extensively represented in patients who undergo chemotherapy, as an effect of systemic therapy. A true challenge in the differential diagnosis is in distinguishing osteomyelitis from bone neoplasms. The diagnosis of Ewing's sarcoma, for example, can be doubtful and the respective images difficult to interpret. Conventional radiology will show elements common to both entities, such as bone disruption, aggressive parosteal reaction, and lack of osteoid matrix proliferation. Subacute and chronic osteomyelitis, as seen on MRI, can demonstrate bone disruption with extension to the periostium or even to subcutaneous tissues, as well as the presence of an intraosseous and/or extraosseus granulation tissue with enhancement after gadolinium administration [4].

18.3.2 Soft Tissues

The possible causes of abnormal muscle signal intensity are multiple: trauma, infection, autoimmune disorders, inflammation, neoplasms, neurologic disorders, iatrogenic causes, and accessory muscles. Signal intensity due to alterations in muscles occur in three settings: muscle edema, fatty infiltration, and mass effect. Muscle edema can be found in association with polymyositis, dermatomyositis, minor muscular lesions, infectious myositis, radiation therapy, subacute denervation, compartment syndrome, the early stages of myositis ossificans, rabdomyolysis, and during a sickle cell crisis [5].

Fatty infiltration is seen with chronic denervation, chronic disuse, after heavy muscle injuries with tendon avulsion, and in case of chronic treatment with corticosteroids.

Mass effect is typical of tumors, intramuscular abscesses, myonecrosis, traumatic lesions, myositis ossificans, sarcoidosis, and parasitic infections. Muscle-tendon injuries include strains, tendon avulsions, and hematomas. In first-degree strains, only edema can be found, without structural alterations inside the muscle. Otherwise, in major strains, the association of hematoma with edema can mimic a neoplasm with characteristics of biological aggressiveness. Contusions are distinguished by the presence of intramuscular edema without a clear mass effect. The radiological features of heterotopic post-traumatic and post-surgical ossifications, such as myositis ossificans, are similar to those of tumors with mineralized matrix (parosteal osteosarcoma) and their aspect depends on the maturity of the lesion. Also, muscular hematomas can mimic soft-tissues neoplasm with variable bleeding inside. Clearly, being aware of a previous trauma is fundamental to a correct diagnosis, but in the absence of such information the MRI signal characteristics can be helpful to confirm a diagnostic suspicion. The presence of signal hyperintensity on T1 fat-saturated sequences is suggestive for methemoglobin residues, and thus for hematoma. If gadolinium is administered, there will be no enhancement at that level, while in case of tumor there will be evidence of nodular areas of enhancement inside the lesion [6].

The presence of accessory muscles, especially at the knee and ankle, is less than rare. Attention should be paid to the potential finding of an intra-articular muscle of the knee, such as an accessory soleus muscle (Fig. 18.3), an accessory flexor hallucis longus, and a peroneus quartus of the ankle, as they can mimic the presence of a soft tissue mass.

18.3.3 Joints

Shoulder MRI is widely used for impingement and impingement-related instability evaluations. The radiologist should be familiar with the normal anatomy of the shoulder and its variants, as well as with the prevalence of the various anomalies of the shoulder. One of the most common anatomical variants is seen in the glenoid labrum. In the literature, the glenoid labrum has been described as triangular, rounded, spiculated, notched, or flat, or it may be absent. However, the three main anatomical variants of the labrum are: (1) the

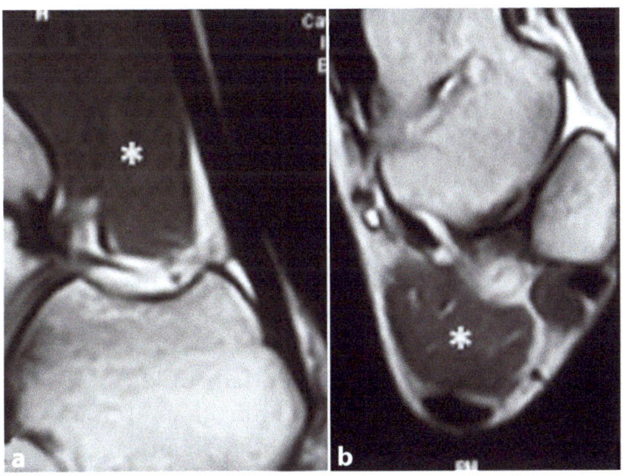

Fig. 18.3 The presence of an accessory soleus muscle (*asterisk*) at the ankle is readily documented on SE T1-weighted MRI both on the sagittal (**a**) and the axial (**b**) scan planes

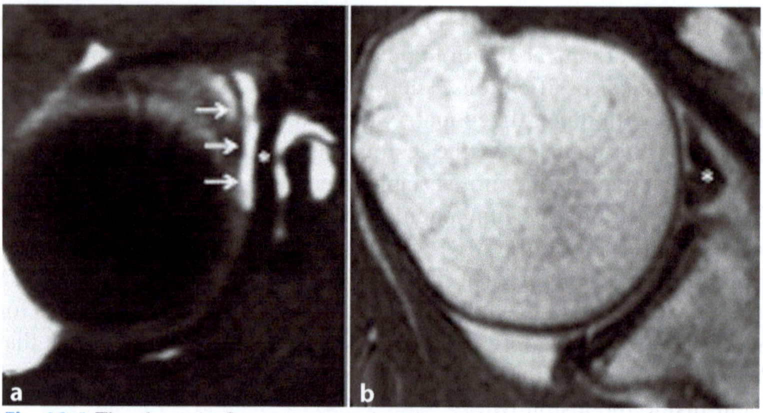

Fig. 18.4 The absence of an anterosuperior glenoid labrum (*arrows*), referred to as a "Buford complex," is well evident on the arthro-MRI proton-density (PD)-saturated sagittal scan planes (**a**). A hypertrophic middle glenohumeral ligament (*asterisk*) is also present and is well depicted on the arthro-MRI PD axial scan plane (**b**)

presence of a sublabral recess, characterized by the presence of a synovial reflection medially and inferiorly located at the apex of the glenoid tuberosity, producing a loose connection of the glenoid labrum at the top of the tubercle. Unlike superior labrum anterior to posterior (SLAP) lesions, in this portion of the labrum the sublabral recess extends only medially; it is of minor extent and directed towards the glenoid cartilage. (2) A sublabral foramen is a focal detachment of the labrum from the surrounding glenoid, more frequently located between 1 and 3 o'clock, anteriorly to the biceps anchor. (3) In the anatomical variant known as the Buford complex, the anterosuperior part of the labrum is absent, while the other parts are normally represented. This variant is also associated with a compensatory hypertrophy of the middle glenohumeral ligament, the "string aspect." Due to the absence of the anterosuperior part of the labrum, a Buford complex may be misdiagnosed as a SLAP lesion (Fig. 18.4).

The anatomical variants involving the labrum include those of the labrum-biceps complex. The long head of the biceps and superior glenohumeral ligament have a common labral insertion, the "labrum-biceps complex." Among the variants of insertion on the glenoid labrum, there are three types of biceps anchor. Types 2 and 3 may mimic a disruption of the labrum's insertion from its natural site and therefore be confused with a SLAP lesion.

The os acromialis variant may be confused with a fracture of the distal part of the acromion. At the insertional level of the coraco-acromial ligament, this can mimic a caudally directed osteophyte [7, 8].

According to our experience, the most important pitfalls of knee MRI are concentrated on the correct interpretation and identification of traumatic lesions. Meniscal tears are often complex and of doubtful significance for at

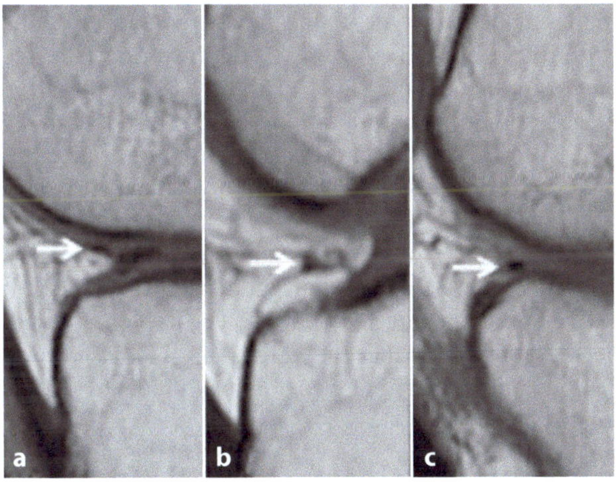

Fig. 18.5 The transverse meniscal ligament (*arrows*) of the knee is readily depicted on MRI sagittal PD contiguous scans from the lateral to the medial (a-c) aspect of the knee

least two reasons: because of the complex anatomy of that area and the presence of particular tissue components that can produce an area of altered signal, mimicking a lesion. A typical example is the transverse meniscal ligament, which connects the anterior horn of the medial and lateral menisci. It has a round appearance on sagittal scans (Fig. 18.5).

The transverse ligament has low signal intensity, as does every ligament, and it can mimic a meniscal tear or a free meniscal fragment, especially at its insertion. The posterior accessory meniscal-femoral ligament (Wrisberg ligament) joins the posterior horn of the lateral meniscus to the medial femoral condyle at its intercondylar side. It typically emerges from the dorsal side of the posterior cruciate ligament (PCL) and can simulate, because of its origin, an external meniscal tear. The anterior accessory meniscal femoral ligament (Humprey ligament), like its posterior counterpart, has the same critical interpretation and is located on the ventral side of the PCL. Interpretation doubts posed by these ligaments can be solved by comparing the sagittal images with images acquired along an axial plane passing through the area of interest, which will demonstrate them much clearly. The oblique meniscus-meniscal ligament (OMML) derives from the anterior horn of the meniscus. It extends through the intercondylar notch, passing between the ligaments of the central pivot and inserting on the posterior horn of the contralateral meniscus. The function of the OMML is still unknown and its presence does not have pathologic consequences. Its importance derives from the possibility of its being mistaken for a bucket-handle injury, particularly on sagittal images. Evidence of a double PCL is indicative of a bucket-handle lesion of the medial meniscus but this can be mimicked by anatomical structures in the intercondylar notch [9-11].

The abnormal insertion of the medial meniscus onto the anterior cruciate ligament (ACL) may lead to the appearance of a pitfall; three different subgroups of insertion are distinguished. In type 1, the most frequent type, the insertion is at the inferior third of the ACL. In type 2, the insertion is at the middle third of the ACL and in type 3 at the superior third, or directly at the intercondylar notch. This insertional structure might be confused with an infrapatellar plica (if there is insertion in the intercondylar notch), or an anterior horn tear (insertion on the inferior third of the ACL), or with an ACL partial tear (insertion on the middle third of the ACL) [12].

Meniscal "flounce," in which there is a single symmetrical fold along the free edge of the meniscus, is considered a normal variant of meniscal position; its origin is controversial. True predisposing factors have yet to be identified, even though studies in the literature show that the valgus and increased joint mobility caused by ligamentous injuries or joint effusion may predispose to its formation [13].

Diagnostic errors more frequently occur in evaluations of the acetabular labrum of the hip. A groove in the posterior-inferior labrum is a common anatomical variant. When this groove is not recognized as a normal finding, it may result in a diagnostic error, especially when the diagnosis is based on MRI arthrography (arthro-MRI) images. Unfortunately, studies conducted with the use of arthro-MRI are controversial. Some researchers have suggested the presence of a sublabral groove as a common finding. More recent studies, in fact, have identified sublabral recesses in the posterior part of the acetabular labrum. Those notches are typically located at the 8 o'clock position, as shown by the interposition of contrast medium, and have a regular and linear morphology. Partial separation of the labrum and the absence of perilabral anomalies are characteristic for the presence of a sublabral recess. In the analysis of MRI results, anatomical variants of the anterior half of the acetabular labrum are much more radiologically relevant, as the majority of pathological alterations occur in that region of the joint [14, 15].

Femoral-acetabular impingement is a common cause of hip pain in young adults. In these patients arthro-MRI often shows degenerative changes or tears in the labrum that generally occur in its superior-anterior part. Based on our experience, we find that two imaging criteria are highly useful in the differentiation of normal recesses from labral tears: (1) The passage of contrast medium involving the upper half of the front labrum should be considered as an injury. (2) Recesses are characterized by their anterior-inferior location, linear shape, and the partial separation of the labrum in the absence of perilabral anomalies [16].

Recent MRI developments, especially in terms of higher spatial and contrast resolution, allow a more precise display of smaller and complex anatomical structures, such as those of the proximal wrist. There is a series of pitfalls that may cause diagnostic challenges, especially with respect to injuries of the triangular fibrocartilage complex (TFCC). The TFCC's ulnar insertion is made up of two distinct sheets separated by the ligament subcruentum, which is composed of fibrovascular tissue. This insertion usually has intermediate signal intensity on T1- and T2-weighted images and sometimes shows internal streaking. The TFCC radial insertion bends around the ulnar side of the radius, producing a linear zone of high signal intensity that must not be confused with an injury [17]. At imaging, the TFCC of the carpus is a hypointense structure in all pulse sequences. However, the radial and ulnar insertions of the TFCC are often of medium to high signal intensity, and thus a potential imaging pitfall.

Wrist and metacarpophalangeal joint in patients with rheumatoid arthritis are a source of many pitfalls that may be encountered on MRI. In the study of rheumatic diseases, erosions can be difficult to distinguish from focal regions of bone marrow edema, particularly on T1-weighted images, as they are seen as areas of low signal intensity [18].

References

1. Davies AM, Pettersson H (1998) Orthopedic imaging, techniques and applications. Springer-Verlag, Heidelberg
2. Peh WCG, Chan JHM (2001) Artifacts in musculoskeletal magnetic resonance imaging: identification and correction. Skeletal Radiol 30:179-191
3. Stacy GS, Dixon LB (2007) Pitfalls in MR image interpretation prompting referrals to an orthopedic oncology clinic. RadioGraphics 27:805-828
4. Herman Kan J (2008) Major pitfalls in musculoskeletal imaging–MRI. Pediatr Radiol 38:S251-S255
5. May DA, Disler DG, Jones EA et al (2000) Abnormal signal intensity in skeletal muscle at MR imaging: patterns, pearls, and pitfalls. RadioGraphics 20:S295-S315
6. Ma LD, Frassica J, Scott WW Jr et al (1995) Differentiation of benign and malignant musculoskeletal tumors: potential pitfalls with MR imaging. RadioGraphic 15:349-366
7. Rdudez J, Zanetti M (2008) Normal anatomy, variants and pitfalls on shoulder MRI. Eur J Radiol 68:25-35
8. Massengill AD, Seeger LL, Yao L (1994) Labrocapsular ligamentous complex of the shoulder: normal anatomy, anatomic variation, and pitfalls of MR imaging and MR arthrography. RadioGraphic 14:1211-1223
9. Tyler P, Datir A, Saifuddin A (2010) Magnetic resonance imaging of anatomical variations in the knee. Part 1: ligamentous and musculotendinous. Skeletal Radiol 39:1161-1173
10. Venkatanarasimha N, Kamath A, Mukherjee K et al (2009) Potential pitfalls of a double PCL sign. Skeletal Radiol 38:735-739
11. Kim EY, Choi S, Ahn JH et al (2008) Atypically thick and high location of the wrisberg ligament in patients with a complete lateral discoid meniscus. Skeletal Radiol 37:827-833
12. Cha JG, Min KD, HAN JK et al (2008) Anomalous insertion of the medial meniscus into the anterior cruciate ligament: the MR appearance. Br J Radiol 81:20-24
13. Park JS, Ryu KN, Yoon KH (2006) Meniscal flounce on knee MRI: correlation with meniscal locations after positional changes. AJR 187:364-370
14. Czerny C, Hofmann S, Urban M et al (1999) MR arthrography of the adult acetabular capsular-labral complex: correlation with surgery and anatomy. AJR 173:345-349
15. Dinauer PA, Murphy KP, Carroll John F (2004) Sublabral sulcus at the posteroinferior acetabulum: a potential pitfall in MR arthrography diagnosis of acetabular labral tears. AJR 183:1745-1753
16. Studler U, Kalberer F, Leunig M et al (2008) MR arthrography of the hip: differentiation between an anterior sublabral recess as a normal variant and a labral tear. Radiology 249:947-954
17. Pfirrmann CWA, Zanetti M (2005) Variants, pitfalls and asymptomatic findings in wrist and hand imaging. Eur J Radiol 56:286-295
18. McQueen F, Ostergaard M, Peterfy C et al (2005) Pitfalls in scoring MR images of rheumatoid arthritis wrist and metacarpophalangeal joints. Ann Rheum Dis 64:48-55

Errors and Medicolegal Issues in Interventional Radiology

19

Raffaella Niola, Giuseppe de Magistris, and Franco Maglione

19.1 Introduction

"You land a million planes safely, then you have one little mid-air and you never hear the end of it" (Air Traffic Controller, New York TRACON, Westbury Long Island).

Radiology is one of the most rapidly evolving medical specialties, embracing new technologies and incorporating several invasive techniques. Interventional radiology is by far more than a diagnostic area of modern radiology. Several gastrointestinal and vascular diseases may be treated either only by interventional radiological procedures or by a combination of this type of procedure with conventional surgery. Additionally, interventional radiology involves elements of both pre- and post-procedural care. Within the context of this rapid transformation of radiological practice, radiologists have been exposed to a higher litigation risk, while lawsuits and insurance claims involving radiologists have dramatically increased [1].

Involvement by radiologist in all medical malpractice claims varies from 5% to 21% [2-4]. Claims brought against radiologists include problems of errors in case management (cognitive), in technique, or in the actions of the supporting staff [5]. The radiologic problems that have most frequently led to medical malpractice lawsuits have been due to "failure to diagnose," i.e., the oversight of abnormalities or the misinterpretation of radiologic images [5]. Although misdiagnosis, especially in breast cancer, remains the largest category of radiology-related litigation, claims of injuries from complications, most of which are due to angiography, increased in the 20-year period from 1975 to 1995 in Cook County, Illinois, USA [6]. There is also an increasing

R. Niola (✉)
Department of Diagnostic Radiological Imaging, Vascular and Interventional Radiology Unit, "A. Cardarelli" Hospital,
Naples, Italy

L. Romano, A. Pinto (eds.), *Errors in Radiology*, © Springer-Verlag Italia 2012 frequency of legal exposure after the use of interventional procedures in the treatment of breast cancer [7].

Public attention was aroused when the Institute of Medicine published its report *To Err Is Human: Building a Safer Health Care System*, in 1999. In that report, it was estimated that 44,000–98,000 hospitalized Americans died in 1997 as a result of preventable medical errors. This is the equivalent in loss of life to one or two full Boeing 737 aircraft crashes every day of the year. These figures do not include those patients who are injured as a result of medical errors but do not die [8].

There are three areas in which considerations regarding negligence should concern the radiologist involved in interventional procedures of the breast. These include the performance of the procedure itself, obtaining consent for the procedure, and the responsibility for follow-up, communication, and management recommendations, involving the patient, the radiologist, and the referring physician [7].

Following the expansion of endovascular therapy into new areas, such as the repair of abdominal and thoracic aneurysms as well as the treatment of carotid bifurcation disease using interventional radiological techniques, the radiologist has been exposed to additional litigation risk. Although in such procedures radiologists are part of a team of physicians dealing with the patient's problem, the responsibility for malpractice related to the patient's management is equally distributed among all those involved at any stage of the diagnostic and therapeutic process. The problem is even more serious when the proposed therapy is not an established treatment, but rather one that is still under validation and mostly allowed only within the context of multicenter randomized trials.

19.2 Discussion

"Complacency or a false sense of security should not be allowed to develop as a result of long periods without an accident or serious incident. An organization with a good safety record is not necessarily a safe organization. Every accident, no matter how minor, is a failure of the organization." (International Civil Aviation Organization, Accident Prevention Manual). Fileni et al. [9] examined the insurance claims of Italian radiologists over the 1993–2006 period. During the study period, 1,424 claims for alleged malpractice were filed against radiologists covered by insurance policies. Of these claims, most involved radiologists working in the public hospitals system (977 cases; 68.6%). Errors in radiologic techniques and procedures accounted for 11.5% of claims (164 cases), most of which (98 cases) involved interventional radiologic procedures [9]. The interventionalist is likely to become an increasingly frequent defendant by virtue of several factors: the surgical and procedural nature of interventional radiology, the sporadic complications that occur, unrealized expectations by patients, and the occasional need to alter initially planned therapy. Even the technically "successful" case may result in a lawsuit. In this current litigious society, interventional radiologists find themselves vulnerable. In past decades, myelography and arteriography were more frequently implicated. In the Cook County study, between 1955 and 1975, medical lawsuits increased 100-fold, and almost 10% were procedure-related [2]. In another report, from 1986, over 30% of malpractice cases against California radiologists were brought because of complications of arteriography, myelography, or intravenous administration of contrast material [3]. Among the complications of arteriography, those related to the arterial puncture site include hematoma, dissection, thrombosis, arteriovenous fistula, and pseudoaneurysm. Although rare, puncture site injuries may cause serious sequelae and can lead to death [10]. The incidence of serious injury resulting from arterial puncture using the Seldinger technique has remained remarkably stable for the past 35 years [11]. The common femoral artery is the safest puncture site, with an incidence of severe complications of < 0.5%. Complications at the axillary and translumbar sites are somewhat more likely, with an incidence of 1.7% and 0.6%, respectively [10]. Although other complications, such as arterial dissection or occlusion, can occur with femoral puncture, bleeding is the most common serious complication. Femoral puncture is safest in the common femoral artery, and punctures either too high or too low are more likely to result in hematoma and pseudoaneurysm. Fluoroscopic localization before puncture can help ensure entry into the vessel over the lower half of the femoral head, which is the ideal site.

More recently, in interventional radiology, the types of procedures that more often prompt or contribute to litigation include: percutaneous biliary drainage (Fig. 19.1), percutaneous nephrostolithotomy, abscess drainage, pancreatic drainage, biopsy, contrast material administration, embolization, stent placement (Figs.19.2, 19.3), and central venous catheter placement. The most common acute complications of central venous catheter placement include misplacement of the catheter, pneumothorax, and arterial puncture. In their review of complications arising from the performance of these procedures, Mansfield et al. [12] found that the best predictor of a complication was failure to complete the procedure on the initial attempt. Patients in whom catheter placement was not achieved on the first attempt, even if the central venous catheter was successfully placed on a repeated attempt by either the same or another physician, had a complication rate of 8% [13]. Other predictors of complications were prior surgery or radiation therapy at the site of placement and patients at the extremes of body mass. Less experienced physician have a statistically significant decreased success rate and more complications. To reduce the complications rate, some authors [12] recommend that if prior surgery or radiotherapy has taken place on one side of the body, the opposite side should be used. They also recommend the use of real-time sonography in performing these procedures.

Interventional neuroradiology represents a high-risk, high-yield field. The patient has an average stroke risk of 5–8% and a mortality risk of 1–2% in very

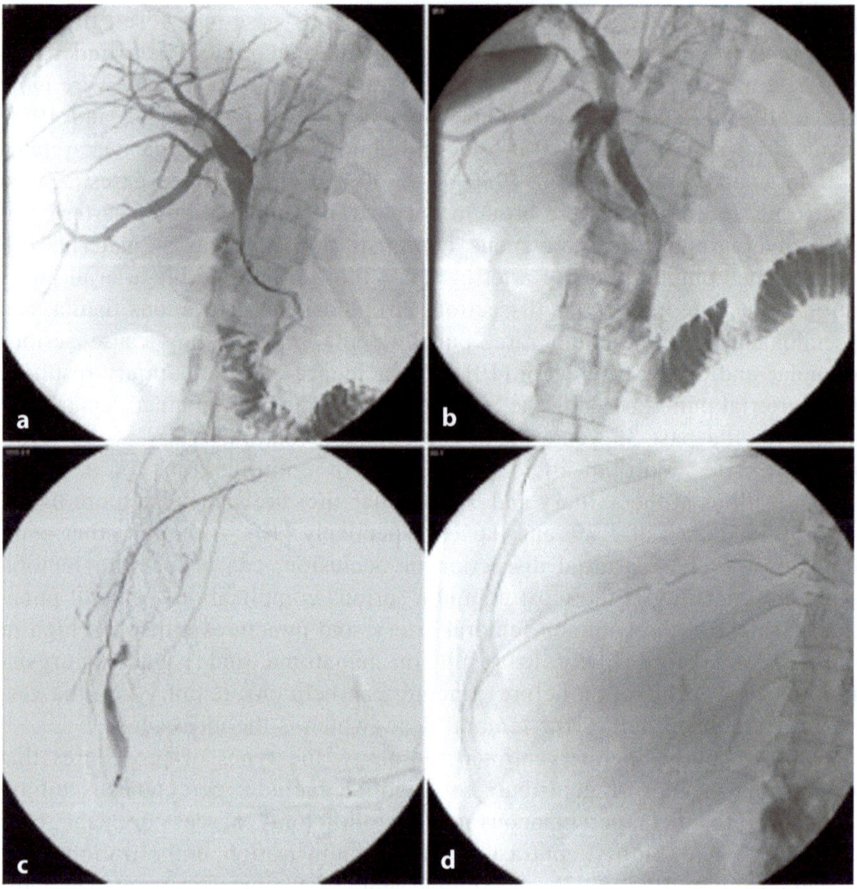

Fig. 19.1 **a** Percutaneous biliary drainage in an obstruction of the proximal third of the common bile duct. **b** Graft placement shows patency, with reflux of bile into the duodenum. **c** The patient was returned to the operating room 6 h later due to shock. **d** Multiple intercostal arteries showed lesions, which were percutaneously embolized

Error: Damage to the hepatic or intercostal artery during a biliary procedure is not an "error" but a serious and avoidable complication. In this case, the first error was the choice of a very supporting but, at the same time, very strong and stiff sheath with which to support the introduction of the graft, and then to remove it without the inner tapered cannula. The second error was not to leave the "sentinel intra-stent" catheter connected to a drainage bag. In fact, if this had been done, the blood would have oozed out immediately, permitting very quick recognition of the problem and thus its treatment, thereby avoiding the shock and the multiple sequelae, including the death of the patient after 20 days on the ICU

experienced hands. Risks escalate with interventions above the skull base, where the thin-walled vessels are small and delicate; their location in the subarachnoid space complicates the situation further. They float freely in cerebrospinal fluid, unsupported by bone or muscle, making them susceptible to

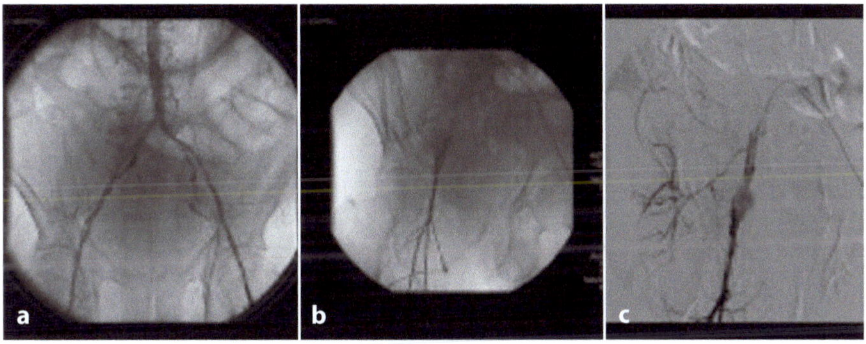

Fig. 19.2 a Aortography via the common left femoral artery, showing free contrast medium in the proximal third of an external iliac calcified artery, due to an iatrogenic lesion. **b** An attempt at graft placement via the common right femoral artery. **c** The final angiogram shows a very poor result, with free contrast still evident

Error: The extremely calcified, yet insulted (due to the iatrogenic lesion after the first puncture for a hepatic chemoembolization procedure) artery should have been surgically approached at the first attempt. Instead, two overlapping grafts of small diameter were placed, without resolution of the problem. The patient underwent surgery 5–6 h after the interventional procedure, went into shock, and died 24 h later in the ICU due to hypotension and heart failure. The mismanagement resulted in high cost, loss of time (interventional radiology in place of an immediate surgery), and the death of the patient

tearing. Mistakes here are deadly. Although extracranial vessels are more robust, they are still friable and susceptible to rupture or dissection. A sense of the acceptable amount of force (good and bad resistance) increases with experience [14].

Informed consent for interventional procedures is a relatively frequent source of legal problems as well. The radiologist performing interventional radiology procedures must properly inform the patient. This includes information about the procedure, the alternatives, and the potential benefits as well as the risks. Informed consent is waived only for mental incompetence, documented patient desire not to be informed, an emergency situation, or if information would induce undue mental anguish (the latter is used in psychiatric situations only) [5]. Radiologists must discuss their own procedures with patients; informed consent for radiologic procedures cannot be left to clinicians [5]. Moreover, the patient should be informed if the proposed procedure is a new therapy still under investigation and without available scientific evidence regarding the long-term benefits over conventional surgery. In such cases, more than the usual amount of time should be spent to provide thorough information and to make sure that patient's understanding of the risks is adequate [15]. Moreover, because interventional radiology is procedural in nature, the ratio of case management problems comprising lawsuits against interventional radiologists may be more akin to that found with surgical specialities.

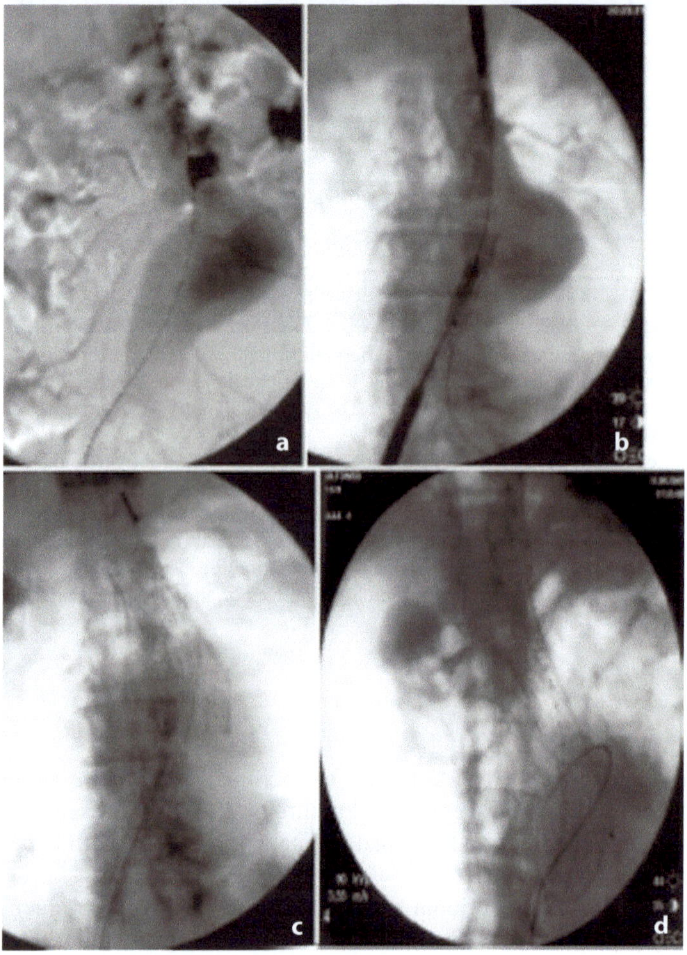

Fig. 19.3 **a** Aortography with pigtail pre-placement of an aortic endoprosthesis for endovascular treatment of an abdominal aortic aneurysm (EVAR). **b** Release of the main body of the device. **c** The gate of the device, on the left, is opened in the aneurysmal sac. **d** The loop of the wire during the multiple attempts at catheterization of the gate

Error: The gravest mistake was the choice of the device. The size was incorrect (based on an a CT interpretation error), as it was too small given the size of the aneurysm. Thus, the gate was opened in the sac, such that its catheterization was impossible. After multiple attempts, during an axillary approach, the goal was to push the wire from "above" and capture it from "below," thereby permitting the device to walk along it, but this too was unsuccessful. In fact, sclerosis of the aorta and the arteries together with the size of the aneurysm guaranteed the failure of the procedure. A conversion to an aorto-uni-iliac endoprosthesis was subsequently performed, but the patient died 48 h later in the ICU. The first procedure was very long and exhaustive for the surgeons and the anesthesia too long for the patient. The costs were very high for the hospital and the end was unsuccessful, including the death of the patient

Note: Safety rounds are devoted to improving patient safety by eliminating sources of preventable medical error [16].

As a fellow in interventional radiology, the physician can expect the institution, as employer, to purchase professional liability insurance. Upon completion of training, the interventional radiologist should verify the existence of tail insurance for all prior acts of potential malpractice. In Illinois, the professional liability insurance policy covers claims that are filed during the year covered under the policy. In determining the appropriate amount of insurance coverage, the interventional radiologist needs to consider the jurisdiction in which he or she practices and the types of procedures performed. The more complicated and risky the procedures, the greater the need for higher insurance coverage [17].

Finally it should be emphasized that being named in a lawsuit does not mean that the radiologist has done anything wrong. A bad outcome of a procedure is not in itself grounds for a lawsuit and does not prove negligence. Nonetheless, the anxiety of being named in a medical malpractice lawsuit purportedly contributes to the physician's subsequent perceived decrease in job satisfaction compared with the satisfaction experienced previously. The rise in medicolegal involvement of an ever-increasing number of physicians, and in particular interventional radiologists, underlines the importance of obtaining written informed consent. The need for setting guidelines and for continuous education from professional societies is urgent. In the rapidly changing environment of radiological practice, measures to ensure safety and professional protection are mandatory.

The Joint Commission on the Accreditation of Healthcare Organizations (JCAHO) accredits these organizations on the basis of evaluations of the quality and safety of care. As part of this emphasis, the JCAHO promotes national patient safety goals and has established a sentinel-event policy calling for the identification, reporting, evaluation, and prevention of sentinel events. According to the JCAHO, a sentinel event is "an unexpected occurrence involving death or serious physical or psychological injury, or the risk thereof" [18]. The terms sentinel event and medical error are not synonymous; not all sentinel events occur because of an error and not all errors result in sentinel events. The JCAHO requires that all sentinel events be investigated by using root cause analysis and that the results of the investigation be reported to it. Root cause analysis is a powerful tool for analyzing system failures and is equally applicable to actual adverse events and to "close calls" (potential adverse events) [19].

In addition, we must make the transition from the old culture of blame ("you screwed up") to a culture of safety ("let's find out what the problem is and fix the system"). An essential component of a culture of safety is sharing and disseminating experience with sentinel events.

References

1. Marchant J (2001) Rising malpractice threat prompts caution. Diagn Imag Eur 17:2624-2639
2. Berlin L (1986) Malpractice and radiologists, update 1986: an 11.5-year perspective. AJR 147:1291-1298
3. Spring DB, Tennenhouse DJ (1986) Radiology malpractice lawsuits: California jury verdicts. Radiology 159:11-814
4. Hamer MM, Morlock F, Foley HT et al (1987) Medical malpractice in diagnostic radiology: claims, compensation, and patient injury. Radiology 164:263-266
5. van Sonnenberg E, Barton JB, Wittich GR (1993) Radiology and the law, with an emphasis on interventional radiology. Radiology 187:297-303
6. Berlin L, Berlin JW (1995) Malpractice and radiologists in Cook County, IL: trends in years of litigation. AJR 165:781-788
7. Brenner RJ (1995) Interventional procedures of the breast: medicolegal considerations. Radiology 195:611-615
8. Kohn LT, Corrigan JM, Donaldson MS (eds) (1999) To err is human: building a safer health care system. National Academy Press, Washington, DC
9. Fileni A, Magnavita N, Mirk P et al (2010) Radiologic malpractice litigation risk in Italy: an observational study over a 14-year period. AJR 194:1040-1046
10. Spies JB, Berlin L (1998) Complications of femoral artery puncture. AJR 170:9-11
11. Waugh JR, Sacharias N (1992) Arterographic complications in the DSA era. Radiology 182:243-246
12. Mansfield PF, Hohn DC, Fornage BD et al (1994) Complications and failures of subclavian-vein catheterization. N Engl J Med 331:1735-1738
13. Spies JB, Berlin L (1997) Complications of central venous catheter placement. AJR 169:339-341
14. Chewning R, Wyse G, Murphy K (2008) Neurointervention for the peripheral radiologist: tips and tricks. Semin Intervent Radiol 25:42-47
15. Mavroforou A, Giannoukas A, Mavrophoros D et al (2002) Physicians' liability in interventional radiology and endovascular therapy. Eur J Radiol 46:240-243
16. Miller DL (2007) Safety in interventional radiology. J Vasc Interv Radiol 18:1-3
17. Hill GQ, Smouse HB (2006) Lessons learned on how to protect an interventional radiologist against malpractice claims. Semin Intervent Radiol 23:315-318
18. Joint Commission on Accreditation of Healthcare Organizations. Sentinel event policy and procedures. http://www. Joint commission.org/SentinelEvents/ Policy and Procedures/. Accessed October 12, 2006
19. Stecker MS (2007) Root cause analysis. J Vasc Interv Radiol 18:5-8

Errors in Radiology Reporting

20

Fabio Pinto, Stefania Romano, and Ciro Acampora

20.1 Introduction

What is an error in the medical field? An error is a mistake made in the process of care that results in (or has the potential to result in) harm to patients. Mistakes include the failure of a planned action to be completed as intended or the use of a wrong plan to achieve an aim. They can be the result of an action that is taken (error of commission) or of one that is not taken (error of omission) [1].

In the clinical routine, a malpractice claim arises when a patient believes that improper medical care has resulted in bodily harm. An error in the interpretation of a radiograph represents an example of a general type of malpractice claim in radiology. The main reason for studying medical errors is to try to prevent them. Reducing errors will improve patient care, may reduce costs, and will enhance the reputation of the hospital. In addition to economic and social effects, malpractice lawsuits often have direct effects on a physician's health. For the physician(s) involved in the claim, litigation for alleged malpractice is often associated with feelings of guilt and isolation. Medical professionals who have committed a severe error are likely to experience a reduction in the quality of life and an increase in the frequency of burnout. Perceived stress is associated with an increase in the number of errors committed in the subsequent period, thus creating a vicious cycle whereby errors lead to stress, which in turn leads to new errors. Accordingly, there is the need to analyze the extent and causes of the various types of errors, which would also help to identify the most effective measures in terms of clinical risk management. This chapter discusses the potential errors in radiologic reporting

F. Pinto (✉)
Department of Diagnostic Radiological Imaging, "A. Cardarelli" Hospital,
Naples, Italy

and provides a classification of the main potential errors in the diagnostic field.

20.2 Radiologic Reporting

Radiologic reporting is a fundamental part of a set of activities, steps, or tasks that integrate people and disparate systems to achieve a common goal. The radiological operative cycle consists of the following steps: (1) initial scheduled appointment; (2) reception of the patients on the day of the exam; (3) informed consent; (4) execution of the radiologic exam; (5) image analysis and report elaboration; (6) report communication/delivery of the report; (7) compilation of the exam file: medical images of a patient are permanent and can be archived, distributed, and displayed and are thus subject to repeated review and reconsideration.

Although in the last few years there have been dramatic innovations in medical imaging and information system technologies, the radiologic report has remained stagnant: nevertheless, it is still an important element with which radiologists are judged by their clinical colleagues [2]. Three or four decades ago, radiologic investigations focused on the pictorial representation of anatomic and, to a lesser extent, physiologic information. Within a few decades, PACS systems became available, changing not only radiological documentation but the structure of radiology practices as well. These revolutionary changes in telecommunications, like all innovations, also brought unintended consequences. Since radiologic images can be electronically transferred, there is less need for face-to-face consultation between the referring physician and the imaging physician [2, 3]. In a traditional film-based setting, the radiologist is often positioned close to where the images are collected and assembled, in the expectation of imminent interpretation. In this context, consultations are likely to occur every time the referring physician enters the reading area to see the patient's film. As the common meeting ground becomes supplanted by the wide dispersion of computer monitors, there is less incentive for the physician to visit the radiologist's domain, even if it is not far away. Moreover, in the majority of Western institutions, not only can the electronic images be quickly sent, but the radiologist's report can be made promptly available in typed, digitally signed form. Consequently, there is the risk that the radiologist will become an increasingly disembodied voice, providing expertise without personality and regarded more as a colorless technician than as a congenial professional colleague able to offer valuable advice through conversation. In this atmosphere, radiologists have begun to refine and redefine their service deliverables, with the radiology report as the most valuable element. Accordingly, in this era of cost containment in health care, the radiologic report must represent, for the radiologist, a sort of golden nugget to be preserved in a safe bank, in that it is one of the most important indicators documenting the pivotal role of this professional in the patient's care and management.

20.3 Classification of Errors in Radiology

Errors in radiology can be divided into four main groups [4]: (1) observer errors, (2) errors in interpretation, (3) failure to suggest the next appropriate diagnostic procedure, and (4) failure to communicate.

20.3.1 Observer Errors

Kundel et al. described three types of observer error, related to scanning, recognition, and decision-making [5]. Scanning errors are the result of the radiologist's failure to fixate on the area of the lesion. Recognition errors involve fixating on the area of the lesion, yet failing to detect the lesion. Decision-making errors are the most common, accounting for about 45% of all observer errors. They are due to incorrect interpretation of a malignant lesion as a normal structure. Moreover, failures of abnormality detection in film reading (i.e., perceptual errors) are subject to psychophysiological factors of human visual perception. Perceptual errors are mainly related to multiple psychophysiological factors, including level of observer alertness, observer fatigue, duration of the observation task, any distracting factors, and conspicuity of the abnormality [6]; an additional source of error results from the influence that a prior radiology report has over another radiologist. This type of perceptual error occurs because the radiologist reads the previous report before looking at the films. If the first radiologist missed something, the next radiologist will be likely to miss it as well.

20.3.2 Errors in Interpretation

There are many reasons why radiologists become involved in medico-legal problems following an error in identifying or interpreting abnormalities. Factors such as clinical history, the presence or absence of previous studies, index of suspicion, the presence of an abnormality, the reading room environment, and the level of vigilance of the interpreter are various sources of error. Eye position studies have determined that obvious abnormalities on a radiograph are detected first and decrease vigilance for unrelated and subtle findings [7].

20.3.3 Failure To Suggest the Next Appropriate Diagnostic Procedure

The American College of Radiology (ACR) "Practice Guideline for Communication of Diagnostic Imaging Findings"[8] states that "follow-up or additional diagnostic studies to clarify or confirm the impression should be suggested when appropriate." The words "when appropriate" are not defined, and thus the circumstances under which radiologists should suggest additional radiologic studies are left to the radiologist's own judgment [9].

20.3.4 Failure to Communicate

Not only is the radiologist asked to render an official interpretation, but he or she is also responsible for communicating these findings directly to the referring physician. Errors in communication are the fourth most frequent allegation against radiologists in medical malpractice claims [10]. Failure to communicate is one area in which the radiologist can take a direct role in reducing the risk of malpractice. When communication is not documented, the radiologist risks losing a lawsuit when there are adverse or unexpected clinical outcomes.

20.4 Malpractice Issues

Radiologists are most frequently sued in malpractice lawsuits involving breast and lung cancers, multiple trauma patients and obstetric ultrasound examinations [11].

Mammography has become the most prevalent procedure involved in malpractice lawsuits filed against radiologists [12]. Early detection of lung cancer at a surgically curable stage is difficult with conventional screening methods: missed lung cancer remains a serious medico-legal issue despite widespread awareness of the problem by radiologists. Patients with multiple injuries often require a series of radiographs to examine all injured sites. The frequency of missed lesions in such patients is high: based on trauma registries, error rates are about 2% [11]. Performing obstetric sonography carries significant medico-legal risk, because missing a detectable fetal abnormality due to negligence often results in the largest indemnification payments in medical malpractice. Whether radiologists perform the examination themselves or rely on a technologist to obtain the images, it is the radiologist who is responsible for the quality of the examination and, in case of diagnostic error, will not be able to claim malpractice immunity because he/she is not a "sonographic specialist."

As for the radiology report, we stress that it is still largely the basis upon which radiologists are judged by their clinical colleagues. Nevertheless, a number of errors still occur, including examination of the wrong patient, incorrect examination performed on a patient, and wrong side of the patient examined. A common cause of incidents related to the wrong patient examined is the misidentification of a patient with the same name as one who is intended to undergo a specific procedure, or a patient responding to the wrong name. In order to reduce these kinds of mistakes, their extent and causes must be analyzed as a first step in identifying the most effective measures in terms of clinical risk management.

A modern organization of the radiology department is advocated in order to minimize psychological and external factors (fatigue, frustration, boredom, unfavorable working environment, noise), all of which contribute to increasing errors in the radiologist's reports.

20.5 Communication

As stated by the ACR Council more than two decades ago, "communication is a critical component of the art and science of medicine and is especially important in diagnostic radiology" [13].

20.5.1 Communication between Radiologists and Patients

The radiologist plays a pivotal role in the care and management of injury and illness in adult and young patients [14]. Although the primary role of the radiologist is to assist in establishing a correct diagnosis, his or her responsibility goes well beyond simple detection and documentation. Communication is crucial in assuring the delivery of quality and safe health care. Lines of communication are most easily recognized between the radiologist and the patient's health-care providers, but they are also becoming increasingly important between the radiologist and the patient him/herself. Radiologists must be familiar with either local or national practice guidelines related to the care of the patient in the standard work-up as well in the emergency setting, with respect to both the construction of the radiology report and the appropriate communication of the results of various studies. Familiarity with these aspects of the radiologists' responsibilities maximizes the chance of successful outcomes and minimizes the frequency of malpractice claims.

20.5.2 Communication of Findings to Referring Physician

The standard of communication between the radiologist and the referring clinician has become an important issue, although the written radiologic report remains the most important means of communication between them [15]. Traditionally, radiologists maintained that their duty to communicate results did not extend beyond dictating and signing their reports. Nowadays, in the USA as well as in Europe, radiologists are asked to ensure that reports be communicated to the referring clinician, particularly when an urgent or unexpected diagnosis is made. A diagnosis provided by a written report does not conclude the responsibilities of the radiologist: direct communication, either face-to-face or by telephone, represents a necessary adjunct, particularly for emergent or for unusual and unexpected findings [13]. Every radiologist should be aware that, as stated by the ACR, "if there are urgent or significant unexpected findings, radiologists should communicate directly with the referring physician."

20.6 Conclusions

In the coming years, radiologists should focus on adopting a radiologic report with a more uniform style and structure. This would provide a more consistent service to all the different stakeholders, including the clinician (who acts on the report), the administrator (who is tasked with analyzing reports), the patient (who is the main party in the recorded data), and the payer (who determines the economic value of the report). Radiology-related litigation occurs most often because of objective or subjective patient injuries. Obviously, radiologists do not intend to injure patients. In the longer term, if diagnostic errors are to be reduced, the care system must allow patients to be seen by better trained doctors. Ideally, the legal system should guarantee the compensation of injured persons without creating an atmosphere of distrust between the patient and the radiologist. Radiologic malpractice, in the future, will probably be affected by several factors: new imaging techniques, innovations in the processing of radiologic images, new standards published by scientific societies, and clinical guidelines issued by medical professional organizations.

We need to develop a safety culture within the radiology departments where, every time we come across an error made by a colleague, we bring that error to his or her attention in a sensitive and constructive fashion. A radiology safety culture will only exist when the radiologist who made the error views such feedback positively, as a learning experience.

References

1. Pronovost PJ, Thompson DA, Holzmueller CG et al (2005) Defining and measuring patient safety. Crit Care Clin 21:1-19
2. Reiner BI (2009) The challenges, opportunities, and imperative of structured reporting in medical imaging. J Digit Imaging 22:562-568
3. Baker SR, Festa S (1999) The use of teleradiology in an emergency setting with speculation on the near future. Radiol Clin North Am 37:1035-1044
4. Pinto A, Brunese L (2010) Spectrum of diagnostic errors in radiology. World J Radiol 28:377-383
5. Kundel HL, Nodine CF, Carmody D (1978) Visual scanning, pattern recognition and decision-making in pulmonary nodule detection. Invest Radiol 13:175-181
6. Pitman AG (2006) Perceptual error and the culture of open disclosure in Australian radiology. Australian Radiol 50:206-211
7. Samuel S, Kundel HL, Nodine CF, Toto LC (1995) Mechanism of satisfaction of search: eye position recordings in the reading of chest radiographs. Radiology 194:895-902
8. American College of Radiology (2005) ACR practice guideline for communication of diagnostic imaging findings. Practice guideline & technical standards. In ACR (ed) American College of Radiology 2005. ACR, Reston, VA, pp 5-9
9. Berlin L (2005) Errors of omission. AJR Am J Roentgenol 185:1416-1421

10. Harrigal CL, Erly WK (2007) On-call radiology: community standards and current trends. Semin Ultrasound CT MR 28:85-93
11. Enderson BL, Reath DB, Meadors J et al (1990) The tertiary trauma survey: a prospective study of missed injury. J Trauma 30:666-669
12. Berlin L (2001) Dot size, lead time, fallibility, and impact on survival: continuing controversies in mammography. AJR Am J Roentgenol 176:1123-1130
13. Kline TJ, Kline TS (1992) Radiologists, communication, and Resolution 5: a medicolegal issue. Radiology 184:131-134
14. Berlin L (2008) Standards for radiology interpretation and reporting in the emergency setting. Pediatr Radiol 38:639-644
15. ESR (2011) Good practice for radiological reporting. Guidelines from the European Society of Radiology (ESR). Insight Imaging 2:93-96

Errors in Radiology: A Biostatistical Framework

21

Francesco Sardanelli and Giovanni Di Leo

21.1 Introduction

An error in radiology is an event commonly thought of in association with a malpractice claim by a patient. However, this is only a relatively weak association. Not all errors can be judged as malpractice. The majority of errors do not determine harm to patients, while a minority of them may cause relevant harm, including fatal consequences. For example, for emergency computed tomography (CT), the discrepancy rate between the initial report and the secondary interpretation is 6–27% but a change in patient management occurs in only 1–5% of these cases; the corresponding values for review of cross-sectional imaging in oncology are 12–19% and 3–9%, respectively [1]. Errors are part of our human and professional life. We expect errors, even though we try to keep the error rate as low as possible. To deal with errors is a matter of numbers and statistics, beginning with the calculation of an error rate. Error analysis is of paramount relevance, both for the learning process and for strategies aimed at reducing the error rate [2]. This is the rationale for attempts to outline a biostatistical framework for errors in radiology.

People usually consider a missed abnormality, typically a cancer or a fracture, as the unique relevant error, i.e., the false-negative. Conversely, to report an abnormality not really present or assigning to a benign irrelevant finding a serious clinical meaning is commonly thought of as a minor error, i.e., the false-positive. The use of these two "bad" terms (false-negative and false-positive) and of their "good" counterparts (true-negative and true-positive) opens a window on the large world of the measures of diagnostic performance, when a standard of reference is available. This is the main mission of biostatistics

F. Sardanelli (✉)
Department of Medical and Surgical Sciences, University of Milan; Radiology Unit,
"San Donato" Hospital IRCCS,
San Donato Milanese (MI), Italy

in diagnostic radiology. In fact, a complete absence of both false-negatives and false-positives is not possible in the real world, if one applies a test on a sufficiently large series of patients representative of a disease spectrum. We would not trust in an article reporting the 100% accuracy of a diagnostic test. In practice, errors cannot be entirely eliminated from diagnosis. This is true not only for radiology and pathology [3] (the latter remaining a predominantly image-based diagnosis), but also for analytical laboratory testing [4].

Disagreement is another way to think about errors. One radiologist may disagree with another radiologist in reporting on a radiogram. On the other hand, one radiologist may disagree with her/himself in reporting on the same radiogram at two different times, or if the patient repeats the examination with the same technical parameters. This is the great challenge of intra- and inter-observer variability, that is well described by quoting the English poet Alexander Pope who in 1732 said: *Who shall decide when doctors disagree?* [5a]. We will see below how other sources of variability influence reproducibility [6]. Notably, in statistics, *observational error* is not a mistake but a way to identify the *residual*, i.e., the difference between repeated observed values. Why is this kind of *error* not a mistake? The answer is that variability is an inherent part of the things being measured and of the measurement process.

Finally, we should consider *errors in radiological studies*, i.e., errors in radiological research. As part of medical science, diagnostic radiology should not be considered only in terms of its performance, but also as a step in the pathway to clinical treatment and outcome, even though levels of efficacy higher than those of technical or diagnostic performance are uncommon in radiological research [7]. However, also these studies may have relevant limitations in terms of scientific quality. They can show a not negligible rate of methodological flaws–even those studies published in high-ranking journals–which heavily limit their generalizability. These flaws have to be carefully considered by our community, especially by its academic component.

This chapter outlines the general principles related to the measure of diagnostic performance and reproducibility, and summarizes the most important errors in radiological research.

21.2 Measuring the Inaccuracy of Diagnostic Tests

The definition and classification of errors in diagnostic radiology are extensively discussed in other chapters of this book. Briefly, the failure of a radiologist to report on an abnormality can be explained by different reasons, mainly poor technique, perceptual errors (such as scanning, detection, and satisfaction of search), and interpretation errors (under-reading) [1, 8], resulting in false-negative cases. As mentioned above, the radiologist may also report on a non-existing abnormality (or a benign finding without clinical significance) as a positive finding calling for further assessment, and resulting in false-positive cases.

The radiologist's diagnostic performance can be regarded as divided in the following two aspects:

1. The *intrinsic quality*, i.e., the radiologist's skill and the quality of the entire diagnostic process (including technological level of equipment/software and global team's performance), as rated by sensitivity and specificity (and reproducibility as well);
2. The *clinical value*, i.e., the reliability of the radiological reports from the viewpoint of the patient and the referring physician, as rated by positive and negative predictive values (PPV and NPV, respectively).

Of course these two aspects are strictly related to each other. To quantify the diagnostic performance we need to define a radiologist's outcome against a reference standard. That may be done using the definitions showed in Table 21.1. The figures of true-positive (TP), false positive (FP), true-negative (TN), and false-negative (FN) can be used to calculate the measures of diagnostic performance listed in Table 21.2.

A complete description of these measures is beyond the aim of this chapter. Here we wish to underline that, if sensitivity and specificity are considered by radiologists to be measures of their performance, the counterparts may be described in terms of the *complement to 100% of sensitivity and specificity*, i.e., the *FN rate* and the *FP rate*. For example, if one radiologist has 90% sensitivity and 75% specificity, then the error rate is 10% and 25%, respectively.

This is true from the radiologist's viewpoint. Vice versa, the error rate perceived by patients and referring physicians is the complement to 100% of the predictive values or accuracy, i.e.:

- Inaccuracy of the positive results (IPR) = (1 – PPV), the probability for a positive result to be wrong;
- Inaccuracy of the negative results (INR) = (1 – NPV), the probability for a negative result to be wrong;
- Global inaccuracy (GI), or accuracy error = (1 – accuracy), the probability for a result to be wrong.

These three measures could be added to the Table 21.2. Importantly, sensitivity and specificity concern affected or unaffected subjects, separately, and

Table 21.1 Two-by-two contingency table for the comparison between the results of a diagnostic test and those of a reference standard in a series of subjects

		Reference standard Affected	 Unaffected	 Total
Diagnostic test	Positive	True positives (TP)	False positives (FP)	All positives (TP + FP)
	Negative	False negatives (FN)	True negatives (TN)	All negatives (FN + TN)
	Total	All affected (TP + FN)	All unaffected (FP +TN)	Grand total (TP +FN + FP + TN)

Table 21.2 Measures of diagnostic performance

Measure	Definition	Formula	Interval	Dependence on disease prevalence
1. Sensitivity or true positive rate	Ability to identify the presence of disease	TP/(TP+FN)	0.0–1.0 (0–100%)	No
2. Specificity or true negative rate	Ability to identify the absence of disease	VN/(VN+FP)	0.0–1.0 (0–100%)	No
3. Positive predictive value (PPV)	Reliability of the positive result	TP/(TP+FP)	0.0–1.0 (0–100%)	Yes
4. Negative predictive value (NPV)	Reliability of the negative result	TN/(TN+FN)	0.0–1.0 (0–100%)	Yes
5. False negative rate	Proportion between FN and all affected	FN/(FN+TP) = (1 – Sensitivity)	0.0–1.0 (0–100%)	No
6. False positive rate	Proportion between FP and all unaffected	FP/(FP+TN) = (1 – Specificity)	0.0–1.0 (0–100%)	No
7. Global accuracy	Probability of a true result (at a given cutoff)	(TP+TN)/(TP+TN+FP+FN)	0.0–1.0 (0–100%)	Yes
8. Positive likelihood ratio (LR+)	Increase in disease probability when the result is positive	Sensitivity/(1 – Specificity)	1.0–∞	No
9. Negative likelihood ratio (LR-)	Decrease in disease probability when the result is negative	(1 – Sensitivity)/Specificity	0.0–1.0	No
10. Diagnostic odds ratio	Discriminating power	(TP TN)/(FP FN) = LR+/LR-	0.0–∞	No
11. Area under the curve (AUC) at receiver operating characteristic (ROC) analysis[a]	Probability of a true result (considering different cutoffs)	Sum of areas of trapezoids in the ROC space	0.0–1.0	No
12. Youden's index (*J* statistics)	Maximal potential effectiveness (at the optimal cutoff)	1 – (FN rate + FP rate)	-1.0–1.0	No

[a]ROC analysis can be performed only for diagnostic tests based on continuous or, at least, ordinal variables. AUC is an integral of an unknown function, approximated by a sum of trapezoids.

the same holds for the FN and FP rates. Consequently, the proportion of affected vs. unaffected subjects, or between affected subjects and the total number of subjects (i.e., the disease prevalence) does not influence the measure. This is not the case for predictive values and accuracy nor for the three error measures mentioned above. They concern a mixture of affected and unaffected subjects (predictive values and inaccuracies of positive and negative results) or the total sample (global accuracy and inaccuracy). Therefore, these measures are influenced by *disease prevalence.* For mathematical reasons, this influence is relatively small for both global accuracy (which ranges between the sensitivity and specificity) and global inaccuracy (which ranges between the FN and FP rates), but dramatically large for predictive values and for inaccuracies of positive or negative results. Figure 21.1 shows inaccuracies as a function of the disease prevalence.

Thus, we must understand that given our *intrinsic quality* (sensitivity and specificity), the *perceived quality* of our work (predictive values and global accuracy) depends on the disease prevalence. The same holds for the *lack of quality* (*errors*, i.e., *inaccuracies*). We can do our best to reduce errors but disease prevalence influences our error rates.

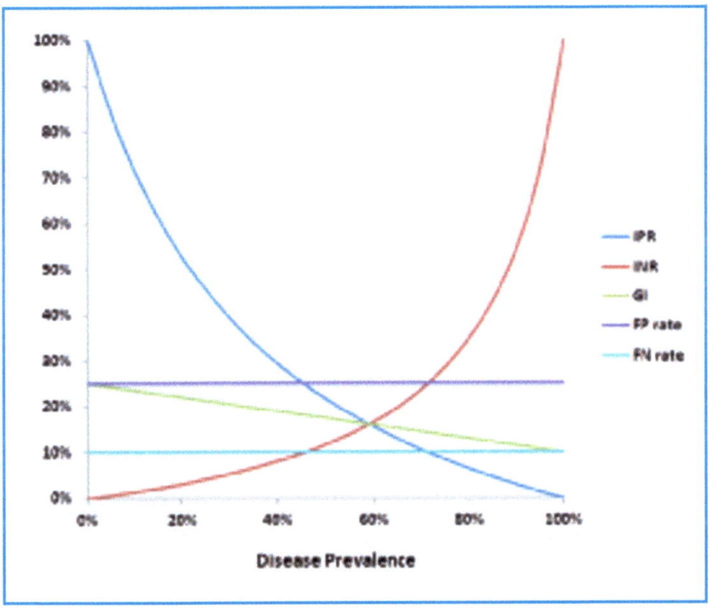

Fig. 21.1 Distribution of the inaccuracy of positive result (IPR), inaccuracy of negative result (INR), and global inaccuracy (GI) as a function of disease prevalence (sensitivity and specificity being constant at 90% and 75%, respectively). Note that IPR and INR range from 0% to 100% according to two different curves while GI decreases linearly from 25% (the FP rate) to 10% (the FN rate). At a disease prevalence of about 60% the three inaccuracies tend to be equal (about 16%). The error rates perceived by patients and referring physicians–IPR, INR, and GI–are the complements to 100% of predictive values and global accuracy (see text)

To further clarify, consider the breast imaging examples shown in Table 21.3. First, in screening mammography in women at average risk of breast cancer (biannual invitation of asymptomatic women from 49 to 69 years of age), we hypothesize a biannual cancer incidence of 0.6%. With a 75% sensitivity (reasonable for screening mammography), if 5% of the screened women are recalled for further imaging, the global inaccuracy is 4.7%. But it is unequally distributed: 91.0% for the positive results; 0.2% for the negative results. Second, in MRI screening of high-risk women (BRCA1/2 mutation carriers), based on an annual cancer incidence of 3.0% (tenfold that of the previous example) and 90% sensitivity: if 10% of the screened women are recalled for further imaging, the global inaccuracy is 6.6%, distributed as 70.0% for the positive results and 0.3% for the negative results. Third, in diagnostic mammography in women with a palpable lump, based on a 20% cancer incidence: if further imaging is requested for 33.3% of them, global inaccuracy goes up to 22.0%, distributed as 34.5% for the positive results and 4.8% for the negative results. To note, here the request of further imaging after a negative diagnostic mammography (commonly an ultrasound examination) is considered as

Table 21.3 Diagnostic performance and error rates for screening mammography in average-risk women, screening MRI in high-risk women, and diagnostic mammography in women with a palpable lump

	Screening mammography in average risk	Screening breast MRI in high risk	Diagnostic mammography for palpable lump
Population and results			
Disease prevalence	0.6%	3.0%	20.0%
True positives	45	270	3,800
True negatives	9,485	9,070	4,000
False positives	455	630	2,000
False negatives	15	30	200
Total	10,000	10,000	10,000
Diagnostic performance			
Sensitivity	75.0%	90.0%	95.0%
Specificity	95.4%	93.5%	66.7%
Positive predictive value	9.0%	30.0%	65.5%
Negative predictive value	99.8%	99.7%	95.2%
Global accuracy	95.3%	93.4%	78.0%
Error rates			
False negative rate	25.0%	10.0%	5.0%
False positive rate	4.6%	6.5%	33.3%
Inaccuracy of positive result	91.0%	70.0%	34.5%
Inaccuracy of negative result	0.2%	0.3%	4.8%
Global inaccuracy	4.7%	6.6%	22.0%

a "recall," i.e. as a positive mammogram, in order to make the comparison with the two screening scenarios possible. Anyway, the highest inaccuracy for the positive results is observed when the disease prevalence is the lowest (screening mammography), and the highest inaccuracy for the negative results when the disease prevalence is the highest (diagnostic mammography).

The take home message here is that *patient selection is crucial for the accuracy (and inaccuracy) of radiology*. To know the disease prevalence in the population we are studying is extremely important.

In clinical radiology, knowledge of the clinical history and the precise clinical question (or the site of a clinical abnormality) can change the pre-test probability and lead the radiologist not only to avoid scanning and detection errors but also to change her/his judgment on detected abnormalities, avoiding interpretation errors. If the radiologist knows that the clinical suspicion is high, she/he instinctively changes (i.e., reduces) the cutoff along the ROC curve, accepting a reduction in specificity in exchange for a higher sensitivity. In fact, a higher disease prevalence implies higher PPVs and lower NPVs; in other words, a higher probability of inaccuracy of the negative results and a lower probability of inaccuracy of the positive results. All of this can be explained in terms of Bayesian theory, likelihood ratios, and by using graphs of conditional probabilities [5b].

Finally, we should distinguish among per-lesion, per-segment, per-organ, and per-patient analysis of diagnostic performance. In this regard, when a diagnostic procedure is initially introduced in clinical research, per-lesion analysis is useful. When we test the value of this procedure for clinical practice, per-patient analysis should be used. The definitions in Table 21.1 are applicable for all these analyses.

21.3 Reproducibility

Differently from accuracy, reproducibility does not concern with the true value but with the capability of a diagnostic test to replicate the same value if the measurement is repeated by the same reader or by a different one.

Reproducibility in radiology should be differently evaluated depending on the type of the variable under consideration. On one side, we have categorical variables: nominal, such as the dichotomic result of a diagnostic test (positive/negative), or ordinal (e.g., the 1-to-5 Breast Reporting and Data System (BI-RADS) scale) [9]. These kind of variables are qualitative even when standardized descriptors are used, as is the case with the BI-RADS. On the other side, we have interval and continuous variables, such as the CT density (in Hounsfield units), the longest diameter of a tumor, or the ejection fraction of a cardiac ventricle. From the reader's point of view, the numerical values of continuous variables are obtained by mean of "instruments," i.e., technical systems sensitive to the quantity to be measured (many of them are now available as software algorithms implemented on computers). However, even if the use of a technical instrument may let us believe that the measurement is an objective process, this process does not proceed by itself; rather it needs the observer's intervention. This intervention may apply at any level and surely impacts on the observed value. For example, the measurement of a vessel diameter based on an US, CT, or MR image requires that the observer place a ruler between two distant points on the image of the vessel wall. The repetition of this action rarely provides the same value as the one previously obtained. Furthermore, an independent observer may perform this measurement by placing the ruler at another level of the vessel, on another slice, or including/excluding wall thickness. Therefore, as for categorical variables, the measurement of continuous variables is characterized by intra- and interobserver variability [6].

Reproducibility and variability are two complementary concepts: the larger the variability, the lower the reproducibility, and vice versa. Moreover, intra- and interobserver variability are only two of the several sources of the total variability for a measurement made on medical images. In the case of a patient who repeats an imaging examination after chemotherapy for a tumor, at two different imaging centers, the total variability associated with the measurement of the tumor in terms of longest diameter or volume will consist of a weighted sum of the following:

a. The intraobserver variability of the radiologist who performed the measurement before treatment;
b. The intraobserver variability of the radiologist who performed the measurement after treatment;
c. The interobserver variability between those two radiologists;
d. The interstudy variability, due to the repetition of the examination;
e. The inter-instrumentation variability, due to the use of two different machines;
f. The biological variability, due to changes in the patient's status during the time elapsed between the two examinations, the effect of treatment being a part—and a potentially extremely relevant part—of this variability.

Why do we need to know the variability of measurements of categorical and continuous variables? The answer is: we need to know the reliability around a measured value before making decisions based on those measurements. If we observe a difference between the tumor diameter or volume measured before and after a treatment, can we establish that the patient's status has really changed? Or is that difference within the expected variability? Of course, the only way to answer that question is to know the variability, which in turn allows us to define *the least significant change* (i.e., the minimal difference we can consider as a real change).

In theory, a way to estimate the measurement variability is to repeat a measurement many times, calculating the mean value and the 95% confidence interval. However, this approach has three important limitations. First, it no longer holds if the measurements are made by different observers, adding interobserver variability. Second, in clinical practice there is little or no time available for repeating the same measurement. Third, it allows for estimating the variability associated with a particular value (or patient); but that variability cannot be applied to all possible values (or patient). Therefore, it is more practical to conduct a preliminary analysis of intra- and interobserver variability.

Statistics for estimating intra- and interobserver variability depend on the type of the measured variable: Cohen k is used for categorical variables [10] and Bland-Altman analysis for continuous variables [11]. Details on these methods can be found in the literature [5c, 10, 11]. The main difference between them can be summarized as follows:

- Cohen k provides a coefficient of agreement that lies within the range [-1, 1], where $k = 1$ indicates total agreement, $k = 0$ no agreement, and $k = -1$ total disagreement;
- Bland-Altman analysis results in values expressed with the same measurement units as the measured variable: *bias* or systematic mean error, and *coefficient of repeatability*, which is a method to calculate the least significant change.

Intra- and interobserver variability may be estimated in parallel. In clinical settings, a suitable protocol include two readers (R1, R2) with similar, possibly average-to-high, experience in the measurement under evaluation. R1 measures the variable of interest twice while only one measurement is made by R2 (or vice versa). The intraobserver variability is estimated using the couples of values obtained by R1, while the interobserver variability is estimated using the first value obtained by R1 and the only value obtained by R2. Notably, if R1 and R2 have different levels of experience, interobserver reproducibility is underestimated, i.e. variability becomes larger. Moreover, reproducibility is commonly higher when evaluated in healthy volunteers and lower when evaluated in real patients, as typically happens in cardiac imaging [11].

Especially when dealing with continuous variables, we need to know the reproducibility in order to allow informed clinical decision-making. Radiology is becoming increasingly quantitative, demanding high levels of reproducibility. The numbers and percentages from tumor diameters determined on the images already serve as surrogate end-points for randomized controlled trials (RCTs) in oncology [12]. Left ventricular ejection fraction on cardiac MR imaging is decisive in the indication for surgical ventricular restoration, as shown in clinical trials [13]. In day-to-day clinical practice, the results of bone mineral densitometry obtained with dual energy X-ray absorption guide decision-making for the therapy of osteoporosis [14]. These are not special cases, but are paradigms for the future. To be informed as to our *measure error*, and not our mistakes, is crucial for quantitative radiology.

21.4 Errors in Radiological Research

Errors can burden not only clinical radiology but also radiological research. As evidence-based radiology (EBR) is increasingly advocated for better use of imaging in clinical practice, we should keep in mind that the evidence corre-

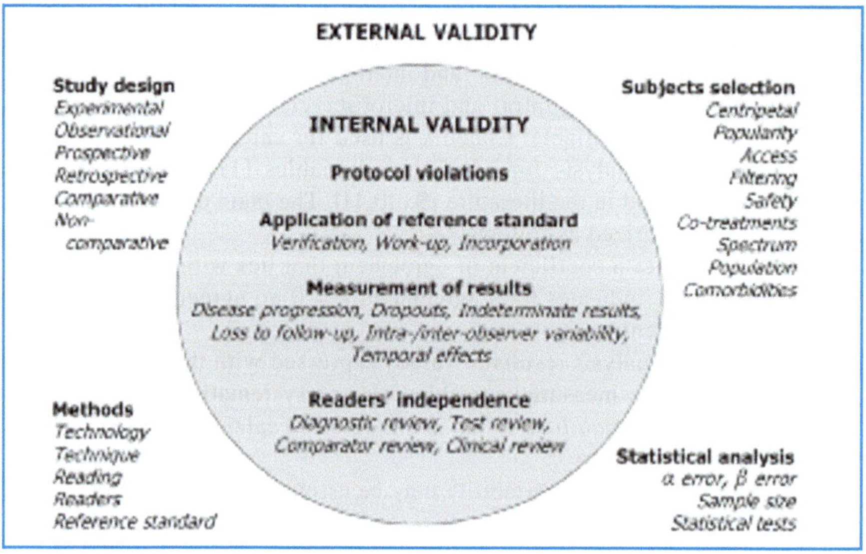

Fig. 21.2 Sources of bias in the studies on diagnostic performance. To apply the results of a study to clinical practice, it must have internal validity, i.e., absence of substantial errors in the methods used in the study, and external validity, i.e., generalizability to other settings (From [5d])

sponds primarily to the quality of the original studies, but also to the quality of secondary studies on radiology, such as meta-analyses, evidence-based guidelines, cost-effectiveness analysis, etc. [15]. Regardless, the quality of the original studies is the key point.

Often, errors encountered in clinical (and preclinical) research are *biases*, namely, systematic distortions. A list of the most important sources of bias for radiological studies on diagnostic performance is represented in Fig. 21.2. Here we wish to distinguish between biases influencing the *external validity* of a study, that is the applicability of its results to clinical practice, and biases influencing the *internal validity* of a study, that is its inherent coherence. The former are mainly due to the *selection of subjects and choice of techniques, leading to lack of generalizability.* The latter are due to errors in the methods used in the study. Both external and internal validity are related concepts: *the internal validity is a necessary but not sufficient condition in order that a study has external validity* [5d].

However, while a lack of generalizability has a negative effect on the external validity, the study can still retain its internal validity. Conversely, errors in performing the study have a negative effect primarily on internal validity and secondarily on external validity. The lack of internal validity makes the results themselves not reliable. In that case, the question about the external validity (i.e., the application of the results to clinical practice) makes no sense. As a consequence, only the results of a study not flawed by errors in planning and performance can be applied to clinical practice [16].

Multiple errors can occur in planning and/or performing a study. Consider the reference standard: one error is the planned use of an inadequate reference standard (imperfect reference standard bias); a different error is performing the study with the incorrect use of the planned reference standard. In other words, we can incorrectly perform the study by choosing incorrect rules or by applying correct rules incorrectly (while also adding errors in the application of already incorrect rules). There is probably only one right way to conduct a study correctly, but there are infinite ways to introduce errors that make a study useless. A bias in performing a study can be due to:

1. Defects in protocol application
2. Unforeseen events or events due to insufficient protocol specification
3. Protocol methods implying errors in performing the study

Errors related to items 2 and 3, may be due, in turn, to errors in planning. In fact, if we have many protocol violations, the study protocol was probably theoretically correct but only partially applicable. In other words, biases in performing a study frequently have their ultimate origin in planning errors, i.e., in the protocol. Details on each of the source of bias can be found elsewhere [5d,16,17].

What is the rate of methodological errors in radiological studies? In 1995, Reid et al. [18] analyzed 112 articles regarding diagnostic tests published from 1978 to1993 in four important medical journals. Authors found that over 80% of the studies had relevant biases resulting in flawed estimates of diagnostic performance. For example, only 27% of the studies reported the disease spectrum of the patients; only 46% of the studies had no work-up bias; only 38% had no review bias; only 11% reported the confidence intervals associated with the point estimates; only 22% reported the frequency of indeterminate results and how they were managed; only 23% of the studies reported data on reproducibility.

In 2003, detailed rules guiding the preparation of a good-quality original article on diagnostic performance were defined by Bossuyt et al. [19]. The extremely useful checklist of 25 recommendations should be acquired by all authors. The paper is entitled: *Towards complete and accurate reporting of studies of diagnostic accuracy: the STARD initiative*. STARD is an acronym for Standards for Reporting of Diagnostic Accuracy. In 2005, Smidt et al. [20] used the 25-item STARD checklist to evaluate 124 articles on diagnostic performance published in 12 journals with an impact factor of 4 or higher: only 41% of articles reported on more than 50% of the STARD items, no articles more than 80%. A flow chart of the study was presented in only two articles. The mean number of reported STARD items was 11.9. The authors concluded that "Quality of reporting in diagnostic accuracy articles published in 2000 is less than optimal, even in journals with high impact factor." While adoption of the STARD requisites will improve the quality of radiological studies, the process remains very slow [21].

Articles reporting on the results of systematic reviews or meta-analyses on diagnostic radiology should evaluate the study validity for specific issues, as pointed out by Dodd et al. [22]: detailed imaging methods; level of excellence of both imaging and the reference standard; adequacy of technology generation; level of ionizing radiation; viewing conditions; etc. Shared rules were published in 2003 [23], validated in 2006 [24], and recently modified in 2011 [25].

21.5 Conclusions

To learn from errors is a key process in human life. However, errors in medicine, and especially in radiology, are not only those that one is able to avoid after having acknowledged them the first time they occur. Rather, diagnostic reasoning is intrinsically probabilistic, not deterministic. Evidence-based medicine developed from practical medicine, from clinical epidemiology, not from galenic, causative, theoretical medicine [15]. Thus, at least some of our errors are due to unavoidable sources of variability not only in the reading process but also in image production and, especially, in the biology we try to reproduce through images.

A certain degree of uncertainty is inherent to the practice of medicine, and by extension, to the practice of radiology. In the diagnostic pathway we should try to reduce this uncertainty, but the context remains that of probability, not absolute causality. The word *probability* is not an ancient one. The concept was introduced not before the 16th century, when Girolamo Cardano began to analyze games of chance, but only in the subsequent century it was further developed, when Pierre de Fermat and Blaise Pascal exchanged their famous letters on problem of points [26]. These letters formed the basis of the theory of probability. Statistical methods for treating probability have been developed during the last two centuries and advanced techniques for dealing with multiple diagnostic tests, especially when they are performed on the same subjects, are still being developed and discussed.

As we have shown, methods for measuring the uncertainty of diagnosis (hence, the error rate associated with a report) are based on statistics. We can try to achieve greater and greater confidence with the clinical use of imaging modalities, but a *confidence interval*, even if narrow, will show that a probability is always associated with our efforts.

References

1. FitzGerald R (2005) Radiological error: analysis, standard setting, targeted instruction and teamworking. Eur Radiol 15:1760-1767
2. Pinto A, Acampora C, Pinto F et al (2011) Learning from diagnostic errors: a good way to improve education in radiology. Eur J Radiol 78:372-376
3. Nottingham J, Anderson M (1999) Errors in radiology and pathology. Lancet 354:1560
4. Plebani M (2010) The detection and prevention of errors in laboratory medicine. Ann Clin Biochem 47:101-110

5. Sardanelli F, Di Leo G (2009). Biostatistics for radiologists. Springer-Verlag, Milan, pp 125 (a), pp 32-40 (b), pp 125-140 (c), 165-179 (d)
6. Di Leo G (2011) Challenges in estimating reproducibility of imaging modalities. World J Methodol 1:12-14
7. Sardanelli F, Hunink MG, Gilbert FJ et al (2010) Evidence-based radiology: why and how? Eur Radiol 20:1-15
8. Pinto A, Brunese L (2010) Spectrum of diagnostic errors in radiology. World J Radiol 2:377-3839. In American College of Radiology (ACR) (2003). Breast Imaging Reporting and Data System (BI-RADS) Atlas. 4th ed. Reston, VA
9. Cohen J (1960) A coefficient of agreement for nominal scales. Educ Psychol Meas 20:37-46
10. Bland JM, Altman DG (1986) Statistical methods for assessing agreement between two methods of clinical measurement. Lancet 1:307-310
11. Sardanelli F, Quarenghi M, Di Leo G et al (2008) Segmentation of cardiac cine MR images of left and right ventricles: interactive semiautomated methods and manual contouring by two readers with different education and experience. J Magn Reson Imaging 27:785-792
12. Sardanelli F, Esseridou A, Del Sole A, Sconfienza LM (2012) Response to treatment: The role of imaging. In: Aglietta M, Regge D (eds) Imaging tumor response to treatment. Springer-Verlag, Milan
13. Jones RH, Velazquez EJ, Michler RE, et al; STICH Hypothesis 2 Investigators (2009) Coronary bypass surgery with or without surgical ventricular reconstruction. N Engl J Med 360:1705-1717
14. Hans DB, Shepherd JA, Schwartz EN et al (2008) Peripheral dual-energy X-ray absorptiometry in the management of osteoporosis: the 2007 ISCD Official Positions. J Clin Densitom 11:188-206
15. Sardanelli F (2012) Evidence-based radiology and its relation to quality. In: Abujudeh HH, Bruno MA (eds) Quality and safety in radiology. Oxford University Press, New York, Chapter 27
16. Kelly S, Berry E, Roderick P, et al (1997) The identification of bias in studies of the diagnostic performance of imaging modalities. Br J Radiol 70:1028-1035
17. Sica GT (2006) Bias in research studies. Radiology 238:780-789
18. Reid MC, Lachs MS, Feinstein AR (1995) Use of methodological standards in diagnostic test research. Getting better but still not good. JAMA 274:645-651
19. Bossuyt PM, Reitsma JB, Bruns DE et al (2003) Towards complete and accurate reporting of studies of diagnostic accuracy: The STARD initiative. Radiology 226:24-28
20. Smidt N, Rutjes AW, van der Windt DA et al (2005) Quality of reporting of diagnostic accuracy studies. Radiology 235:347-353
21. Wilczynski NL (2008) Quality of reporting of diagnostic accuracy studies: no change since STARD statement publication--before-and-after study. Radiology 248:817-823
22. Dodd JD, MacEneaney PM, Malone DE (2004) Evidence-based radiology: how to quickly assess the validity and strength of publications in the diagnostic radiology literature. Eur Radiol 14:915-922
23. Whiting P, Rutjes AW, Reitsma JB et al (2003) The development of QUADAS: a tool for the quality assessment of studies of diagnostic accuracy included in systematic reviews. BMC Med Res Methodol 3:25
24. Whiting PF, Weswood ME, Rutjes AW et al (2006) Evaluation of QUADAS, a tool for the quality assessment of diagnostic accuracy studies. BMC Med Res Methodol 6:9
25. Whiting PF, Rutjes AW, Westwood ME et al (2011) QUADAS-2: a revised tool for the quality assessment of diagnostic accuracy studies. Ann Intern Med 155:529-536
26. Devlin K (2008) The unfinished game: Pascal, Fermat, and the seventeenth-century letter that made the world modern. Basic Books, New York, NY

Child Abuse: Imaging and Legal Aspects

22

Claudio Defilippi and Roberta Cotti

22.1 Introduction

In 1860, Ambroise Tardieu described in small children a series of traumatic lesions with common characteristics indicating physical maltreatment: 55% of these cases involved children younger than 5 years, and 30% were under 1 year [1]. In 1946, Caffey reported the frequent association of central nervous system injuries with bony lesions. Since then, various terms have been used in reference to this constellation of symptoms, such as Ambroise-Tardieu syndrome, Caffey-Silverman syndrome, parent-infant trauma syndrome, battered child syndrome, and non-accidental-injury (NAI) [2, 3].

The radiologist may be the first to suspect the diagnosis of child abuse, based on radiological findings (although required for different clinical questions). Thus, radiologists should be on the lookout for unexplained injuries in children whose gravity is discrepant with respect to the clinical history reported and they should document with high-quality images all possible injuries in these cases. For this purpose, the radiologist needs to be familiar with (and, if not, should research) the typical radiological aspects of child abuse and of the diseases that may be confused with it.

In the first phase of the evaluation, this means checking for the presence of traumatic lesions, followed by developing and applying the most appropriate care, aimed at reducing the physical damage. There are also risk-benefits to consider with respect to radiation exposure versus the importance of documenting NAI. Even if the images are of potential legal value, the clinician must consider the child's radiation exposure that will result from the examination. Thus, it is up to the radiologist to recommend the most appropriate investigation, one that will achieve the best results with the lowest radiation dose.

R. Cotti (✉)
Radiology Unit, "Regina Margherita" Children's Hospital,
Turin, Italy

22.2 Radiology in Suspected Child Abuse

First-level imaging is represented by conventional radiography (CR), obtaining specific high-quality radiographs (Table 22.1) rather than large-format or wide projection radiographs ("babygrams"). While bone scintigraphy has a high sensitivity, especially in cases with poor clinical findings, the technique is burdened by a low specificity for metaphyseal lesions. The latter are highly specific for NAI.

Sonography is useful if an abdominal trauma is suspected in non-critical stable patients or, as additional imaging for soft tissues and joints. It also supplements the evaluation of metaphyseal fragments involving the cartilaginous component or, in the acute phase, of epiphyseal detachment (in the absence of signs of ossification of the epiphyseal growth nucleus), as these are not easily detectable with CR.

Multidetector computed tomography (MDCT) with contrast medium is required for suspected abdominal trauma in critical but stable patients.

Finally, CT and MRI are essential in patients with head and spinal cord trauma. As second-level imaging they could be used in particular cases of joint and bone injuries (e.g., facial bone fractures).

Table 22.1 Conventional radiology projections in NAI

Full skeletal survey: • L-L projection skull, cervical • A-P projection thoraco-abdominal • A-P projection pelvis + legs • A-P projection arms • L-L projection thoracic-lumbar-sacral spine

22.3 Typical Injuries in Child Abuse

Abdominal injuries in abused children are less common than musculoskeletal and craniocerebral injuries; however, they carry high mortality and morbidity rates [4]. Any abdominal injury pattern may be observed following physical abuse and none is specific for abuse. Nevertheless, a high index of suspicion should be maintained for every case of pancreatic, hollow viscus, and solid-organ injuries, especially when there has been a delay in seeking help or there is a history of trauma to the child or siblings, young age, undernourishment, ecchymosis, or a non-plausible explanation for the injuries based on the provided history and the psychomotor condition of the child.

Abdominal trauma due to abuse can go unrecognized for various reasons.

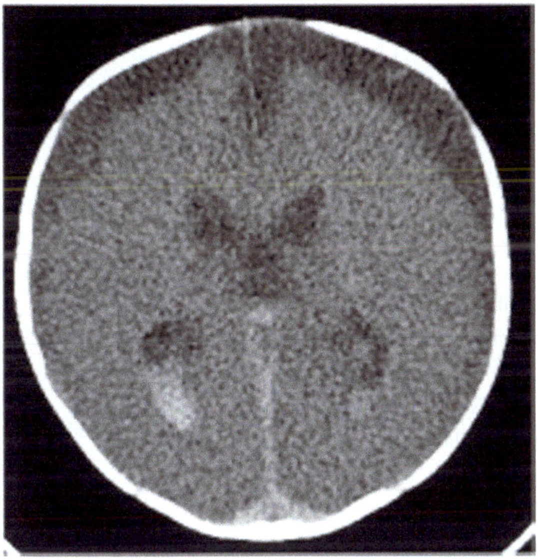

Fig. 22.1 Shaken baby: diffuse brain hypodensity, poor differentiation between white and gray matter, subdural fronto-temporal fluid collections, subdural and subarachnoid hemorrhages

External bruising may be absent in a quarter of cases, due to increased pliability of the abdominal wall, even following severe intra-abdominal injuries.

Abusive head trauma is a significant cause of severe brain injury in infants; shaking alone will cause the characteristic injuries. Violent shaking subjects the infant's head to acceleration-deceleration and rotational forces that create differential movement of the brain within the cranial compartment. This typically results in subdural, subarachnoid, and retinal hemorrhages, often associated with hypoxic-ischemic injury. CT of the brain is often the first examination for patients with acute head injury in order to demonstrate subdural hematoma (Fig. 22.1), which provides one of the diagnostic clues of child abuse.

However, in very young children there is also a state of benign enlargement of the subarachnoid space (BESS), which is not pathognomonic for child abuse. Moreover, BESS may be accompanied by spontaneous subdural hematomas.

22.3.1 Bone Fractures in Child Abuse

Skeletal lesions occur in only 50% of abuse cases, but when present often lead to a correct diagnosis. In our institution, we consider four levels of specificity for skeletal lesions (Table 22.2).

Usually, there is at least a diaphyseal fracture of the long bones of the limbs (humerus, femur). This lesion, even if not specific, can nonetheless show a

Table 22.2 Specificity degree of skeletal lesions in NAI

Grade 0/1	Non-specific; low specificity
Isolated diaphyseal fracture of long bones of the limbs (1)	
Fracture of the middle third of the clavicle: with (0) or without (1) callus	
Isolated rib fracture: with (0) or without (1) callus	
Linear skull fracture (0)	
Subperiosteal new bone formation (SNBF) (0)	
Grade 2	**Middle specificity**
Isolated diaphyseal not-recent fracture that has not received care	
Unilateral and bilateral synchronous multiple fractures	
Multiple synchronous rib fractures of the middle and anterior arches	
Vertebral body fracture in the newborn/infant	
Epiphyseal detachment in a not newborn child	
Tubular bone fractures of the hands and foot in a baby not yet walking	
Diaphyseal cortical hyperostosis signs	
Complex fracture of the skull	
Grade ¾	**High/Very high specificity**
Multiple non-synchronous fractures (4)	
Multiple rib fractures of the posterior arch (4)	
Any kind of metaphyseal fracture (4)	
Fractures of the distal third of the clavicle (3)	
Fractures of femoral neck and of the ileal-ischio-pubic branches (3])	
Fractures of the scapula, sternum, vertebral apophyses (3)	

peculiar repair process indicative of a lack of care, such as an irregular, coarse and exuberant callus.

Skull fractures are very frequent in NAI, but they have no characteristics that should raise suspicion of a non-accidental origin. Skull fractures in particular cannot be back-dated with certainty, since there is no callus formation.

Sometimes the anatomical sites of certain fractures may in themselves suggest NAI, for example, the shoulder girdle (Fig. 22.2a). Also, some sites are unlikely in children who do not walk yet (Fig. 22.2b), such as the fingers and toes, femoral neck, and ileal-ischio-pubic branches; the vertebral body is rarely affected in accidental trauma [5].

Some fractures are highly suspicious to be not-accidental, given their location and the radiographic characteristics of the anatomy, e.g., rib fractures [6] that are multiple, date back to different episodes, and marked by exuberant callus formation (Fig. 22.3). These injuries will cause stiffness of the chest, respiratory failure, infections, and can even lead to death. Fractures located on the midaxillary line cannot be distinguished from, for example, those

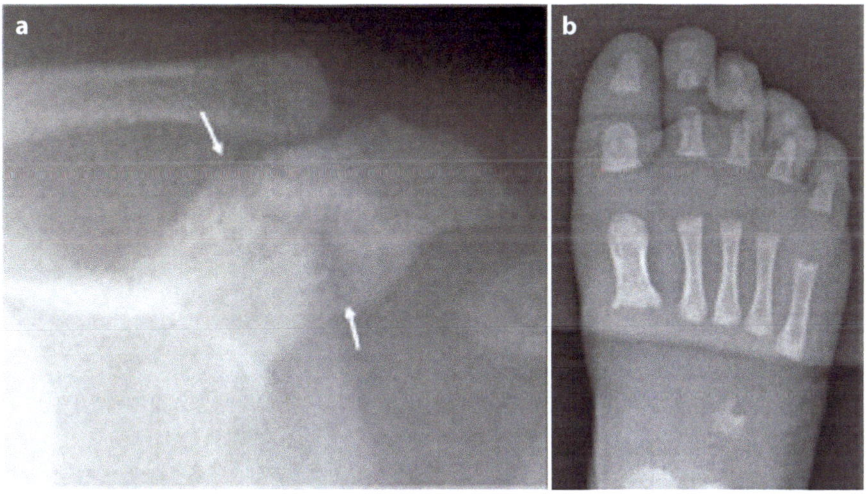

Fig. 22.2 **a** Fracture of the acromion (*arrows*). **b** Traumatic fragmentation of the proximal metaphysis of the first metatarsus

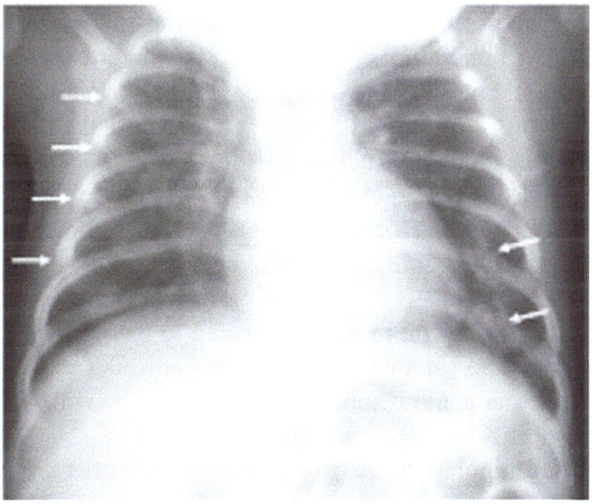

Fig. 22.3 NAI: rib fractures (*arrows*)

determined by resuscitation maneuvers (often cited to justify the radiographic findings), but other types can only be the result of a violent action, namely, rib fractures located on the posterior arch and fragmentations of the chondro-costal junction [7].

Metaphyseal lesions are specific [8], result in poor clinical and physical findings (they are never the cause of early hospitalization and can hardly be

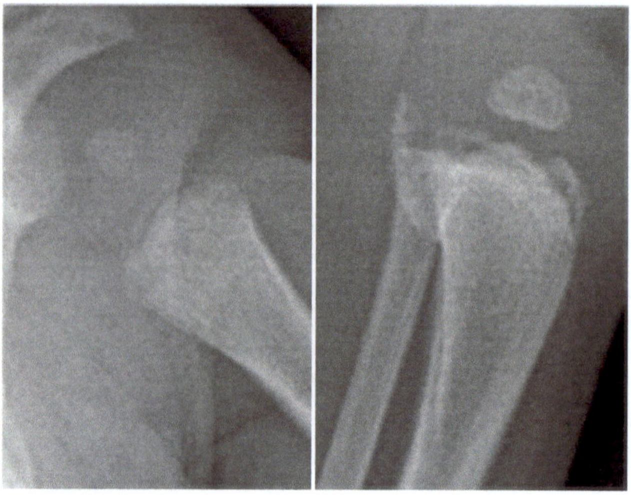

Fig. 22.4 Bucket-handle fractures

suspected by those who care for the child). Especially in young children (less than 3 years), metaphyseal fragmentations are very suspicious as they are frequently the result of a shaking and/or compression trauma. The injuries are related to the underlying anatomy: in a young child, the periosteum covers the metaphysis, is closely attached to the physis, and merges with the perichondrium. Thus, metaphyseal fragmentation produces two very characteristic findings: "corner lesions" and "bucket handle fractures" (Fig. 22.4). The most severe forms of fragmentations result in a metaphyseal cup-shaped deformation. The slow healing process (many weeks or months) leads to permanent changes in the limbs, such as curvatures and length differences.

Metaphyseal hemorrhage due to traumatic fragmentation invades the periosteum, which covers the metaphysis and is intimately connected to the perichondrium. The result is dissection and neo-osteogenesis. Repeated episodes extend the dissection and the periosteal osteogenic response to the diaphysis, with the subsequent appearance of outer cortical hyperostosis (Fig. 22.5a) [9].

The evolution of repeated and ignored subperiosteal bleeding causes large meta-diaphyseal sleeves [10]. However, these are also a late radiographic expression of epiphyseal detachment. Indeed, a Salter-Harris fracture type I can result from birth and lack of care, not only from NAI.

22.3.2 Bone Fracture Dating

The dating of bone lesions is the fundamental task of the radiologist, since based on radiological characteristics it is often possible to establish the approximate the age of the fracture. Multiple such injuries dating back to

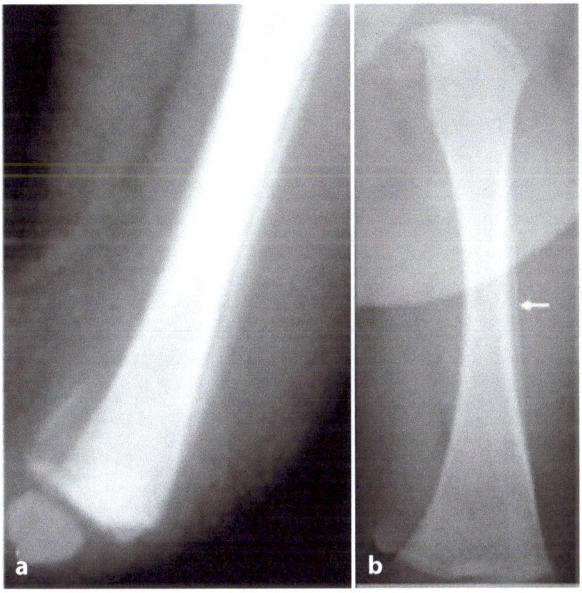

Fig. 22.5 a Meta-diaphyseal sleeves. **b** Physiological subperiosteal new bone formation

different episodes and accounted for by far-fetched excuses provide a high suspicion of physical abuse.

Metaphyseal fractures can be dated with some precision, which makes them even more important for the diagnosis of NAI.

22.4 Differential Diagnosis

Numerous clinical situations comprise the differential diagnosis, including almost all diseases that, in children between the ages of 1 month and 3 years, result in skeletal manifestations, such as shaft fractures, subperiosteal new bone formation (SNBF), metaphyseal abnormalities, and osteopenia [11] (Table 22.3).

22.4.1 Physiological SNBF

In the child, the periosteum has a very thick germinal layer; it is highly vascularized but quite lax. Thus, as a result of mechanical stress it slips onto the fibrous layer, bleeds, and reacts by producing cortical bone. This condition can be the result of a violent action, but also of inadequate care.

Diaphyseal periosteal bends (see Fig. 22.5b) are very common, especially in the femur, and are either an expression of normal bone physiology or secondary to para-physiological processes.

Table 22.3 Differential diagnoses of the bony lesions in NAI

	Rickets	Neonatal dismetabolic bone disease	Congenital syphilis	Leukemia	Prosta-glandin E1 treatment	Scurvy	Vitamin A toxicity	Vitamin E deficiency	Caffey's disease	Menke's syndrome	Osteogenesis imperfecta
Shaft fractures	+	+	-	-	-	-	-		-	-	+
Subperiosteal new bone formation	+	+	+	+	+	++	+	-	++	+	-
Metaphyseal abnormalities	+	+	++	+	-	+	-	-	-	+	-
Osteopenia	++	++	-	+	-	+/-	-	-	-	+/-	++
Intracranial hematomas	-	-	-	+	-	-	-	++	-	++	+/-
Comments	Tabes; serological evaluations metabolic panel	Prematurity; impaired metabolism of calcium/ phosphate	History, serology, pseudopa-ralysis, Wimber-ger's sign	Rare in the newborn; hematolo-gical data; bone marrow analysis; hemorrhagic manifesta-tions	-	Over 6 months of age	-	- -	Involve-ment of the scapula, clavicle, jaw as well as the long bones of the limbs	Males with copper serum deficiency, wormian bones, abnorma-lities of the hair, tortuous intracranial vessels	Bell aspect of the thorax, thin ribs, horizontal cotyloid roofs; blue sclerae

22.4.2 Birth Fracture

Proximal chondro-epiphyseal detachment of the humerus is one of the most frequent forms of birth fracture (pseudo-obstetric paralysis). Fractures of the clavicle and of the femoral and humeral shafts are also common childbirth-related injuries.

In the clavicle, a birth fracture is typically located in the middle third, while a non-accidental fracture is more frequent in the distal third (Figs. 22.6, 22.7).

Posterior arch fractures of the ribs are seen less frequently.

Importantly, birth fractures are synchronous, with early and exuberant callus formation (7–10 days).

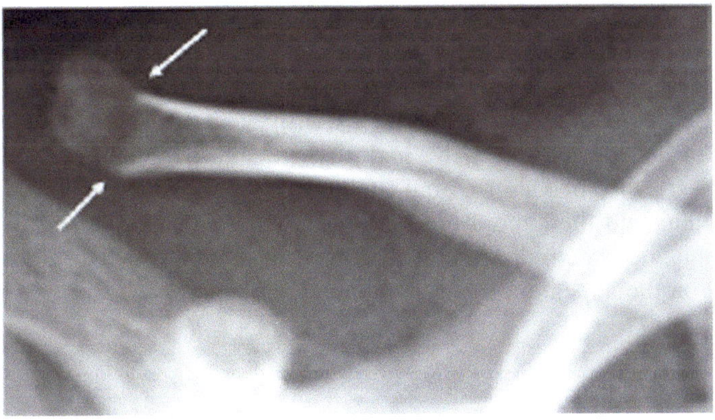

Fig. 22.6 NAI: distal third of the clavicle (*arrows*)

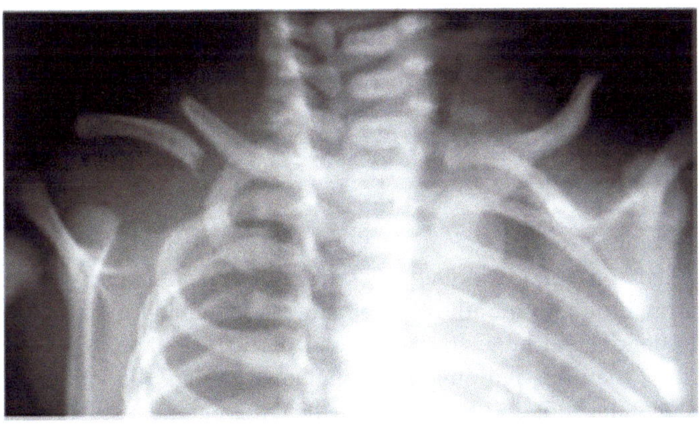

Fig. 22.7 NAI: recent fracture of the right clavicle and birth fracture of the left clavicle

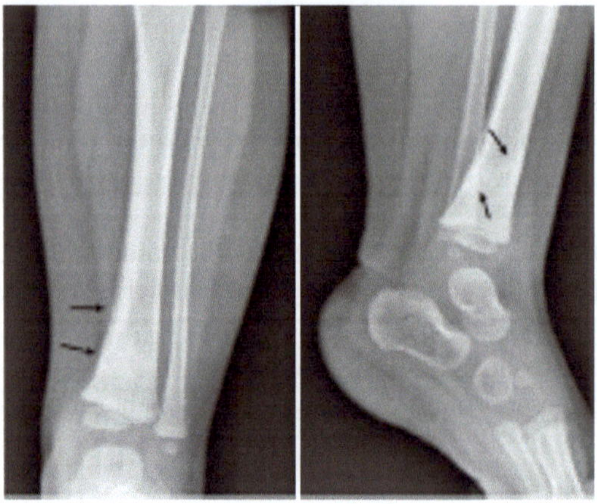

Fig. 22.8 Toddler's fracture of the tibia (*arrows*)

22.4.3 Toddler's Fracture

The child who is learning to walk often presents with typical traumatic bone lesions localized in the lower limbs. The majority are spiral fractures of the distal tibia, buckle fracture of the proximal tibia or first metatarsus, and fractures of the calcaneus and the cuboid bone. These fractures, accompanied by few clinical findings, become radiographically apparent only a few days after the trauma, based on the appearance of reparative phenomena (Fig. 22.8).

22.4.4 Osteogenesis Imperfecta

Defective osteogenesis is a connective-tissue disorder resulting from abnormal type I collagen synthesis. Its presentation is extremely varied. However, fractures (Fig. 22.9) are a feature of this disease, which, accordingly, must be considered in all cases of suspected NAI. The location, number, and date of the fractures, and the likelihood of the explanation should be determined [12].

22.4.5 Infantile Cortical Hyperostosis (Roske-De Toni-Caffey-Silverman Syndrome)

The triad of lesions comprises soft-tissue swelling, cortical bone lesions, and irritable behavior. The condition is already present in utero and an early diagnosis is possible around the 5th month of pregnancy, by antenatal ultrasonography. Layers of subperiosteal bone formation and cortical thickening of the long bones, especially the tibia and ulna, mandibulae, scapulae, ilia, and ribs, characterize the skeletal lesion. The condition heals spontaneously during infancy and does not require medical intervention (Fig. 22.10).

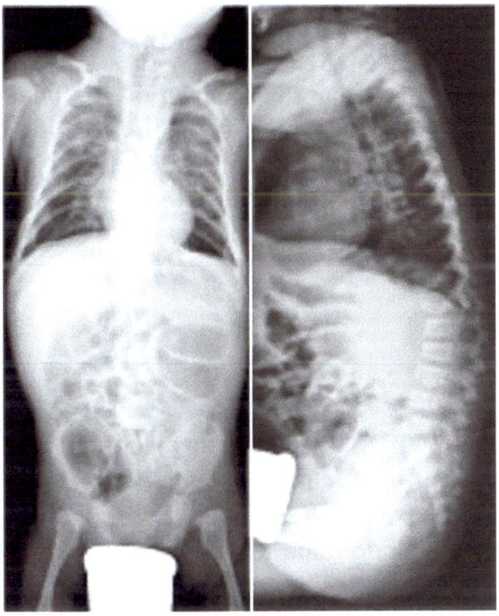

Fig. 22.9 Osteogenesis imperfecta: multiple, non-synchronous rib and vertebral fractures

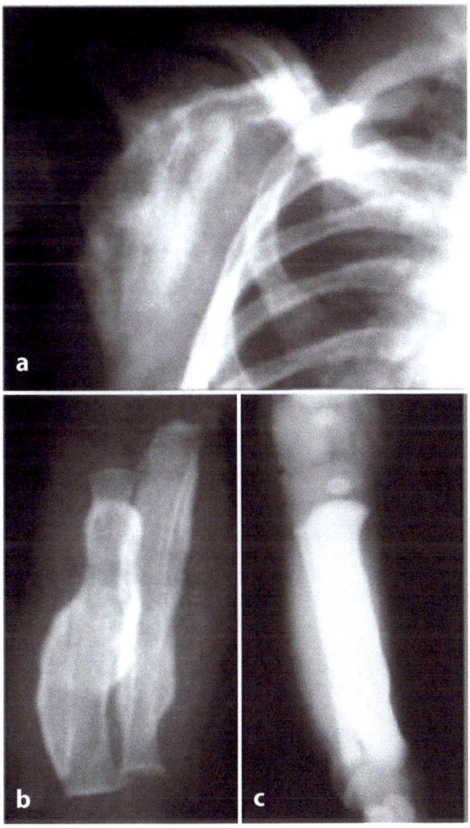

Fig. 22.10 Caffey's disease: cortical hyperostosis of the scapula, the clavicle (a) and the long bonesof the forearm (b) and leg (c)

22.4.6 Menkes' Syndrome

This is a progressive neurodegenerative disease due to a congenital, X-linked recessive defect in copper metabolism, essential to the formation of bone, nerve tissue, and other body structures. Neurological deficits, seizures, subdural hematomas, metaphyseal fragmentation, anterior rib defects, and fractures of the long bones are classical features of Menkes' disease, but these are also common findings in child abuse.

22.4.7 Neonatal Dismetabolic Bone Disease

Prematurity is the principal cause of the NDBD. Since nowadays more premature infants survive,an increased number of these cases are seen. Infants with NDBD have a diffuse decrease in bone density, metaphyseal alterations, and fractures of the long bones. The causes include bone disease of prematurity and copper deficiency (Fig. 22.11).

By contrast, the condition known as temporary brittle bone disease is not diagnosed based on clinical evidence, although the defense in child abuse cases frequently mentions this disease during trial proceedings [13].

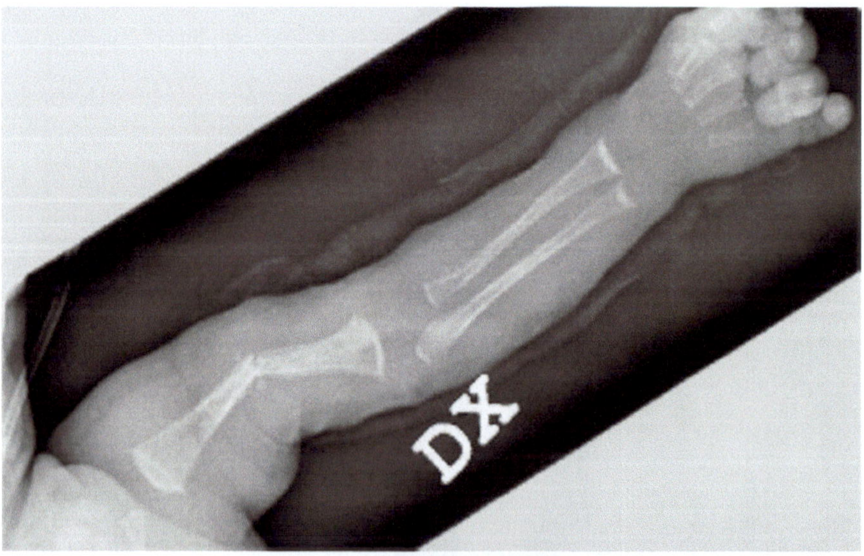

Fig. 22.11 Neonatal dismetabolic bone disease: humeral fracture

22.4.8 Rickets

The high rate of emigration throughout the developing world has been accompanied by the re-emergence of many diseases, including rickets. If the pregnant mother has a vitamin D deficiency, her child will have one as well, with its continuation in the neonate in the absence of a dietary supplement. In a retrospective evaluation of all suspected cases of NAI over a period of 20 years, Paterson et al. identified only four cases of rickets. This small number may have been due to the fact that rickets is too rarely considered among the differential diagnoses of NAI [14].

22.4.9 Congenital Syphilis

In these children, the bones most frequently affected are the tibia, femur, and ulna. The destructive lesions are painful and accompanied by the hypomobility of the affected limbs, a condition known as pseudoparalysis of Parrot. Another characteristic finding on the radiograph is symmetrical erosive changes at the proximal metaphyses of both tibias (Wimberger's sign) (Fig. 22.12).

22.4.10 Bone Dysostosis with Bone Fragility

Many rare forms of dysplasia are associated with bone fragility and/or metaphyseal lesions, but they are part of a spectrum of other diseases not only skeletal ones. Among these, are metaphyseal dysplasia of the Jansen type, osteopetrosis, mucolipidosis type II, and hypophosphatasia.

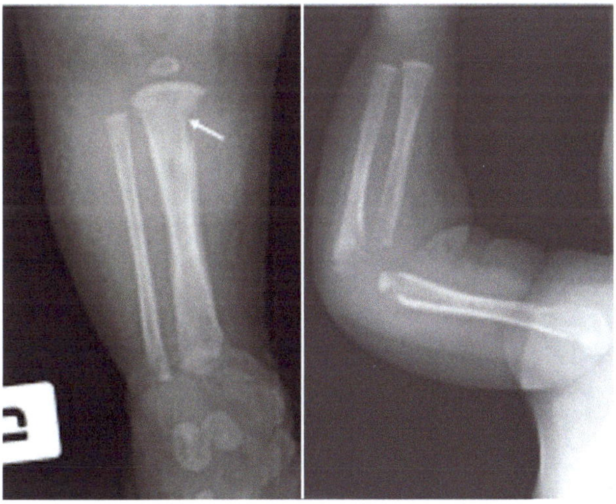

Fig. 22.12 Congenital syphilis: erosive changes at the elbow and shin; Wimberger's sign is present (*arrow*)

References

1. Tardieu A (1860) Etude médico-légale sur les sévices et mauvais traitements exercés sur des enfants. Annales d'hygiène publique et de médecine légale. Paris 13:361-398
2. Caffey J (1946) Multiple fractures in the long bones of infants suffering from chronic subdural hematoma. AJR 56:163-173
3. Kempe CH, Silverman FN, Steele BF et al (1962) The battered-child syndrome. J Am Med Assoc 181:17-24
4. Lane WG, Dubowitz H, Langenberg P (2009) Screening for occult abdominal trauma in children with suspected physical abuse. Pediatrics 124:1595-1602
5. Sonika A, Stein-Wexlera R, Rogersb KK et al (2010) Follow-up skeletal surveys for suspected non-accidental trauma: Can a more limited survey be performed without compromising diagnostic information? Child Abuse Negl 34:804-806
6. Anilkumar A, Fender L J, Broderick NJ et al (2006) The role of the follow-up chest radiograph in suspected non-accidental injury. Pediatr Radiol 36:216-218
7. Williams RL, Connolly PT (2004) In children undergoing chest radiography what is the specificity of rib fractures for the non-accidental injury? Arch Dis Child 89:490-492
8. American Academy of Pediatrics (2009) Diagnostic imaging of child abuse. Section on Radiology. Pediatrics 123:1430-1435
9. Ruess L, O'Connor SC, Quinn WJ et al (2003) An animal model for the classic metaphyseal lesion of child abuse. Pediatr Radiol 33:s112
10. Martino F, Defilippi C, Caudana R (2010) Imaging of pediatric bone and joint trauma. Chapt. 11, Springer Verlag Italia, pp 187-202
11. Carty H, Pierce A (2002) Non-accidental injury: a retrospective analysis of a large cohort. Eur Radiol 12:2919-2925
12. Paterson CR, Burns J, McAllion SJ (1993) Osteogenesis imperfecta: the distinction from child abuse and the recognition of a variant form. Amer J Med Genet 45:87-192
13. Mendelson KL (2005) Critical review of "temporary brittle bone disease." Pediatr Radiol 35:1036-1040
14. Paterson CR (2009) Vitamin D deficiency rickets and allegations of non-accidental injury. Acta Paediatrica 98:2008-2012

Retained Intra-abdominal Surgical Sponges: Critical Issues

23

Nicola Gagliardi, Nicoletta Pignatelli di Spinazzola, and Ciro Stavolo

23.1 Introduction

Intra-abdominal retained surgical foreign bodies are still a significant problem, with an incidence between 0.3 and 1.0 per 1000 abdominal operations [1]. In most cases they are surgical sponges, referred to as a gossypiboma. The term "gossypiboma" is derived from the Latin word *gossypium*, meaning cotton, and the Swahili word *boma*, meaning place of concealment [2]. More recently, with the increasing use of sponges made of synthetic material, as retained objects they are referred to as a textiloma or cottonoid [3].

Gossypibomas are not frequently reported because of legal and ethical concerns but their presence must be detected in order to avoid their attendant complications. They are most frequently observed in obese patients, during emergency operations, and following laparoscopic interventions [4]. In most countries, surgical sponges contain radio-opaque marking filaments, which facilitate their detection by standard abdominal radiography and on computed tomography (CT) images. Older sponges do not always include such markers such that they can be very difficult to identify on standard radiography and CT [5]. However, delays in the diagnosis of gossypibomas could increase morbidity and mortality.

23.2 Complications

Gossypiboma can present as a pseudotumoral, occlusive, or septic syndrome, although the exact clinical symptoms depend on the site and type of complica-

N. Gagliardi (✉)
Department of Diagnostic Radiological Imaging, "A. Cardarelli" Hospital, Naples, Italy

tion resulting from the presence of the sponges. The diagnosis may prove challenging because gossypiboma can mimic a benign or malignant soft-tissue tumor in the abdomen and pelvis [6]. Consequently, there are often erroneous biopsy attempts and unnecessary manipulations. Patients may present with nonspecific abdominal pain and intestinal obstruction, a palpable mass, nausea, vomiting, gastrointestinal hemorrhage, abdominal distension, and pain [4, 7].

Gossypibomas may become symptomatic at any time, from immediately postoperatively to several months after surgery. While the sponge remains in the body, it may be extruded externally through a fistulous track or internally into the rectum, vagina, bladder, or intestinal lumen [8, 9]. Indeed, in the early stage the surgical sponges can in some cases cause infection or abscess formation, and in others adhesions, encapsulation, and granuloma formation. Eventually, intestinal fistulas may develop, with the sponges completely migrating into the ileum, resulting in intestinal obstruction [10].

Because retained sponges often mimic tumors, both clinically and radiologically, and their manifestations and complications are so variable diagnosis is often delayed and patient morbidity is significant [11]. The presence of a gossypiboma usually necessitates reoperation, for the treatment of complications and retrieval of the sponge.

23.3 Radiological Findings

The diagnosis of gossypiboma is based on the many characteristic radiological findings specific for the various methods. Nevertheless, there is a high risk of error because these findings may be unusual and are often dissimilar. Accordingly, and given the legal implications of this diagnosis, it is essential that the radiologist is familiar with and is able to assess the main signs pointing to a gossypiboma.

23.3.1 Standard Radiography

This is the most commonly used method to detect retained surgical sponges. If there is a radio-opaque marker in the sponge, the diagnosis can be made easily, whereas if the sponge is radiolucent diagnosis is difficult (Fig. 23.1). In some cases, standard abdominal radiography will reveal an area of fine opacity suggesting a soft-tissue mass with small gas bubbles in and around the structure, but the relationship between the lesion and the abdominal structures cannot be determined [12]. In others, the typical appearance of a retained sponge with a whirl-like pattern of radio-opaque thread is seen on the radiograph. However, this finding is not always present [4, 5].

If the gossypiboma has resulted in fistula formation, the administration of oral contrast material may help in its identification and thus the correct diagnosis [13].

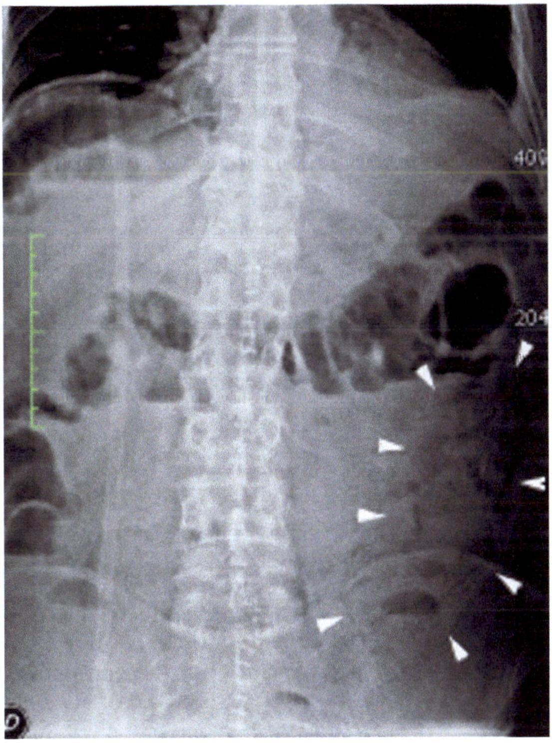

Fig. 23.1 Gossypiboma: radiolucent material (surgical drape) is seen on the left side (*arrowheads*)

In cases of a suspected abdominal retained sponge immediately after surgery, standard radiography can be performed in the operating theatre, with the patient still under anesthesia.

23.3.2 Ultrasound

An intra-abdominal retained sponge can often be detected sonographically. Its characteristic appearance is a hyper-reflective and well-delineated lesion with wavy internal echo, a hypoechoic ring, and a strong posterior shadow [4, 14].

At ultrasound, gossypibomas may present as a mass of cystic or solid type. The former consists of a cystic lesion with a winding echogenic bundle, and the latter as a complex structured mass with hyper- and hypoechoic areas (Fig. 23.2a, b) [15]. The pattern of acoustic shadowing changes with the direction of the ultrasound beam but is caused by the material itself, indicating calcified regions or a pocket of air. The sonographic detection of a mass with high echoes casting acoustic shadows should alert radiologists to the likelihood of a retained surgical sponge.

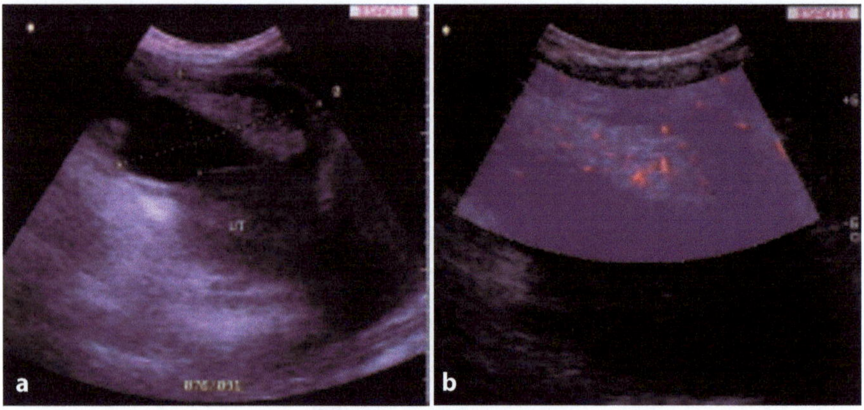

Fig. 23.2 a An abdominal mass of complex structure (gossypiboma) adherent to the anterior peritoneum. b Power Doppler scan shows the small signals from the vascular coating

23.3.3 Computed Tomography

Gossypibomas and their possible complications are best identified on CT. Most authors describe a well-circumscribed masses with a thick wall, with or without gas, showing calcification or wall enhancement after the administration of contrast medium [5, 16].

The internal structure may be whirl-like or spongiform due to the presence of gas trapped in the meshes of the sponge (Fig. 23.3). It may be of low density or complex, with both low density and wavy, striped, or spotted high-density areas [17]. The radio-opaque marker strip, if present, is seen as a thin metallic density in the mass (Fig. 23.4).

The typical spongiform pattern with gas bubbles is the most specific CT sign for the detection of gossypiboma (Fig. 23.5a, b), although, rarely, a long-

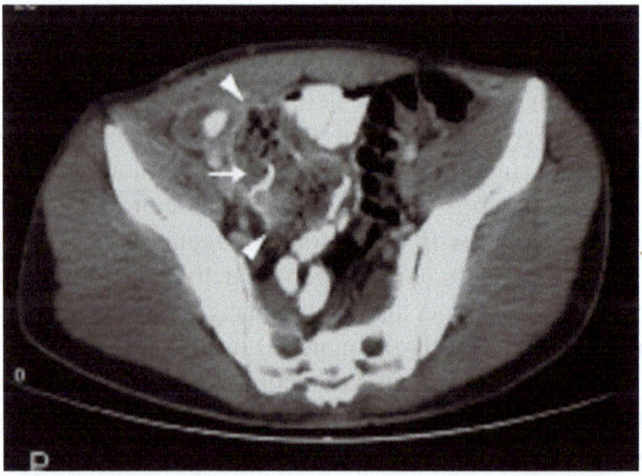

Fig. 23.3 Gossypiboma in the right iliac fossa after hemicolectomy, with a spongiform pattern (*white arrowheads*) and a radio-opaque marker (*white arrow*)

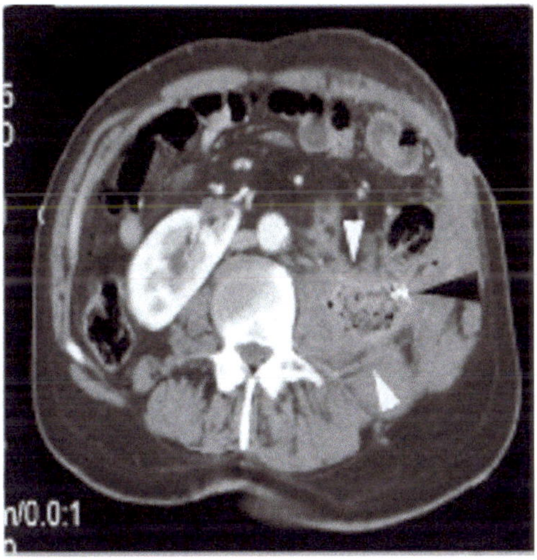

Fig. 23.4 Gossypiboma in the left renal space after nephrectomy, with a spongiform pattern (*white arrowheads*) and radio-opaque marker (*black arrowhead*)

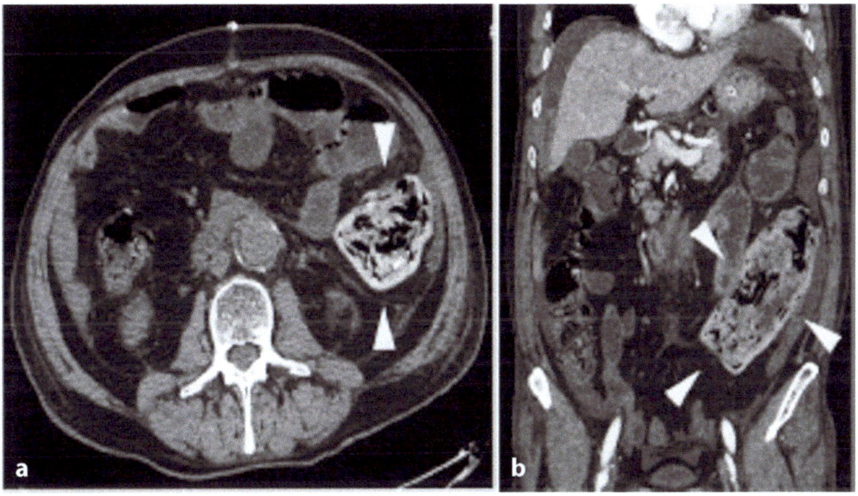

Fig. 23.5 Same case as in Fig. 23.1. **a**, **b** Gossypiboma, from a surgical drape, without a radio-opaque marker. Note the spongiform pattern and the presence of gas bubbles on the left side (*white arrowheads*)

lasting gossypiboma will resemble a cystic mass bounded by a calcified ring. The reticulated and calcified appearance of the internal portion of the mass is due to the gradual calcification along the fibers of the surgical gauze [18].

Nonetheless, the variable appearance of retained surgical sponges (Fig. 23.6a, b) can lead to diagnostic misinterpretations. Since it is not anticipated, a gossypiboma is frequently misdiagnosed, potentially resulting in unnecessary surgical procedures [11, 19].

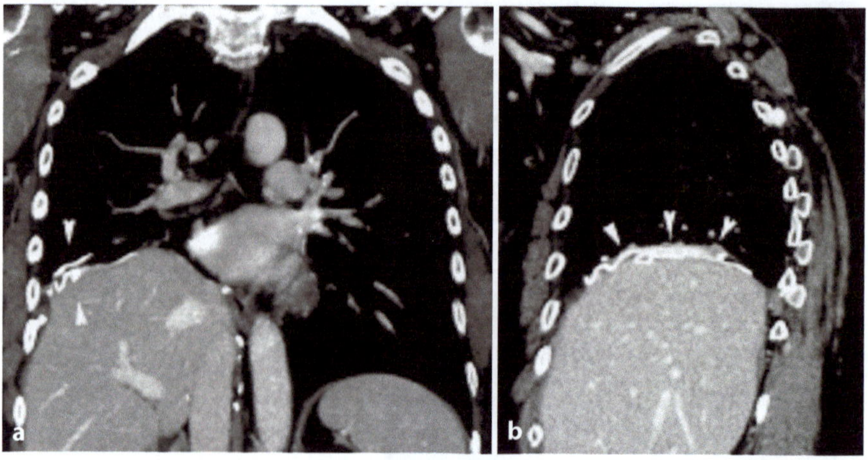

Fig. 23.6 a, b Gossypibomain the right sub-diaphragmatic space is visible only with the aid of the radio-opaque marker (*white arrowheads*)

23.3.4 Magnetic Resonance Imaging

To date, only a few reports of the MRI appearance of gossypiboma in the abdomen and pelvis have been published. On MRI, the signal intensity of any mass will vary according to its histologic composition, stage, and fluid content. A retained sponge is typically seen as a soft-tissue-density mass with a thick well-defined capsule; on T2-weighted imaging it has a whorled internal configuration [6, 20].

23.4 Diagnosis of Gossypiboma: Ethical and Legal Concerns

The symptoms of gossypiboma are nonspecific and may first appear years after surgery. It should be considered in the differential diagnosis of any patient with postoperative unresolved or unusual problems. Indeed, if a gossypiboma is suspected, the patient should undergo imaging based on a multi-technique approach [4, 5].

Foreign bodies retained in the peritoneal cavity after surgeries are rarely documented, owing to medical, legal, and other reasons that can jeopardize the reputation of a surgeon amongst his or her professional colleagues and the public at large [21].

How should the radiologist proceed when a gossypiboma is found? Is he or she required to report the case, thereby fulfilling his or her professional responsibility? Or should the damage to the surgeon be taken into account and the case therefore not reported?

Reporting may be exhaustive, requiring a detailed description of the lesion, its relationship with surrounding structures, and any complications, without using "gossypiboma" or a similar word. Will this later be viewed as an omission aimed at safeguarding the surgeon?

In our opinion, a complete and correct report allowing surgical intervention in order to protect the patient from the consequences of any kind of professional failure is warranted. This implies the need for the radiologist to take the responsibility associated with this difficult diagnosis, in order to avoid any legal ramifications.

References

1. Stawicki SP, Evans DC, Cipolla J et al (2009) Retained surgical foreign bodies: a comprehensive review of risks and preventive strategies. Scand J Surg 98:8-17
2. Jain M, Jain R, Sawhney S (1995) Gossypiboma: ultrasound guided removal. J Clin Ultrasound 23:321-323
3. Kernagis LY, Siegelman ES, Torigian DA (2009) Case 145: Retained Sponge. Radiology 251: 608-611
4. Manzella A, Borba Filho P, Albuquerque E et al (2009) Imaging of gossypibomas: pictorial review. AJR 193: S94-S101
5. O'Connor AR, Coakley FV, Meng MV et al (2003) Imaging of retained surgical sponges in the abdomen and pelvis. AJR 180:481-489
6. Kim CK, Park BK, Ha H (2007) Gossypiboma in abdomen and pelvis: MRI findings in four patients. AJR 189:814-817
7. Gencosmanoglu R, Inceoglu R (2003) An unusual cause of small bowel obstruction: gossypiboma case report BMC Surg 3:6
8. Cheng TC, Chou ASB, Jeng CM et al (2007) Computed tomography findings of gossypiboma. J Chin Med Assoc 70:565-569
9. Godara R, Marwah S, Karwasara RK et al (2006) Spontaneous transmural migration of surgical sponges. Asian J Surg 29:44-45
10. Haegeman S, Maleux G, Heye S et al (2008) Texiloma complicated by abscess formation, three years after surgical repair of abdominal aortic aneurysm. JBR BTR 91:51-53
11. Kopka L, Fisher U, Gross AJ et al (1996) CT of retained surgical sponges (textilomas): pitfalls in detection and evalutation. J Computed Assist Tomogr 20:919-923
12. Parasad S, Krishnan A, Limidi J et al (1999) Imaging features of gossypiboma: report of two cases. JPGM 45:18-19
13. Kaiser CW, Friedman S, Spurling KP et al (1996) The retained surgical sponge. Ann Surg 224:79-84
14. Ersoy H, Saygili OB, Yildirim T (2004) Abdominal gossypiboma: ultrasonography and computerized tomography findings. Turk J Gastroenterol 15:65-66
15. Murphy CF, Stunell H, Torreggiani WC (2008) Diagnosis of gossypiboma of the abdomen and pelvis. Am J Roentgenol 190:W382
16. Tzu Chieh Cheng, Andy Shau Bin Chou, Chin Ming Jeng et al (2007) Computed tomography findings of gossypiboma. J Chin Med Assoc 70:565-569
17. Kiernan F, Joyce M, Byrnes CK et al (2008) Gossypiboma: a case report and review of the literature. Ir J Med Sci 177:389-391
18. Lu YY, Cheung YC, Ko SF et al (2005) Calcified reticulate ring sign: a characteristic feature of gossypiboma on computed tomography. World J Gastroenterol 11:4927-4929
19. Sun HS, Chen SL, Kuo CC et al (2007) Gossypiboma retained surgical sponge. J Chin Med Assoc 70:511-513
20. Kim CK, Park BK, Ha H (2007) Gossypiboma in abdomen and pelvis: MRI findings in four patients. AJR 189:814-817
21. Shyung LR, Chang WH, Lin SC et al (2005) Report of gossypiboma from the standpoint in medicine and law. World J Gastroenterol 11:1248-1249

Foreign Body Ingestion and Rectal Foreign Body Insertion: Diagnostic Challenges

24

Antonio Pinto, Amelia Sparano, and Teresa Cinque

24.1 Introduction

Foreign body (FB) ingestions are common in children and mentally handicapped adults. Typical examples include children swallowing coins and mentally handicapped adults swallowing razor blades and silverware. A correlation has been found between age groups and specific types of ingested objects. Coins, toys, crayons, and ballpoint pen caps are most often ingested during childhood, while adults tend to have problem with meat and bones. Moreover, psychiatric patients and prison inmates may ingest such unlikely objects as spoons and razor blades. Fortunately, the vast majority of all swallowed objects pass through the gastrointestinal (GI) tract without problem [1]. The remainder may become lodged in the esophagus or other locations in the GI tract, placing the patient at risk for developing significant complications such as obstruction, aspiration, bleeding, perforation, fistulization, sepsis, and even death [1]. Elongated or sharp objects, such as needles, eating utensils, bobby pins, or razor blades, are more likely to lodge at areas of narrowing (from bowel adhesions or strictures) or to impinge at regions of anatomic acute angulation. The duodenal loop, duodenojejunal junction, appendix, and ileocecal valve region are predisposed to impaction from these types of objects. There is a greater than 90% chance that a FB will be passed spontaneously once it reaches the stomach. However, objects larger than 2 cm in diameter may lodge at the pylorus, whereas objects longer than 6 cm may become entrapped either at the pylorus or at the C-curve of the duodenum, between the first, second, and third parts of the duodenum, and rarely pass beyond that point [2, 3]. Otherwise, the only remaining obstacle hindering passage of the

A. Pinto (✉)
Department of Diagnostic Radiological Imaging, "A. Cardarelli" Hospital, Naples, Italy

FB is the ileocecal valve. Rarely, a FB becomes entrapped in a Meckel's diverticulum or at the sigmoid S-curve, which is more flexible than the duodenal C-curve since it is not fixed in the retroperitoneum and hence more readily allows passage of the FB [4].

Foreign body insertions are seen in four broad categories of patients: children, mentally handicapped or mentally retarded persons, adults with unusual sexual behavior, and children or adults with predisposing factors or injurious situational problems. Surprisingly, most FBs inserted into the rectum do not cause significant injury even if they are large, sharp, or pointed. Common rectal FBs that result from medical procedures going awry include thermometers, rectal tubes, anal packs, light covers, enema tips and covers, suppository wrappers, and oral or topical medication used inappropriately in the rectum [1].

24.2 Appearance of Foreign Bodies on Radiographs

The radiological visualization of FBs depends on their radiopacity (Fig. 24.1). Metal objects with a relatively high atomic weight are readily visible on plain films, where they are intensely radiopaque regardless of their volume. Almost all objects composed of plastic and most thin aluminum objects, such as pull tabs on cans, are not radiopaque. Aluminum is of low radiodensity, which makes visualization on radiographs difficult [5]. The atomic numbers of soft

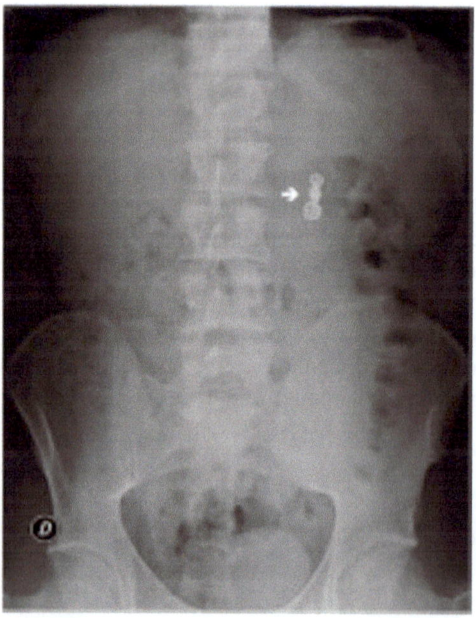

Fig. 24.1 Plain abdominal film shows an ingested radiopaque foreign body (*arrow*)

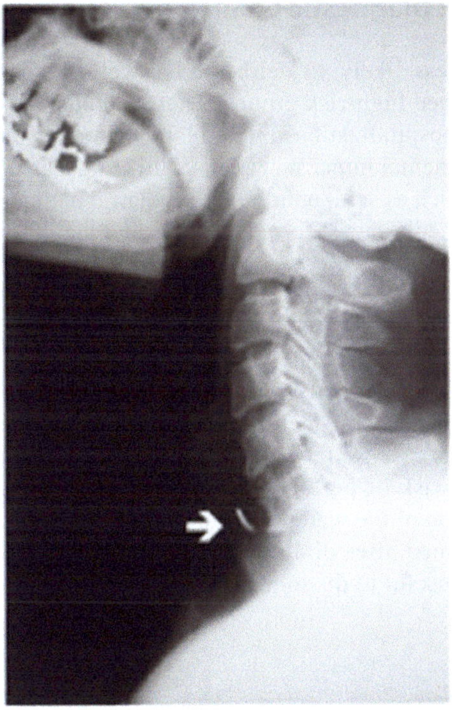

Fig. 24.2 Lateral plain film shows the presence of a radiopaque foreign body (chicken bone) (*arrow*) anterior to the body of C6

tissue and aluminum (7.5 and 13, respectively) are similar [6]. On the other hand, all chicken bones (Fig. 24.2) and most meat bones are opaque on radiographs, whereas the majority of fish bones are not, although some fish bones are readily evident [1]. Glass is always radiopaque, and its radiopacity does not depend on its content of lead or other metals. Glass FB, whether ingested, inserted into a body cavity, or deposited in the soft tissues of an extremity by an injury, should always be detectable on radiographs. This detectability obviously depends on the size of the object. Submillimeter pieces of glass buried deep in the soft tissue of an obese person may not be visible. However, any substantial piece of glass 1–2 mm or larger should generally be visible. Ingested aluminum objects are not easily detected on radiographs [1]. Children, mentally incapacitated adults, and suicidal individuals may knowingly or inadvertently ingest poisonous substances. Most medications and toxic agents are probably not opaque enough to be easily detected by routine imaging methods. However, many metals and their compounds are sufficiently opaque to be seen on abdominal radiographs. These substances include barium, lead, arsenic, bismuth, thorium, and iodine compounds.

24.3 Foreign Body Ingestion: Diagnostic Challenges

In contrast to children, adults are less likely to deliberately swallow non-digestible objects except in well-defined high-risk groups. These include prisoners seeking secondary gain from hospitalization, individuals attempting to smuggle illicit drugs, and those with mental impairment caused by drugs, alcohol, dementia, or psychiatric illness such as schizophrenia. Psychiatric patients and prisoners are more prone to repeatedly ingest foreign objects and therefore should be monitored carefully.

In case of suspected FB ingestion, antero-posterior and lateral chest, lateral neck and abdominal radiographs should be obtained for confirmation or exclusion. The two projections radiographs are mandatory because some FB, especially those of discoid shape, can be seen only in one projection, remaining undetectable in the others. If oral contrast medium is administered, the sensitivity increases (Fig. 24.3). In this case, water-soluble contrast-medium is preferable to barium, given the high risk of perforation. In the absence of a clear sign of extraluminal extravasation of the water-soluble contrast-medium, additional radiographs can be performed after oral administration of barium. Plain films of the esophagus are also useful to distinguish coins from the more dangerous button batteries.

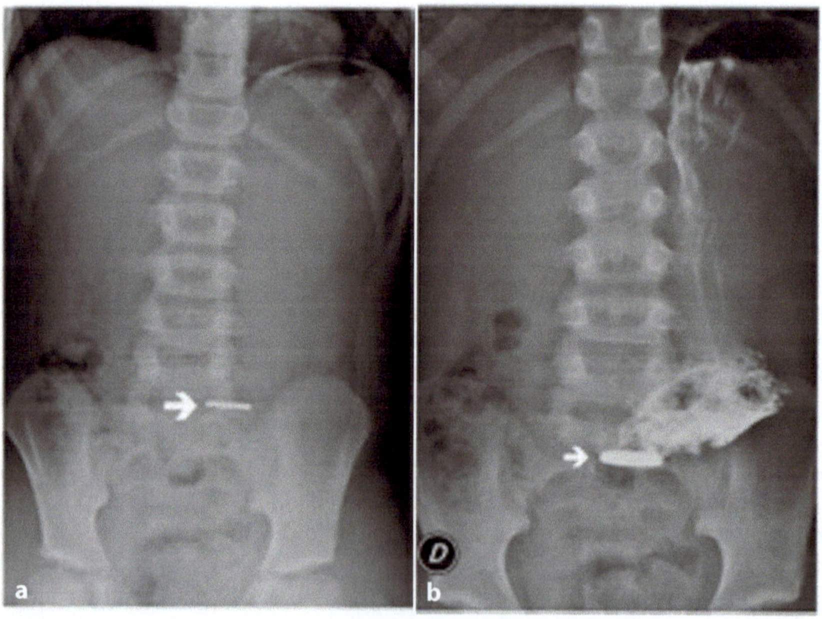

Fig. 24.3 A plain abdominal film (**a**) performed in a child who ingested a coin confirmed the presence of a radio-opaque foreign body (*arrow*). The exact location of the ingested foreign body is demonstrated after oral administration of gastrografin (**b**).

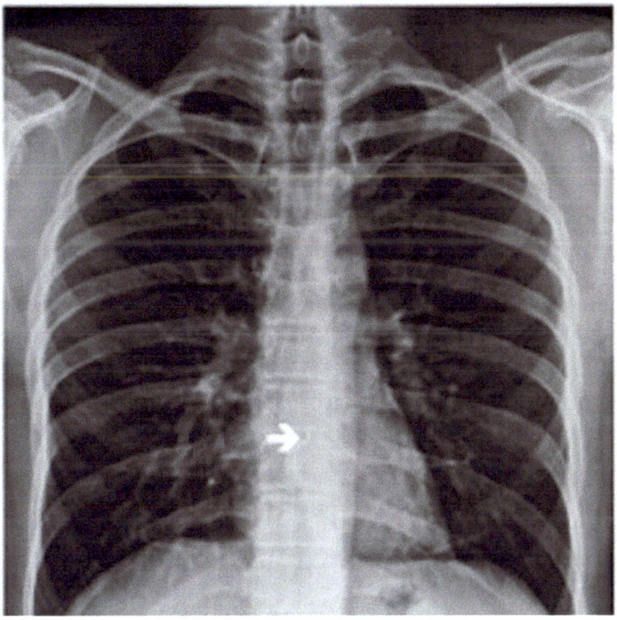

Fig. 24.4 Chest plain film: a small ingested foreign body (*arrow*) located in the distal thoracic esophagus was missed. The patient did not report an adequate history

It has been recommended that infants and children with suspected FB ingestion undergo radiographic examination from the base of the skull to the anus, to evaluate for more than one foreign object [7]. Commercially available handheld metal detectors have a 98%-100% sensitivity in detecting and localizing ingested coins in the esophagus [8, 9]. This technique is potentially useful in limiting radiation exposure in children who are asymptomatic or have a questionable history.

Multidetector row computed tomography (MDCT) is rarely needed to diagnose FBs, but occasionally it is used to detect ingested objects that are missed by other modalities. MDCT is also helpful in the detection of FB complications, such as perforation, fistula, or abscess [10]. It is important to remember that failure to demonstrate a FB radiographically does not preclude its presence.

The diagnosis of an ingested FB is often overlooked in those patients who cannot report an adequate history (Fig. 24.4) or who have swallowed objects that are not inherently opaque. When sharp or pointed FBs (e.g., metallic objects, animal or fish bones, and toothpicks) are ingested, the risk of perforation is higher than with blunt FBs [1]. Therefore, patients who have ingested a sharp or pointed object require urgent treatment. If the patient does not receive timely and appropriate treatment, the object can cause serious conditions, such as esophageal perforation with resultant fatal mediastinitis or intestinal perforation with associated peritonitis. Other complications of FB ingestion include hemorrhage, bowel obstruction, perforation, and erosion into adjacent viscera. Hemorrhage occurs when the FB injures the mucosa or lodges in a region close to a visceral artery, such as an object in the pylorus eroding into the gastroduodenal artery. Bowel obstruction can also occur when the FB is bigger than any of the narrow anatomical areas of the intestinal tract mentioned above, hence lodging at that site and causing obstruction, with possible progression to hemorrhage when followed by erosion into an artery or injury of the mucosa. The FB may perforate freely in the peritoneum or extraperitoneally when it reaches the distal rectum; these patients will present with abscess and rectal bleeding [4].

Key factors influencing patient management include the type of object, its physical characteristics, the location of the object, the time elapsed since its ingestion, associated medical conditions, the presence or absence of symptoms, and evidence of complications, such as complete obstruction or perforation.

Two interesting phenomena occur that help protect the bowel wall from injury during FB passage. The first is related to axial flow and a tendency for sharp objects to be turned in the intestine so that the sharper end trails down the lumen. Second, once the foreign object reaches the colon, it becomes surrounded by fecal material, which aids in bowel wall protection [7].

24.4 Rectal Foreign Body Insertions: Diagnostic Challenges

Retained colorectal foreign bodies may pose a risk of serious morbidity. Affected individuals will often have made several unsuccessful attempts to remove the object themselves, resulting in further delay of medical care and potentially increasing the risk of complications. FBs can be introduced into the rectum for diagnostic and therapeutic procedures, self-administered treatment, autoeroticism, accidental introduction, and criminal assault [11-13]. A foreign body inside the anorectal area has various causes, which will determine treatment, as will the symptoms, and the severity of the anorectal damage [14, 15]. The type of FB varies with the pathway for insertion. Peroral FBs are usually animal bones, fish bones, fish hooks, or tooth-picks that have been swallowed by patients who are inattentive or drunken [14]. In patients with mental illnesses, numerous unexpected FBs are reported [11, 15]. In cases in which the FB was inserted through the anus, a sexual purpose is reported to be the most common cause [11, 16]. Foreign bodies inserted into the rectum to enhance sexual stimulation are a common cause of rectal injuries. As with FBs in the upper GI tract, the types of objects introduced through the anus are unlimited [17]: vibrators, rubber phallus, vegetables (carrots, zucchini, corn cob), fruit (apple, banana), stones, wire, toothbrush, screwdrivers, rodents, cans, bottles, and jars are but a few of the retained rectal objects reported [17, 18]. Diagnostic problems can occur with trans-anal rectal injuries, because of the natural hesitancy of the patient to describe what might have been a very embarrassing and socially unacceptable incident (Fig. 24.5). Trans-anal high hydrostatic pressure may cause severe colorectal injury, necessitating resection of the blown

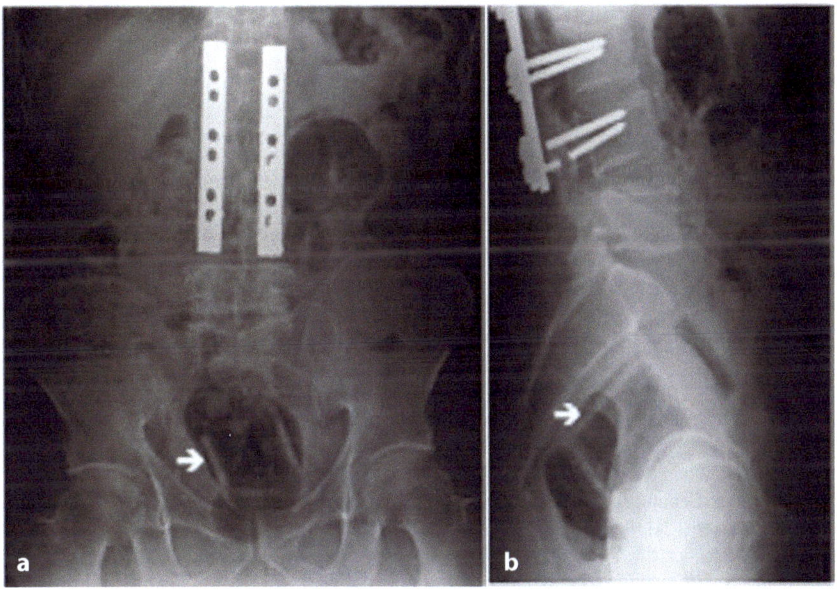

Fig. 24.5 Radiographs of a 48-year-old man with a foreign body (**a**, **b**, *arrows*) inserted into his rectum. He denied having done so

injured segment. The firm lateral support of the rectum makes the rectosigmoid junction the first part to be hit by the pressure column, which acts as a solid body as it opens the anal sphincter [19].

24.5 Conclusions

Foreign body ingestion is most commonly seen in children, alcoholics, people with mental health problems and people wearing dental prostheses. Most foreign bodies will traverse the gastrointestinal tract uneventfully – but between 10 and 20% will fail to pass. Complications occur in fewer than 1% of cases. The diagnosis of an ingested FB is often overlooked in those patients who cannot report an adequate history or who have swallowed objects that are not inherently opaque.

In case of suspected FB ingestion, antero-posterior and lateral chest, lateral neck and abdominal radiographs should be obtained for confirmation or exclusion. The FB radiological visualization depends on the object's radiopacity. Metal objects with a relatively high atomic weight are readily visible on plain films, as they are intensely radiopaque regardless of their volume. Rectal FBs present a difficult diagnostic and management dilemma. A foreign body inside the anorectal area has various causes, which will determine treatment, as will the symptoms, and the severity of the anorectal damage. Diagnostic problems can occur with trans-anal rectal injuries, because of the natural hesitancy of the patient to describe what might have been a very embarrassing and socially unacceptable incident.

References

1. Hunter TB, Taljanovic MS (2003) Foreign bodies. RadioGraphics 23:731-757
2. Koch H (1977) Operative endoscopy. Gastrointest Endosc 24:65-68
3. Velitchkov NG, Grigorov GI, Losanoff JE et al (1996) Ingested foreign bodies of the gastrointestinal tract: retrospective analysis of 542 cases. World J Surg 20:1001-1005
4. Goh BK, Chow PK, Quah HM et al (2006) Perforation of the gastrointestinal tract secondary to ingestion of foreign bodies. World J Surg 30:372-377
5. Conners GP (2000) Finding aluminum foreign bodies. Pediatr Rev 21:172
6. Stewart GD, Lakshmi MV, Jackson A (1994) Aluminum ring pulls: an invisible foreign body. J Accid Emerg Med 11:201-203
7. Smith MT, Wong RKH (2007) Foreign bodies. Gastrointest Endoscopy Clin N Am 17:361-382
8. Bassett KE, Schunk JE, Logan L (1999) Localizing ingested coins with a metal detector. Am J Emerg Med 17:338-341
9. Gooden EA, Forte V, Papsin B (2000) Use of a commercially available metal detector for the localization of metallic foreign body ingestion in children. J Otolaryngol 29:218-220
10. Pinto A, Muzj C, Stavolo C et al (2004) Pictorial essay: foreign body of the gastrointestinal tract in emergency radiology. Radiol Med 107:145-152
11. Clarke DL, Buccimazza I, Anderson FA et al (2005) Colorectal foreign bodies. Colorectal Dis 7:98-103
12. Losanoff JE, Kjossev KT (1999) Rectal "oven mitt": the importance of considering a serious underlying injury. J Emerg Med 17:31-33
13. Orr CJ, Clark MA, Hawley DA et al (1995) Fatal anorectal injuries: a series of four cases. J Forensic Sci 40:219-221
14. Choi KD (1990) Foreign bodies in the anorectum: report of five cases and a review of literature. J Korean Soc Coloproctol 6:55-62
15. Yaman M, Deitel M, Burul CJ et al (1993) Foreign bodies in the rectum. Can J Surg 36:173-177
16. Huang WC, Jiang JK, Wang HS et al (2003) Retained rectal foreign bodies. J Chin Med Assoc 66:607-612
17. Lyons MF 2nd, Tsuchida AM (1993) Foreign bodies of the gastrointestinal tract. Med Clin North Am 77:1101-1114
18. Stack LB, Munter DW (1996) Foreign bodies in the gastrointestinal tract. Emerg Med Clin North Am 14:493-521
19. Farbin S, Davisdon P, Shockley L (1996) Perforation of the sigmoid colon by hydrostatic pressure of a public water fountain. J Emerg Med 14:703-706

Radiological and Medico-legal Problems of Body-packing

25

Antonio Pinto, Ciro Stavolo, and Carlo Muzj

25.1 Introduction

We live in a world plagued by illicit drug traffic and drug use, in which the importation of illegal drugs is a major industry. Some of the bit players in this trade are the "mules" or "body-packers" who smuggle drugs past border patrols and Customs by ingesting drug-filled packets or by inserting them into their rectum or vagina.

Over the last two decades, as drug smuggling has increased worldwide, the gastrointestinal (GI) tract has been the increasingly preferred vehicle for the concealed transport of narcotics [1-4].

Body-packing and body-stuffing are the terms employed for intracorporeal concealment of illicit drugs, mainly cocaine and heroine. Body-packers fill their GI tract with large bags (2–8 cm) [5] containing narcotics prior to crossing international borders, in order to retrieve them after arrival at their destination. Their drug bags are generally carefully packed and wrapped in containers designed to transit through the GI tract. On arrival, body-packers pass their contraband, often with the aid of laxatives, cathartics, or enemas. In contrast, body-stuffers, also called mini-packers, are usually street dealers, often drug abusers themselves [6], who either store or unexpectedly and hastily hide one or several small packets of drugs in their body cavities, when prompted by fear of arrest by the police.

In order to escape detection by law enforcement authorities, the packets are swallowed or they are introduced into the vagina or rectal ampulla.

A. Pinto (✉)
Department of Diagnostic Radiological Imaging, "A. Cardarelli" Hospital,
Naples, Italy

25.2 Body-packers, Drugs, and Packets

The general profile of a body-packer is someone who returns from a trip abroad in a location with a history of illicit drug export and who has a history of frequent trips. Of drug couriers, 80% are presumed to be body-packers [7]. When used as a drug courier by a drug organization, body-packers usually wear a shirt and jacket of better quality than the trousers or shoes. They usually do not wear expensive watches or jewelry and differ from business people by the way of conversation [7]. The smuggled drugs are those that yield a high profit, particularly cocaine and heroin but also amphetamines, 3,4-methylene-dioxymethamphetamine ("ecstasy"), marijuana, or hashish. The packaging material is made of high-grade latex, aluminum foil, or condoms [6]. Occasionally, more than one type of drug is ingested. Body-packers usually carry about 1 kg of drug, divided into 50 to 100 packets of 8 to 10 g each, although persons carrying more than 200 packets have been described [4]. Each packet of cocaine, heroin, or amphetamine contains a life-threatening dose of the drug.

McCarron and Wood have described three types of cocaine packets [8]. Type I contains loosely packed cocaine powder covered by two or four layers of condoms or other latex-like material. This packet is highly susceptible to leakage and rupture. Types II and III contain tightly packed cocaine powder or paste. The second type is well wrapped in multiple layers of tubular latex and often gives the impression of having been packed by machine. The third type has a covering of aluminum foil. Some of these early packets were radiolucent [8]. Pidoto et al. [9] recently report a detailed description of the type IV packet: it is constructed by dissolving cocaine hydrochloride in a watery alcohol solution. The resultant dense cocaine paste is introduced into a processing device and, when hardened, is ready for packaging in tubular latex. Preparation is completed by covering the packet with colored paraffin or fiberglass. These packages are always radiopaque and easily identified on abdominal x-ray study, based on their shape and dimensions.

Drug packets, previously varied in size and construction, but are now well crafted, with a precision that suggests the use of an automated process. First, the drug is densely packed into a latex sheath, such as a condom or balloon. This layer is tied at the open end, covered with several other layers of latex, and sealed with a hard wax coating. Aluminum foil, plastic food wrap, carbon paper, or other materials may be incorporated to alter the radiodensity, in an attempt to limit the risk of detection [4].

25.3 Appearance of Drug Packets on Radiological Imaging

Patients suspected of being body-packers require radiographic evaluation. Plain abdominal X-ray is the most widely used radiological tool to detect drug-filled packets of 2–8 cm within the GI tract of body- packers [3, 5, 7].

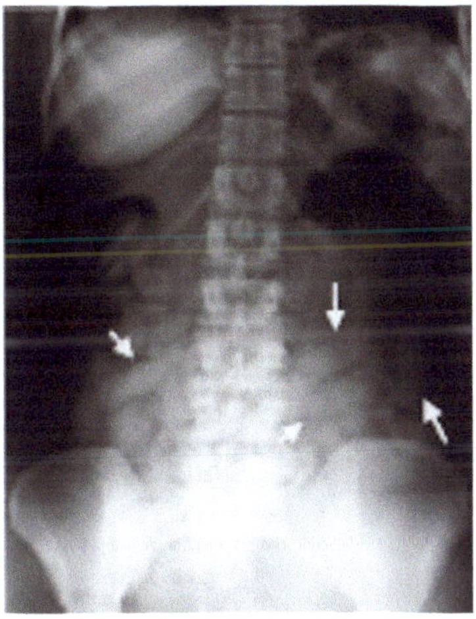

Fig. 25.1 Plain abdominal film showing multiple radiodense foreign bodies (*arrows*) in a 35-year-old body-packer

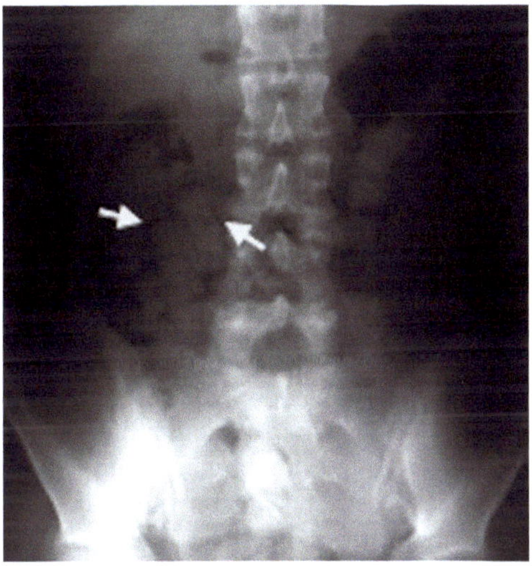

Fig. 25.2 On plain abdominal film, some hyperdense foreign bodies are observed within small bowel loops; the packages are surrounded by a radiolucent rim (*arrows*)

However, due to limited contrast resolution, conventional radiographs (CR) of body-packers reveal the presence of drug containers only in 40–90% of the cases [1, 3, 4, 10-12].

Several specific signs on the abdominal radiograph may suggest the presence of body-packing: multiple radiodense foreign bodies (Fig. 25.1), a "rosette-like finding" formed by air trapped in the knot where a condom is tied [3, 11], and a "double-condom" sign [3, 8, 10] in which air trapped between layers of latex makes the packets more visible (Fig. 25.2). The last finding may also suggest a loss of integrity of the packing material [13]. Nonetheless, up to 60% of these large ingested drug bags may remain undetected. The far smaller cocaine-filled packets ingested by body-stuffers are even more easily

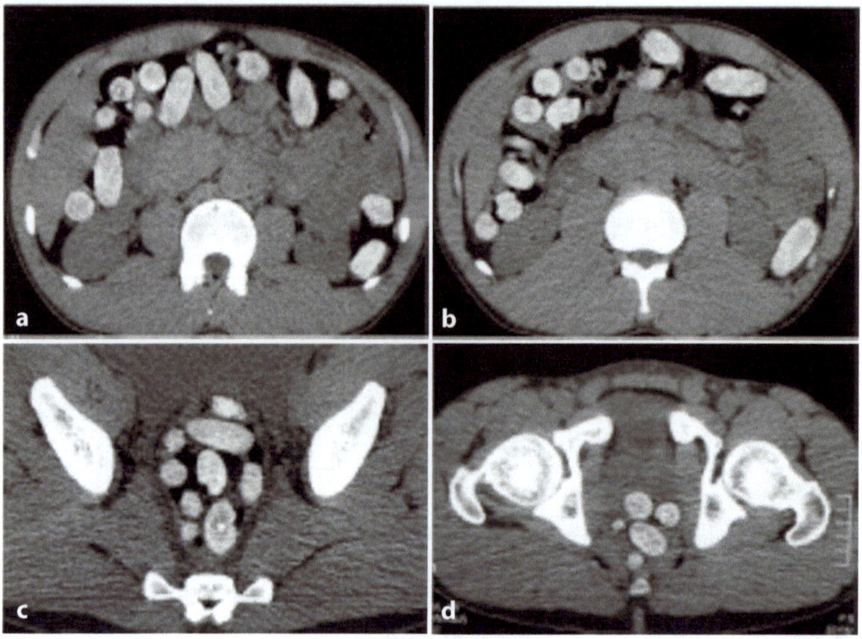

Fig. 25.3 Unenhanced abdominal CT showing multiple hyperdense foreign bodies located in the colonic loops (**a**, **b**) and in the rectum (**c**, **d**)

missed by plain films [6, 8, 11], thus requiring another, more sensitive imaging modality for their detection. False-positive studies may be due to bladder stones inspissated stool, or intra-abdominal calcifications [4]. The reasons for false-negative studies are less well established but may involve the reader's inexperience [14] or the technical quality of the study. Abdominal ultrasound (US) [3] and radiographic studies after oral intestinal opacification with hydrosoluble contrast agents [1] have been used and are recommended for investigation of body-packers. However, for the detection of the smaller cocaine-filled packets, which may be located anywhere in the digestive tract, neither of these methods is considered sufficiently sensitive [7]. Due to its speed and safety, US would seem to be a practical approach in the initial evaluation of body-packers, but there are scant data in support of its use.

Magnetic resonance imaging (MRI) is rarely used as first-line emergency modality, because of its high costs and limited availability. The diagnostic value of Multi-detector row Computed Tomography (MDCT) is better than that of CR, US, or MRI [15]. Schmidt et al. [16] reported the good diagnostic value of unenhanced CT (Fig. 25.3) for the detection of cocaine-filled packets. The radiological appearance of the packets is based on the presence of an air–solid interface: an outer halo of air, representing the wrapped cellophane containing tiny amounts of air trapped during the packing and surrounding the central cocaine [16]. This so-called "double-condom" sign is considered the key feature of drug-filled condoms of body-packers seen on plain films [3, 5, 12] and CT [17]. Other CT signs of cocaine-filled packets are focal areas of high-density [2, 10]. The amount of attenuation depends on the purity of the cocaine and its admixture [3, 7]. Pure cocaine powder is a low-attenuating substance, measuring as little as 200 HU, whereas cocaine stones, crack cocaine (cocaine base 51%), and pressed cocaine powder mixed with another substance are of high density [7]. The density is also determined by how tightly the cocaine is packed as well as the type of wrapping material used [11]. Eng et al. reported one case of a false-negative unenhanced CT of the abdomen in a cocaine body- stuffer [18]. Moreover, Sengupta et al. [19] recommend the simple step of reviewing CT scans of suspected body-packers on altered windowing and standard abdominal windowing in order to improve the detection of fatty drug packages.

25.4 Body-packing: Abdominal Complications

Body-packers may present to health-care providers in three ways: (1) with signs and symptoms of drug toxicity owing to leaking or ruptured packets, (2) with symptoms of GI obstruction or perforation, or (3) asymptomatic, because they fear the consequences of packet rupture or they may already be under arrest. Intoxication after packet rupture can be a challenge in terms of the correct diagnosis if there are no attendants with the intoxicated person who are able to provide information, or if there are no extracorporeal signs of the patient being a drug abuser. Certainly, the risk of intoxication as a drug courier is low compared to the number of body-packers [7].

For all such patients, airway, breathing, and circulation should be secured. Drug packets in the rectum or vagina should be carefully removed, but only if they can be easily grasped with the fingers. Conservative management of asymptomatic patients includes in-patient observation, drug screening, and a liquid diet [4]. Bowel obstruction is commonly reported in body-packers; the level of obstruction is usually at the ileocecal valve; other sites of obstruction are the pylorus and the splenic flexure of the colon. The treatment urgency in patients with impacted cocaine-filled condoms is due to the risk of transmucosal absorption and its potentially lethal consequences. Bowel wall perforation, peritonitis, esophageal obstruction, and esophageal perforation are less frequently noted [4]. Radiologists should be aware that bowel obstruction with all its consecutive complications may be caused by foreign bodies. Careful reading of plain X-ray films of the abdomen and a high skill in conducting US examinations is needed in order to avoid missing the underlying cause of an acute abdomen. If there is any suspicion of drug packets in the intestine, CT may be used as a further diagnostic tool. The number of packets ingested does not appear to correlate with the risk of complications. Patients presenting with symptoms of GI obstruction or perforation should also undergo immediate operative intervention. There is no role for conservative management.

Endoscopic removal of drug packets is contraindicated because of concern for packet rupture during extraction.

Acute drug overdose is a very serious risk to the smuggler if one or more of the condoms should rupture. There have been reports of sudden deaths from massive drug overdoses. But, as noted, considering the large amount of smuggling that no doubt takes place by this means, the complication rate is rare.

25.5 Ethical and Medico-legal Issues

Emergency departments face an increasing number of drug-related health problems, with difficult medico-legal and social consequences. In the wake of the events of September 11, 2001, security at border crossings in the United States has increased dramatically. One of the unintended consequences of this action has been an increase in drug seizures. There are three main reasons why radiologists are confronted with the diagnosis of body-packing: the suspicion that the person being detained is a drug courier; intoxication of the detainee; and mechanical complications suffered by that person due to the packets. Before examining a person presented by a Customs inspector, radiologists must inform themselves as to the medico-legal implications in their country, i.e., whether the use of X-ray, CT, or MRI without a medical indication is legal. This may be different in countries of the European Community. In some countries the detainee has to agree to the possibly harmful examinations; in others, the necessary exams needed to convict a suspected (by Customs) body-packer are allowed, but a judicial injunction may be necessary; therefore, the legal situation should be clear in advance [7].

Faced with this increase in security, drug smugglers have begun using children, older people, and pregnant women as vehicles to transport their cargo. Pregnant women represent a challenge in management, particularly in the event of package rupture. In the pregnant body-packer, a detailed medical history and physical examination are necessary before an appropriate treatment scheme is implemented, as treatment must address the anatomic and physiologic changes of pregnancy, essentially involving two patients. The major risk factor for toxicity is packet construction. Although packets today are usually constructed so as to prevent leakage or rupture [4, 19] in the past they were fabricated from condoms or digits of latex gloves [20] and were therefore prone to leakage and rupture.

Such packets are occasionally still seen. If packet construction is in question, a single abdominal radiograph can help define the character, location, and number of packets [4, 7] while also evaluating the GI tract. Customs and Emergency Department personnel may be hesitant to expose the fetus to radiation out of concern for teratogenicity or liability. However, if a radiograph is medically indicated, the average radiation dose to the fetus from a single abdominal radiograph is approximately 100 mrad [21, 22]. A radiation dose of < 5,000 mrad does not appear to increase the risk of malformations, and the risk of leukemia or malignancy development appears to be low [21, 22]. US is an alternative for detecting packets and correlates with the results of plain radiographs in the non-pregnant body-packer [23], although its efficacy in this setting has not been adequately studied.

Body-packers in legal custody may refuse to undergo invasive (i.e., rectal) examinations and radiography, but they cannot insist on being medically cleared and discharged. Appropriate management is admission for observation. In the unlikely event that a physician is served with a court order to forcibly examine or treat a body-packer, the hospital's legal counsel would most likely seek injunctive relief on the grounds that a physician is the patient's advocate, not an agent of the state.

25.6 Conclusions

Body-packing is the concealment of illicit substances in the human body for the purpose of smuggling. A body-packer usually swallows small packets containing heroin, cocaine, amphetamine, ecstasy, or marijuana. Apart from the social implications of drug smuggling, swallowers put themselves at considerable risk, as rupture of a single packet inside the body may be fatal, depending on the type and concentration of the ingested drug. Radiological diagnosis of packets may depend on the number, size, density, position and air-substance interfaces. Plain abdominal radiograph is the initial method of choice for the detection or exclusion of drug-filled packets within the GI tract of body-packers, although it is sometimes unable to identify the packets. The best imaging modality for revealing foreign bodies is MDCT, which is superior to abdominal radiographs and US in terms of sensitivity, localization, and density characterization.

References

1. Marc B, Baud FJ, Aelion MJ et al (1990) The cocaine body-packer syndrome: evaluation of a method of contrast study of the bowel. J Forensic Sci 35:345-355
2. Cranston PE, Pollack Jr CV, Harrison RB (1992) CT of crack cocaine ingestion. J Comput Assist Tomogr 16:560-563
3. Hierholzer J, Cordes M, Tantow H et al (1995) Drug smuggling by ingested cocaine-filled packages: conventional x-ray and ultrasound. Abdom Imaging 20:333-338
4. Traub SJ, Hoffman RS, Nelson LS (2003) Body packing - the internal concealment of illicit drugs. N Engl J Med 349:2519-2526
5. Pinsky MF, Ducas J, Ruggere MD (1978) Narcotic smuggling: the double condom sign. J Can Assoc Radiol 29:79-81
6. Roberts JR, Price D, Goldfrank L et al (1986) The bodystuffer syndrome: a clandestine form of drug overdose. Am J Emerg Med 4:24-27
7. Hergan K, Kofler K, Oser W (2004) Drug smuggling by body packing: what radiologists should know about it. Eur Radiol 14:736-742
8. McCarron MM, Wood JD (1983) The cocaine "body packer" syndrome: diagnosis and treatment. JAMA 250:1417-1420

9. Pidoto RR, Agliata AM, Bertolini R et al (2002) A new method of packaging cocaine for international traffic and implications for the management of cocaine body packers. J Emerg Med 23:149-153
10. Pollack Jr CV, Biggers DW, Carlton Jr FB et al (1992) Two crack cocaine body stuffers. Ann Emerg Med 21:1370-1380
11. Beerman R, Nunez Jr D,Wetli CV (1986) Radiographic evaluation of the cocaine smuggler. Gastrointest Radiol 11:351-354
12. Sporer KA, Firestone J (1997) Clinical course of crack cocaine body stuffers. Ann Emerg Med 29:596-601
13. McCleave NR (1993) Drug smuggling by bodypackers: detection and removal of internally concealed drugs. Med J Aust 159:750-754
14. Caruana DS, Weinbach B, Goerg D et al (1984) Cocaine-packet ingestion: diagnosis, management, and natural history. Ann Intern Med 100:73-74
15. Gor DM, Kirsch CF, Leen J et al (2001) Radiologic differentiation of intraocular glass: evaluation of imaging techniques, glass types, size, and effect of intraocular hemorrhage. AJR Am J Roentgenol 177:1199-1203
16. Schmidt S, Hugli O, Rizzo E et al (2008) Detection of ingested cocaine-filled packets - Diagnostic value of unenhanced CT. Eur J Radiol 67:133-138
17. Meyers MA (1995) The inside dope: cocaine, condoms, and computed tomography. Abdom Imaging 20:339-340
18. Eng JG, Aks SE, Waldron R et al (1999) False-negative abdominal CT scan in a cocaine body stuffer. Am J Emerg Med 17:702- 704
19. Sengupta A, Page P (2008) Window manipulation in diagnosis of body packing using computed tomography. Emerg Radiol 15:203-205
20. Wetli CV, Mittlemann RE (1981) The "body packer syndrome": toxicity following ingestion of illicit drugs packaged for transportation. J Forensic Sci 26:492-500
21. International Commission on Radiological Protection (2000) Pregnancy and medical radiation. Ann ICRP 30:iii-viii,1-43
22. Cordero DR, Medina C, Helfgott A (2006) Cocaine body packing in pregnancy. Ann Emerg Med 48:323-325
23. Meijer R, Bots ML (2003) Detection of intestinal drug containers by ultrasound scanning: an airport screening tool? Eur Radiol 13:1312-1315

Assessment of Risk in Radiology Using Malpractice RVUs

26

Massimo Cristofaro, Elisa Busi Rizzi, and Vincenzo Schininà

Policymakers and public opinion are concerned about the role of medical malpractice liability in driving up the total cost of medical care. As a result, risk management, a fundamental component of clinical administration, is now the centre of attention of healthcare experts, administrative officers, and operators, as well as representatives of various international groups that have an interest in public health [1]. The available methods for assessing the nature and scale of harm caused by health systems have widely differing purposes, strengths, and limitations and should thus be considered as complementary, by providing different levels of qualitative and quantitative information [1].

There are very few studies in which healthcare providers were interviewed or administrative data or confidential inquiries evaluated, whereas the number of articles on reporting systems or medical record reviews is almost unlimited [2]. Although decision-makers need data on the effectiveness of methods encouraging action or aimed at prevention at the national and local levels, comparative studies may have poor external validity since the results are likely to depend on local conditions [2].

Experts on the management of human error have published conceptual frameworks for causal analyses of harm and errors, James Reason's is the most frequently used. His model describes how errors occur despite the many existing defenses and safeguards. He states that few errors occur as a result of the action of a single individual. Behind the active errors, latent human, team, task, organizational, and institutional conditions result in weaknesses in the system. Thus, in his view, most error events are the result of both active error and systemic weakness [3].

Detailed analysis on the causes and remedies needed to reduce the incidence of malpractice has been under continual analysis [4-11]. Among the various

M. Cristofaro (✉)
Radiology Department, National Institute for Infectious Diseases IRCSS "L. Spallanzani", Rome, Italy

approaches, root cause analysis (RCA) has been widely used to study and identify the causes of an adverse event. On the basis of a conventional RCA, the cause of an adverse event is identified, corrective actions are implemented, and outcome measures are formulated. RCA tends to focus on an event that has already occurred; it is not used to proactively identify potential risks or failures in the system [12-15].

By contrast, healthcare failure mode and effect analysis (FMEA) is a *qualitative* method used to proactively detect risks to the patient in a particular healthcare process and correct potential errors before adverse events occur. The core of the FMEA approach includes the construction of a multidisciplinary team, a diagramming process, the identification of failure mode and causes, and the prioritization of potential risks, decision making, implementation of actions, and measures of outcome [16, 17].

Limited data are available regarding *quantitative* evaluation of the risk of malpractice [18, 19]. To determine radiological risk, in a preventive and quantitative manner, we use malpractice relative value units (MP RVUs). In our opinion, they have the following characteristics as good indicators: appropriateness, accuracy, discriminating capacity, significance, credibility, measurability, precision, and reproducibility [19].

Since January 1, 1992, Medicare has paid for physicians' services under section 1848 of the Social Security Act (the Act), "Payment for Physicians' Services." The Act requires that physician payments be based on national uniform RVUs according to the relative resources used in furnishing a service. Medicare pays physicians for services based on submission of a claim using one or more specific CPT codes. Each code has an RVU assigned to it which, when multiplied by a conversion factor (CF) and a geographical adjustment (GPCI), determines the compensation level for a particular service. The RVU system has the major objective of proposing a model that can evaluate radiological risk in a quantitative manner. For each service, Medicare determines RVUs for three types of resources. Physician-work RVUs account for the time, technical skill and effort, mental effort and judgment, and stress to provide a service. Practice-expense RVUs account for the non-physician clinical and non-clinical labor of the practice, as well as expenses for building space, equipment, and office supplies. Malpractice RVUs are generally the smallest component of the RVU values [20].

All of the RVUs can be downloaded from the CMS web site and are updated annually in addition to being reviewed in depth every 5 years. The MP RVUs are based on malpractice insurance premium data collected from commercial and physician-owned insurers from all the USA.

Malpractice RVUs are derived from a complex mathematical analysis that combines average national insurance premiums, average national insurance premiums for each specialty, and the percentage of procedures for each specialty [13, 14]. Resource-based MP RVUs were implemented in the Physician Fee Schedule (PFS) final rule published November 2, 1999.

The underlying task is to allocate the costs of physician malpractice insurance to a relative value scale in which physicians are compensated based on the procedures they perform. The difficulty is that malpractice insurers do not charge physicians per procedure performed; physicians are typically charged premiums for all services performed over a given period of time, usually a year or more. These premiums are based on certain risk characteristics, such as specialty, surgical involvement, and experience. The solution to this difficulty is to develop malpractice RVUs that take into account an assessment of the relative risk of the procedure. This assessment is made using two methods. The first relies solely on a weighted average of the malpractice premiums of the specialties that perform the procedure; the second uses the analysis of the first but adds work RVUs as an additional measure of risk. Work RVUs are believed to represent a reasonable proxy for risk since they were developed to reflect the time, intensity, and level of experience needed to perform the procedure.

Using this system, we assigned an effective risk index to each radiological procedure in order to obtain an effective quantification that influences the tariffs for remuneration of services and insurance payments [21]. We employed the American Medical Association's Current Procedural Terminology, (CPT), i.e., the HCPCS codes, used by Medicare, and the physician MP RVUs assigned to each procedure, as reported in Medicare's National Physician Fee Schedule (Table 26.1). We considered the ratio of MP RVUs to the number of exams as an index of the insurance risk (MP index) compared to the difficulty index (ratio of work RVUs to the number of exams) used in the literature to evaluate workload [22-24].

In our opinion, the values of MP RVUs are indicative of the risk of malpractice when considered globally and when subgrouped according to radiological methodology. The MP index correlates this risk with the number of exams carried out divided by the methodology. The utilization of the MP RVUs allows for quantification and comparison of radiological risk over various time periods.

In on our experience, traditional radiography (including contrast-enhanced radiological exams, but excluding mammography) carries a low risk of malpractice (MP index = 0.049). Ultrasound exams have an MP index of 0.125 and therefore a higher risk of malpractice. The MP index of CT is 0.434, indicating a relatively high risk of malpractice, whereas MRI has the highest risk of

Table 26.1 Malpractice relative value units (MP RVUs)

CPT HCPCS	Description	MP RVUs
70470	CT head/brain ± contrast medium	0.37
71010	Chest X-ray	0.03
73718	MRI lower extremity	0.36
75600	Contrast X-ray exam of aorta	0.56
76700	US exam, abdominal, complete	0.13
76805	Obstetric US >/= 14 weeks, single fetus	0.14

Table 26.2 Summary of data: Part 1

	Number of exams	MP RVUs	MP index
Traditional radiology	80,374	3,493	0.049
Ultrasonography	74.728	9,841	0.125
CT	30,024	13,823	0.434
MRI	22,908	15,240	0.667
Interventional radiology	1,268	181	0.143
Total	209,302	42,578	0.201

Table 26.2 Summary of data: Part 2

	Number of exams (%)	MP RVUs (%)
Traditional radiology	40.1	8
Ultrasonography	35.2	23.1
CT	13.1	32.1
MRI	11.2	36.2
Interventional radiology	0.4	0.6
Total	100.00	100.00

malpractice, with an MP index of 0.667. For interventional radiology (mainly ultrasound-guided liver biopsies), the MP index is 0.143, which is higher than the index of traditional radiology and ultrasonography (Tables 26.2, 26.3). Knowing the value of the MP index allows the identification of methodologies associated with higher relative risks, which could lead to improved diagnostic protocols and the design of strategies to decrease risk.

The extension of a model based on MP RVUs or other, similar models may have an important role in providing quantitative data for projects in which risk management play a role, including in business. In radiology practice, this would mean determining potential correlations between data obtained in different radiological departments. This approach may also facilitate the formation of contracts with insurance companies using concrete data, providing the basis for programming and the sharing of data regarding risks within the different departments on a national or local level.

References

1. Lakdawalla DN, Seabury SA (2009) The welfare effects of medical malpractice liability. National Bureau of Economic Research MA, USA
2. WHO working group on patient safety (2003) Patient safety : rapid assessment methods for assessing hazards: report of the WHO working group meeting, Geneva, Switzerland, 17-19 December 2002 Geneva, World Health Organization.
3. Reason J (1995) Understanding adverse events: human factors. Quality in Health Care 4:80-89

4. Kohn LT, Corrigan JM, Donaldson MS (1999) To err is human: building a safer health system. National Academy Press, Washington, DC
5. Carroll R (2003) Risk management handbook for health care organizations. Hoboken, NJ
6. Borgstede JP, Zinninger MD (2004) Radiology and patient safety. Acad Radiol 11:322-332
7. Grabert M, Gordon R, Franklin N (2002) Reducing diagnostic errors in medicine: what's the goal? Acad Med 77:981-992
8. Thrall JH (2004) Quality and Safety Revolution in Health Care. Radiology 233:3-6
9. Hillman BJ, Amis ES, Neiman HL (2004) The future quality and safety of medical imaging: proceedings of the third annual ACR forum. J Am Coll Radiol 1:33-39
10. FitzGerald R (2001) Error in radiology. Clin Radiol 56:938-946
11. Richard B, Gunderman KE (2005) Managing risk: threat or opportunity? AJR 185:43-45
12. Joint Commission on Accreditation of Healthcare Organizations (2001) Preventing adverse events in behavioral health care: a system approach to sentinel events. Oakbrook Terrace, IL
13. Leape LL, Bates DW, Cullen DJ et al (1995) Systems analysis of adverse drug events. ADE Prevention Study Group. JAMA 274:35-43
14. Farley DO, Haviland A, Champagne S et al (2008) Adverse-event-reporting practices by US hospitals: results of a national survey. Qual Saf Health Care 17:416-423
15. Melvin C, Bodley R, Booth A et al P (2004) Managing errors in radiology: a working model. Clin Radiol 59:841-845
16. Thornton E, Brook OR, Mendiratta-Lala M et al (2011) Application of failure mode and effect analysis in a radiology department. Radiographics 31:281-293
17. Abujudeh HH, Kaewlai R (2009) Radiology failure mode and effect analysis: what is it? Radiology 252:544-550
18. Dalle Carbonare S, Folli F, Patrini E, Bellazzi R (2009) A methodology for the extraction of quantitative risk indexes from medical injuries compensation claims. Stud Health Technol Inform 150:595-599
19. Cristofaro M, Bellandi G, Squarcione S et al (2007) Assessment of risk in radiology using malpractice RVU. Eur J Radiol 61:367-371
20. Mooriflied JM, MacEwan DW, Sunshine JH (1993) The radiology relative value scale: its delovpment and implication. Radiology 187:316-326
21. Centers for Medicare & Medicaid Services (CMS), HHS. (2010) Final Report on GPCI Malpractice RVUs for the CY 2010 Medicare Physician Fee Schedule Rule. Fed Regist 40040-40709, Washington, DC
22. Conoley PM (2000) Productivity of radiologists in 1997. Estimates based on analysis of resources based relative value units. AJR 175:591-595
23. Bhargavan M, Sunshine JH (2005) Workload of radiologists in the united states in 2002–2003 and trends since 1991–1992. Radiology 236:920-931
24. Cristofaro M, Bibbolino C, Lauria FN et al (2004) Comparison between indicators for the measurement of radiology activity volumes (Italy-USA). Radiol Med 108:426-438

Contrast Media Administration: Safety Issues and Legal Aspects

27

Yousef W. Nielsen, Manal Azzouz, and Henrik S. Thomsen

27.1 Introduction

Contrast media (CM) are commonly used in radiological procedures such as radiography, computed tomography (CT), and magnetic resonance imaging (MRI) to enhance the differences between structures or fluids within the body tissue. There are various types of CM, and their chemical and physical properties determine their specific application.

27.1.1 Iodine-based Contrast Media

Iodine-based contrast media (ICM) increase the absorption of X-rays, leading to better tissue contrast in CT and in conventional radiographic procedures. All iodine agents are based on a tri-iodine benzene ring with three radicals [1]. According to the number of benzene rings, ICM are classified as monomeric and dimeric (Table 27.1). Furthermore, an agent can be ionic or non-ionic. All ICM are water-soluble and they have similar pharmacokinetics, with rapid diffusion to the extracellular space and excretion by the kidneys.

The osmolality of ICM ranges from 300 to 2000 mosm kg^{-1} depending on the concentration and the type of agent. The limit for osmotoxicity is approximately 800 mosm kg^{-1}. Below this level, the importance of osmolality is limited. Osmolality is proportional to iodine content. ICM may be high- or low-osmolar, with an osmolality cut-off of 800 mosm kg^{-1}. Non-ionic ICM are iso-osmolar with blood (300 mosm kg^{-1}).

Y.W. Nielsen (✉)
Department of Diagnostic Radiology, Copenhagen University Hospital,
Herlev, Denmark

Table 27.1 Iodine-based contrast media

Name	Commercial name	Osmolality	Structure
Amidotrizoate	Urografin	High	Monomer
Iothalamate	Conray	High	Monomer
Ioxithalamate	Telebrix	High	Monomer
Ioxaglate	Hexabrix	Low	Dimer
Iohexol	Omnipaque	Low	Monomer
Iopentol	Imagopaque	Low	Monomer
Ioversol	Optiray	Low	Monomer
Iopamidol	Iopamiro	Low	Monomer
Iomeprol	Iomeron	Low	Monomer
Iopromide	Ultravist	Low	Monomer
Ioxilan	Oxilan	Low	Monomer
Iodixanol	Visipaque	Iso	Dimer
Iotrolan	Isovist	Iso	Dimer

27.1.2 Barium Sulfate

Barium sulfate CM are used to visualize the gastrointestinal tract. These agents are water-insoluble with no absorption from the gut.

27.1.3 Gadolinium-based Contrast Media

Gadolinium-based contrast media (GdCM) form a complex between a chelating ligand and the paramagnetic gadolinium. The ligand acts to minimize gadolinium toxicity [2]. Depending on the structure of the ligand, GdCM are classified as macrocyclic or linear. Furthermore, they may be ionic or non-ionic.

In relation to safety, GdCM are divided into three stability classes: Non-ionic linear, ionic linear, and macrocyclic, the latter being the most stable (Table 27.2). GdCM are also classified as non-specific extracellular GdCM and high-relaxivity agents or organ-specific agents. Non-specific, extracellular agents are eliminated by renal excretion. High-relaxivity agents show weak to strong protein binding, and some of them are excreted through the bile and via the kidneys.

27.1.4 Ultrasound Contrast Media

Ultrasound CM produce their effect by their higher backscattering of sound compared with blood, other fluids, and most tissues. The currently available

Table 27.2 Gadolinium-based contrast media

Name	Commercial name	Chelate	Ionicity	NSF risk group	Distribution
Gadodiamide	Omniscan	Linear	Non-ionic	High	Extracellular
Gadovertisamide	Optimark	Linear	Non-ionic	High	Extracellular
Gadopentate dimeglumine	Magnevist	Linear	Ionic	High	Extracellular
Gadobenate dimeglumine	Multihance	Linear	Ionic	Intermediate	Extracellular and liver specific (4%)
Gadoxetate disodium	Primovist, Eovist	Linear	Ionic	Intermediate	Liver specific (50%)
Gadofosveset trisodium	Vasovist, Ablavar	Linear	Ionic	Intermediate	Blood pool agent
Gadoteridol	Gadovist, Gadavist	Macrocyclic	Non-ionic	Low	Extracellular
Gadoteridol	Prohance	Macrocyclic	Non-ionic	Low	Extracellular
Gadoterate meglumine	Dotarem, Magnescope	Macrocyclic	Ionic	Low	Extracellular

agents are based on microbubbles, either octafluoropropane-filled albumin microspheres or sulfur hexafluoride gas in polymer with phospholipid.

27.2 Contrast Media Indications

Radiological examinations are increasingly tailored to fit the individual clinical problems. Accordingly, the decision whether or not to administer a contrast agent has to be addressed on a case-by-case basis. In daily practice, CM facilitate the diagnosis of a wide range of pathologies. However, CM are not physiologically inert such that the potential risk of their administration has to be weighed against the diagnostic and clinical benefits of performing the contrast-enhanced study. Therefore, it is difficult to state general indications for CM. With modern CT, and in particular MRI and ultrasound, it is often possible to answer the clinical question with either an unenhanced examination or by using another imaging modality, should CM administration be contraindicated with the primary imaging modality. It should be borne in mind that a patient is only referred for imaging because of signs and symptoms, e.g., macroscopic hematuria indicating a disease, or to control treatment response, e.g., in cancer patients.

Since CT offers poorer soft-tissue discrimination than either ultrasonography or, in particular, MRI, the use of CM is much more strongly indicated in connection with CT than with the other two modalities; for example, with MRI it is possible to distinguish between the renal medulla and cortex without CM, whereas this is impossible in CT. Sadly, the incidence of adverse reactions is higher after the administration of ICM than after GdCM and it is even less with the use of ultrasound CM. On the other hand, there is no drug except ICM that can be administered in such high amounts (i.e., 1000 ml of 300 mg I/ml) and cause so few side effects.

27.3 Safety Issues

As with other drugs, adverse reactions may follow the administration of CM [3]. An adverse drug reaction can be defined as "A response to a medicinal product that is noxious and unintended and occurs at doses normally used in humans for the prophylaxis, diagnosis, or therapy of disease or for the restoration, correction, or modification of a physiological function." Adverse reactions to CM are classified as non-renal or renal.

27.3.1 Non-renal Adverse Reactions

Non-renal adverse reactions are sub-divided into acute, late, and very late reactions. By definition, an acute reaction occurs within 1 hour of CM injection, a late reaction within 1 hour to 1 week, and very late reactions usually more than 1 week after CM injection.

Acute reactions to CM range from mild to severe. Mild reactions include nausea/mild vomiting, urticaria, and itching. Moderate reactions are severe vomiting, marked urticaria, bronchospasms, facial/laryngeal edema, and vasovagal attacks. Severe reactions are hypotensive shock, respiratory and/or cardiac arrest, and convulsions.

For ICM, a number of risk factors have been identified: previous moderate or severe acute reaction to an ICM, asthma, allergy (requiring medical treatment), and use of high osmolality ionic agents. According to the guidelines on CM from the European Society for Urogenital Radiology (ESUR) the following factors reduce the risk of an acute reaction in all patients: use of a nonionic CM, keeping the patient in the radiology department for 30 min after contrast injection, and having drugs and equipment for resuscitation readily available [4]. In patients with one of the risk factors stated above, an alternative diagnostic test not requiring an ICM should be considered. In patients with a previous reaction, a different ICM should be used. Clinical evidence of the effectiveness of premedication remains limited. There is no documented evidence of a difference in the incidence of acute adverse reactions between the various non-ionic agents.

In general, an acute reaction is significantly less likely with a GdCM than with an ICM; however, there is still a risk of an acute reaction. The risk factors are: previous reactions to a GdCM, asthma, and allergy (requiring medical treatment). Accordingly, another diagnostic test not requiring a GdCM should be considered in patients with a risk factor. Patients with a previous reaction should be examined with a different GdCM. There is no clinical evidence of the effectiveness of premedication to reduce acute reactions following GdCM administration. No prospective study has shown a difference in the incidence of acute adverse reactions between the various GdCM.

Late reactions to ICM were first recognized in the mid 1980s. In the literature, a variety of late symptoms have been described, including nausea, vomiting, headache, musculoskeletal pain, and fever. However, many of these are not related to the administered contrast medium. Skin reactions appear to account for the majority of true late reactions, with most of these being mild to moderate and self-limiting—similar to the skin reactions that occur with many other drugs [5]. Most skin reactions develop within the first 3 days and resolve by 7 days. Despite their apparent pathogenesis, late reactions are not fully understood, as it seems that many are type IV hypersensitivity reactions (T-cell mediated). Risk factors for skin reactions following ICM administration include previous CM reaction, allergy, and interleukin-2 treatment. Although prophylaxis is generally not recommended, patients with a previous serious late adverse reaction may benefit from steroid premedication. Late reactions occur more frequently in response to the non-ionic dimer than to the non-ionic monomers.

For GdCM, nephrogenic systemic fibrosis usually presents after 1 week but may occur earlier.

Very late reactions to ICM are rare but largely consist of thyrotoxicosis. Risk factors are untreated Graves' disease, multinodular goiter, and thyroid autonomy. The risk of CM-induced thyrotoxicosis is especially high in elderly patients and amongst patients living in areas with dietary iodine deficiency. An endocrinologist should monitor high-risk patients. CM-induced thyrotoxicosis does not occur in patients with normal thyroid function.

Importantly, the free iodine from iodine-based CM interferes with thyroidal iodine uptake. Consequently, diagnostic thyroid scintigraphy and radioiodine treatment of thyroid malignancies cannot be carried out for two months following the administration of ICM.

Nephrogenic systemic fibrosis (NSF) is an important very late reaction to the least stable GdCM. The link between NSF and some GdCM was recognized in 2006 [6]. NSF is a severe or even fatal scleroderma-like, fibrosing condition. The initial signs of NSF may be seen as early as hours after exposure to GdCM, but may also occur as late as years after exposure.

Usually, the initial stage of NSF is characterized by sub-acute swelling of the distal parts of the lower extremities. Other symptoms in the initial stage are erythema, pruritus and pain. In the subsequent weeks, severe skin induration occurs and the disease may extend to the thighs, forearms, and lower abdomen. Flexion contractures and constant pain can develop. Involvement of internal organs such as the liver, lungs, and heart may explain the suspected increased mortality of NSF patients.

Patients at higher risk of developing NSF are those with end-stage renal disease corresponding to chronic kidney disease (CKD) stage 4 and 5 (GFR<

30 ml/min). Patients on dialysis, as well as patients with acute kidney insufficiency, are also at increased risk. At lower risk are patients with CKD 3 (GFR 30–59 ml/min) and children under one year due to their immature renal function. However, NSF has never been reported in patients below five years of age. Patients with normal renal function are probably not at risk of NSF. Each time a patient receives an injection of a GdCM, a tiny amount of gadolinium is left in the body, especially in the bones. The residual amount is much higher (> 10 times) for non-ionic linear agents than for the macrocyclic agents. The long-term effects are not known. The least stable agents should be administered in doses < 0.1 mmol/kg body weight to any patient, independent of kidney function [7].

Thus far, it is known that two factors need to be present for the development of NSF: (1) reduced renal function, and (2) exposure to one of the chemically less stable GdCM (i.e., gadodiamide, gadopentate dimeglumine, or gadoversetamide). Release of free Gd^{3+} from the chelated agents is more likely to occur if the contrast agent remains in the body for a long time, for example in patients with renal impairment, including those on dialysis. The release of free Gd^{3+} seems to be the key event among those leading to tissue fibrosis. However, not all high-risk patients exposed to the above-mentioned GdCM develop NSF; rather, certain co-factors triggering the process must be present as well. Although several such factors have been proposed (for example, metabolic acidosis, high dose EPO, hypercoagulability), it remains unclear which is the culprit.

The regulatory rules on the use of GdCM are discussed in Sect. 27.4.

27.3.2 Renal Adverse Reactions

Contrast medium-induced nephropathy (CIN) is defined as a condition in which impairments in renal function (an increase in serum creatinine by > 25% or 44 μmol/l) occur within three days of CM administration, in the absence of alternative etiology.

The incidence of CIN varies between different studies, but it seems to be higher when the CM is administered intra-arterially rather than intravenously. The pathophysiological mechanism of CIN is not known, but a number of risk factors have been identified: estimated GFR < 45 ml/min/1.73m^2 (when the contrast is given intravenously) or < 60 ml/min/1.73m^2 (when the agent is administered intra-arterially), especially secondary to diabetic nephropathy, dehydration, congestive heart failure, gout, age over 70 years, administration of nephrotoxic drugs (e.g., NSAID), use of high osmolality CM, and large doses of CM [8]. In patients with one or more risk factors, a number of preventive strategies can be used: an alternative imaging method not requiring ICM, stopping nephrotoxic drugs at least 24 h before CM administration, hydration with intravenous normal saline (1–1.5 ml/kg body weight per hour) in 6 h before and after the procedure. An alternative protocol is intravenous sodium bicarbonate, 3 ml/kg/h for 1 h before contrast medium administration and 1 ml/kg/h for 6 h afterwards. During the imaging procedure, a low-osmolar or iso-osmolar contrast medium should be used, and in the lowest dose that yields a diagnostic result.

The anti-diabetic drug metformin is excreted unchanged in the urine. In case of renal impairment, either pre-existing or due to CIN, metformin may accumulate in the body and cause metabolic lactate acidosis. To avoid this serious condition, patients with estimated GFR < 45 ml/min/1.73m^2 taking metformin should stop taking the drug 48 h before contrast medium administration and remain off the drug for 48 h after. Metformin should only be restarted if serum creatinine is unchanged. Metformin does not cause renal damage.

27.3.3 Pregnancy and Lactation

Radiographic examinations, including CT, are rarely performed in the pregnant woman due to radiation issues. However, in exceptional cases, when radiographic examination is essential, ICM may be given during pregnancy. As a precaution, thyroid function should be checked in the neonate following administration of ICM to the mother during pregnancy. GdCM administration in pregnant women is contraindicated; if clinically important, the stable agents may be used. No neonatal tests are necessary in such cases.

Breast-feeding may be continued normally when an ICM has been used and when the GdCM is of high stability. If a low stability agent is used, the milk produced within the next 24 h after the examination must be thrown away.

27.4 Contraindications

Contraindications are an important part of product summary and they should be followed. Contraindications may be absolute. In most cases, use of a drug in contraindicated areas can be considered malpractice, except if there are very good reasons for doing so. In general, ICM are contraindicated in patients with untreated hyperthyroidism. Also, documented or suspicion of hypersensitivity to the drug and/or the additives are considered a contraindication. Non-compensated cardiac insufficiency is also listed. High-osmolar ICM should not be used for myelography.

The gadolinium area is much more regulated. There are two reasons for this difference. First, most ICM were approved many years ago, when efficacy studies of the various body regions were not required. With the exception of gadopentetate dimeglumine, which was approved for intravenous injection, documentation of efficacy in various areas of the body (e.g., musculoskeletal, central nervous system and spine, vasculature) is required. Second, a link between some GdCM and the occurrence of NSF has been recognized. Also for GdCM, documented or suspicion of hypersensitivity to the drug and/or the additives is a contraindication. The high risk of NSF-inducing agents (gadoversetamide, gadodiamide, and gadopentetate dimeglumine) excludes their use in patients with GFR < 30 ml/min 1.73 m^2, in newborns less than one month of age, and in patients in the perioperative phase of liver transplantation. These agents may only be administered with precaution in patients with GFR between 30 and 60 ml/min 1.73m^2. In such cases, the lowest amount should be used and any two injections should be given at an interval of at least seven days. Renal function must always be measured prior to the use of these agents.

For the other GdCM, the precautions applicable to patients with GFR below 30 ml/min 1.73 m^2 are applicable; routine laboratory determination of GFR is not required.

27.5 Off-label Uses

The manufacturer must submit specified information on the quality, safety, and efficacy of a drug to the relevant national medical regulatory body before a new medicine can be approved for patient use. If the new medicine is approved, a Marketing Authorization is issued. The summary of product characteristics is the important document, as it reflects the entire regulatory process. It also provides vital information for the prescriber: the precise indication and dosage of the product, instructions for its administration, contraindications, interactions, and possible adverse reactions. As a condition for the approval, the drug may only be marketed for use under the terms outlined in the Marketing Authorization, since these terms reflect the content of the original information submitted by the manufacturer. However, this does not preclude the use of the drug outside the terms of the Marketing Authorization by individual clinicians, so called off-label use [9, 10]. Although the precise definitions have changed over time, in general, off-label drug use is the practice of prescribing drugs outside their authorized indications with respect to dosage, age, indication, or route. For CM, the off-label use of drugs has become an important issue throughout the world due to changes in the policies of the various regulatory bodies. For registration, a certain number of facts has to be forwarded as documentation, whereas for off-label use the documentation varies from randomized trials in a highly ranked journal to a case report presented at a scientific meeting. In many countries, off-label use requires informed consent, but the facts that should be included in the information given to patients are often either not fully provided, or simply may not be available. For example, could a radiologist have informed a patient receiving gadodiamide for conventional angiography about the potential risk of NSF before 2006? Gadobutrol is currently not approved for musculoskeletal MRI but for angiography of the liver and kidney. However, it is the same drug and dose that is used in both instances. In fact, the CM enters unapproved areas of the body, the only difference being where the imaging coil is placed. Nevertheless, use of gadobutrol for musculoskeletal MRI is considered off-label. A Marketing Authorization holder is not allowed to market an unapproved indication, including advising the physician about off-label use. The authorities in the USA have taken several companies to court for marked off-label indications and received billions of dollars in penalties. The same will probably occur in Europe in the future, when the European Medicines Agency has approved most agents on a multistate level. Currently, not all CM list all indications in their product summary.

Registration practice has changed during the last 20 years, as before that a contrast medium could be granted approval for intravenous injection (same as approved for every part of the body). Since then, the authorities require not only safety data but also efficacy data for the various parts of the body. This change opened off-label use in Europe. The price for an indication is high as it requires several studies performed in various centers (multicenter study). Furthermore, why conduct all those studies, when doctors use the agent anyhow? The safety data are the same whether it is a CT of the brain or of the peripheral arteries, but the efficacy data may differ. In addition, the symptoms and signs are not identical from patient to patient, leading to variations in the population studied. In contrast to other areas of medicine, it is of utmost importance for radiology to either document or rule out serious pathology. Randomized trials comparing a contrast agent with saline is not possible as the images will always reveal who was administered the agent and who was not. Also, the technician will always know whether an agent or saline was used.

Malpractice in relation to CM has not been a major issue in Europe, yet. The use of high-osmolar ICM for myelography and of gadodiamide in patients with reduced renal function are only two examples of malpractice. Thus, cases center around patients who have been exposed to an unnecessarily high risk of adverse reactions that could have been avoided by using another, safer agent: a non-ionic ICM for myelography and a macrocyclic GdCM for MRI, respectively.

References

1. Aspelin P (2009) Classification and terminology. In: HS Thomsen, JAW Webb (eds) Contrast media safety issues and ESUR Guidelines, 2nd edn. Springer, Heidelberg
2. Morcos SK (2009) Chelates and stability. In: HS Thomsen, JAW Webb (eds) Contrast media safety issues and ESUR Guidelines, 2nd edn. Springer, Heidelberg
3. Webb JAW (2009) Prevention of acute reactions. In: HS Thomsen, JAW Webb (eds) Contrast media safety issues and ESUR Guidelines, 2nd edn. Springer, Heidelberg
4. Thomsen HS, Morcos SK (2004) Contrast Media Safety Committee of the European Society of Urogenital Radiology. Management of acute adverse reactions to contrast media. Eur Radiol 14:476-81
5. Bellin MF, Stacul F, Webb JAW et al on behalf of the Contrast Media Safety Committee of the European Society of Uroradiology (2011) Late adverse reactions to intravascular iodine based contrast media: an update. Eur Radiol 21:2305-2310
6. Marckmann P, Skov L, Rossen K et al (2006) Nephrogenic systemic fibrosis: suspected causative role of gadodiamide used for contrast-enhanced magnetic resonance imaging. J Am Soc Nephrol 17:2359-2362

7. Thomsen HS (2010) Contrast-enhanced MRI in patients with impaired renal function: recent recommendations to minimize the risk of nephrogenic systemic fibrosis. Solutions in Contrast Imaging 1:1-8
8. Stacul F, van der Molen AJ, Reimer P et al on behalf of the Contrast Media Safety Committee of the European Society of Urogenital Radiology (2011) Contrast induced nephropathy: updated ESUR Contrast Media Safety Committee guidelines. Eur Radiol 21:2527-2541
9. Reimer P, Vosshenrich R (2008) Off-label use of contrast agents. Eur Radiol 18:1096-1101
10. Fairman KA, Curtiss FR (2010) Regulatory actions on the off-label use of prescription drugs: ongoing controversy and contraindication in 2009 and 2010. JMCP 16:629-639

Strategies To Reduce Errors in Radiology 28

Luca Brunese, Alfonso Reginelli, and Ferdinando Caranci

28.1 Introduction

To err may indeed be human; nevertheless, society requires faultless medical professionals. For radiologists, being held to such standards is particularly challenging due to the rapidly advancing science of image acquisition. Errors in medicine have become headline news in recent years. Within radiology, the important progress in demonstrating disease has left error analysis a subject that is often mostly ignored.

The work of diagnostic radiology consists of the complete detection of all abnormalities in an imaging examination and their accurate diagnosis [1]. Failure to diagnose generally leads to medical malpractice lawsuits. The three main categories of claims are misdiagnoses, complications, and miscellaneous [2-4]. Diagnostic errors are often unrecognized or unreported and may result in high patient morbidity. According to some studies, error rates range from an unsurprising 3–5% in general radiological practice [5-7] to shocking figures of 30–90%[5, 8-10] for mammography [11] and the detection of lung cancers [12]. Of course, in general radiological practice many errors are minor and may have little effect on patient outcome [13, 14]; however, litigation against American and European radiologists continues to increase [15, 16], with a missed diagnosis as the most common cause for a legal grievance [15-17] and accounting for up to half of such cases.

L. Brunese (✉)
Department of Health Science, Chair of Radiology, University of Molise,
Campobasso, Italy

28.2 Causes of Error in Radiology

The causes of error in radiology are multifactorial and frequently combined [18, 19]. Poor technique, failure of perception, lack of knowledge, and misjudgment may all play a role [20]. In general, there are four main reasons why radiologists are sued: observer errors, errors in interpretation, failure to suggest the next appropriate procedure, and failure to communicate in a timely and clinically appropriate manner. According to Kundel et al. [21], observer errors can be divided into three types: scanning error, recognition error, and decision-making error. A fourth type of observer error is satisfaction of search error, in which an abnormality is missed due to the more imposing presence of another abnormality [22]. In addition, there are multiple causes of error in interpretation: absence of clinical history, absence of previous studies, the reading room environment, and the level of vigilance of the interpreter [23]. Although optimizing the reporting environment is undoubtedly helpful, it may be impossible to completely eradicate all distractions. Consequently, of equal importance is maintaining a consistent, methodical approach to reporting.

28.3 Timely Communication of Imaging Results

Many types of issues are involved in communication, including substantive aspects of reporting, timeliness, and the ensured receipt of results. According to the ACR practice guidelines for communication of diagnostic imaging findings [24], a diagnosis provided by a written report does not conclude the responsibilities of the radiologist: direct communication is a necessary adjunct, particularly in the presence of emergent or unusual and unexpected findings. The basis for the report should rely on personal commentaries and self-reported trial decisions, as well as non-binding legal opinions [25]. For the radiologist, the duty to report findings is neither static nor avoidable and sometimes requires direct communication beyond the simple issuance of an interpretative report. Direct communication of the radiological report is mandatory in case of findings suggesting the need for immediate medical treatment, conclusions differing form the first interpretation, findings suggesting a dangerous condition, and ambiguous findings [26]. While guidance is available from the ACR guidelines and appellate court decisions regarding the need for direct communication to ensure the receipt of information, there may still be many situations in which verified communication is required on a less urgent basis. Today, technology-based systems incorporate both the urgent and less urgent findings that must be communicated in a more detailed manner than a simple interpretive report. The trail of communication between a radiologist and a treating health care provider as well as that between a health care provider and a patient is a recurrent theme in such initiatives. Indeed, poor communication can determine up to 80% of malpractice lawsuits involving radiologists [27].

Radiology reports are the primary form of communication between the radiologist and the clinician, and they must be structured to allow the easy transfer of information. Moreover, they are important medico-legal documents and, because their accuracy is vital, clinical radiologists must avoid the urge to "hedge their bets" unless absolutely necessary. When a clinician requests a radiological examination, he or she is seeking the opinion of a radiologist, and the sought after informationn should be clearly conveyed, to the extent possible, in the report. The radiological report should be conceived as a method of communicating the expertise and clinical judgment of the radiologist and not as a means of hiding behind obscure and ambiguous language.

28.4 How To Reduce Errors in Radiology

Diagnostic errors can be reduced by improvements both in knowledge and in systems. The former consists of communication of the patient's clinical history, comparison of the current with the previous radiological investigation, and proper selection of the initial and subsequent radiological procedure, all of which can reduce the rate of diagnostic errors [28]. Better system organization consists of improvements in working conditions and in the time available for reporting, equipment modifications to prevent accidental error, double reporting, and regular dialogue between clinicians and radiologists [28]. Double-reading of radiological examinations in an attempt to reduce error rates is a standard practice in mammographic screening. In fact, the literature contains several small studies in which the double-reading of other types of examination yielded similar benefits [29-31]. This idea is worthy of mention, but in reality the workload issues faced by most radiology departments is such that double reporting is beyond their resources. An important goal of error analysis is to create processes aimed at reducing or preventing the occurrence of errors and at minimizing the degree of harm. Diffusion of a peer review process in diagnostic radiology is one approach to responding to this need [32].

There is good evidence that computer-assisted detection (CAD) can improve operator performance in the detection of lung nodules [33] and breast lesions, but programming computers to recognize objects in a diagnostic image is still very difficult and current technology is a long way from being able to compete with humans in terms of speed and accuracy [34]. However, there is another computer-assisted approach that might bear fruit: Instead of assisting in object detection, computers can be used to assist observer performance through what are described as human factor technologies [34].

Retrospective analysis of cases in which an error is felt to have arisen has educational benefit, and an appreciation of the error along with the identification of its possible causal factors enables the appropriate modification (departmental practice, radiological technique, or reporting behavior) such that in the future similar errors might be avoided. Radiologists should organize and attend meetings in which cases involving radiological errors are presented and discussed [35, 36].

Although a missed diagnosis or other form of error may be the most feared event for a radiologist, it can also be one of the best opportunities for learning [37]. Many errors are the result of flawed processes or reasoning that can be rectified if dealt with appropriately [38]. Learning from errors requires a critical appraisal of our own practice and the implementation of change to enhance performance levels. Where quality assurance mechanisms highlight error, it should be personally recorded and reviewed. Moreover, cases in which the diagnosis is not certain should be actively followed through multidisciplinary team meetings involving cooperation amongst the involved departments. Wherever errors are made, they should be seen as learning opportunities, not just individually, but corporately too: for radiology and medical colleagues, radiology trainees, and students. Error meetings are an excellent way of facilitating this process and their value has been well documented [36]. They should be viewed as integral to continuing medical education; accordingly, accredited residency and fellowship programs should be actively involved in their organization. A culture of shared responsibility and teamwork within the radiology department should also be encouraged and supported, as it will enhance individual performance [32, 39] in addition to facilitating a culture of safety through the process of shared learning from mistakes [4]. Nonetheless, there will inevitably be some radiologists who fail to learn from their mistakes and thus almost certainly repeat them. How we deal with these individuals is the subject of ongoing debate, but revalidation may be one means of addressing this thorny issue [40]. Educational programs, morbidity meetings, and a comprehensive and respected root cause analysis process are important for decreasing the likelihood of future diagnostic errors.

28.5 Conclusions

The main reason for studying medical errors is to try to prevent them. Diagnostic errors fall into recurrent patterns. Error traps need to be uncovered and highlighted, in order to prevent repetition of the same mistakes. While probably an inevitable part of radiological practice, errors mostly arise during image interpretation. It seems that increased reliance on cross-sectional imaging and the complexity and sensitivity of these studies make these techniques the most common source of error. Identification and reduction of diagnostic error provides a measure of the efficacy of the healthcare system, as it reduces mortality, morbidity, length of hospital stay, and additional health care costs. Greater openness regarding the incidence of radiological error, as well as the departmental practice of peer support, instead of blame, can help radiologists to learn from their mistakes and to improve their performance.

In the future, radiological malpractice will be affected by several factors: new imaging techniques, innovations in the processing of radiological images, new standards published by scientific societies, as well as revised clinical guidelines issued by medical professional organizations. We need to develop a safety culture within radiology departments in which, every time an error made by a colleague is discovered, it is brought to his or her attention in a sensitive and constructive fashion. A radiology safety culture will only exist when the radiologist who made the error views such feedback positively, as a learning experience. Despite the undeniable importance of learning from errors, many radiologists and institutions do not engage in such practices. However, it is essential that radiologists and radiology departments continue to improve the process of recording and addressing errors. There is no magic solution that will eliminate diagnostic errors in radiology.

References

1. Pitman AG (2006) Perceptual error and the culture of open disclosure in Australian radiology. Australas Radiol 50:206-211
2. Berlin L (1986) Malpractice and radiologists, update 1986: an 11.5-year perspective. AJR Am J Roentgenol 147:1291-1298
3. Spring DB, Tennenhouse DJ (1986) Radiology malpractice lawsuits: California jury verdicts. Radiology 159:811-814
4. Hamer MM, Morlock F, Foley HT et al (1987) Medical malpractice in diagnostic radiology: claims, compensation, and patient injury. Radiology 164:263-266
5. Berlin L (2001) Defending the "missed" radiographic diagnosis. AJR Am J Roentgenol 176:317-322
6. Borgstede JP, Lewis RS, Bhargavan M et al (2004) RADPEER quality assurance program: a multifacility study of interpretive disagreement rates. J Am Coll Radiol 1:59-65
7. Siegle RL, Baram EM, Reuter SR et al (1998) Rates of disagreement in imaging interpretation in a group of community hospitals. Acad Radiol 5:148-154
8. Goddard P, Leslie A, Jones A et al (2001) Error in radiology. Br J Radiol 74:949-951
9. Quekel LG, Kessels AG, Goei R et al (1999) Miss rate of lung cancer on the chest radiograph in clinical practice. Chest 115:720-724
10. Forrest JV, Friedman PJ (1981) Radiologic errors in patients with lung cancer. West J Med 134:485-490
11. Berlin L (1999) The missed breast cancer: perceptions and realities. AJR Am J Roentgenol 173:1161-1167
12. Muhm JR, Miller WE, Fontana RS et al (1983) Lung cancer detected during a screening program using four-month chest radiographs. Radiology 148:609-615
13. Berlin L (2007) Radiologic errors and malpractice: a blurry distinction. AJR Am J Roentgenol 189:517-522
14. Williams SM, Connelly DJ, Wadsworth S et al (2000) Radiological review of accident and emergency radiographs: a 1-year audit. Clin Radiol 55:861-865
15. Berlin L, Berlin J (1995) Malpractice and radiologists in Cook County, IL: trends in 20 years of litigation. AJR Am J Roentgenol 165:781-788
16. Fileni A, Magnavita NA (2006) A 12-year follow-up study of malpractice claims against radiologists in Italy. Radiol Med 111:1009-1022
17. Potchen EJ, Bisesi MA (1990) When is it malpractice to miss lung cancer on chest radiographs? Radiology 175:29-32
18. FitzGerald R. Error in radiology (2001) Clin Radiol 56:938-946
19. Tuddenham WJ (1962) Visual search, image organization, and reader error in roentgen diagnosis: studies of the psychophysiology of roentgen image perception. Radiology 78:694-704

20. Robinson PJA (1997) Radiology's Achilles' heel: error and variation in the interpretation of the Roentgen image. Br J Radiol 70:1085-1098
21. Kundel HL, Nodine CF, Carmody D (1978) Visual scanning, pattern recognition and decision making in pulmonary nodule detection. Invest Radiol 13:175-181
22. Samuel S, Kundel HI, Nodine CF et al (1995) Mechanism of satisfaction of search: eye position recordings in the reading of chest radiographs. Radiology 194:895-902
23. Pinto A, Acampora C, Pinto F et al (2011) Learning from diagnostic errors: A good way to improve education in radiology. Eur J Radiol 78: 372-376
24. American College of Radiology (2005) ACR practice guideline for communication of diagnostic imaging findings. In: Practice guidelines and technical standards 2005. American College of Radiology, Reston, pp 5-9
25. American College of Radiology (2004) Report of the ACR Task Force on Diagnostic Reporting. Annual Meeting and Chapter Leadership Conference, May 10.
26. Brenner RJ (2006) To err is human, to correct divine: the emergence of technology-based communication systems. J Am Coll Radiol 3:340-345
27. Levinson W (1994) Physician-patient communication: a key to malpractice prevention. JAMA 272:1619-1620
28. Goddard P, Leslie A, Jones A et al (2001). Error in radiology. Br J Radiol 74:949-951
29. Newman-Toker DE, Pronovost PJ (2009) Diagnostic errors: the next frontier for patient safety. JAMA 301:1060-1062
30. Newman-Toker DE, Camargo Jr CA, Hsieh YH, et al (2009) Disconnect between charted vestibular diagnoses and emergency department management decisions: a cross-sectional analysis from a nationally representative sample. Acad Emerg Med 16:970-977
31. Pinto A, Brunese L (2010) Spectrum of diagnostic errors in radiology. World J Radiol 2:377-383
32. FitzGerald R (2005) Radiological error: analysis, standard setting, targeted instruction and teamworking. Eur Radiol 15:1760-1767
33. Kakeda S, Moriya J, Sato H et al (2004) Improved detection of lung nodules on chest radiographs using a commercial computer-aided diagnosis system. AJR Am J Roentgenol 182:505-510
34. Schwaninger A (2005) Increasing efficiency in airport security screening. Saf Security Eng 82:405-416
35. The Royal College of Radiologists (2007) Standards for radiology discrepancy meetings. The Royal College of Radiologists, London
36. Espinosa JA, Nolan TW (2000) Reducing errors made by emergency physicians in interpreting radiographs: longitudinal study. BMJ 320:737-740
37. Berlin L (1994) Reporting the "missed" radiologic diagnosis: medicolegal and ethical considerations. Radiology 192:183-187
38. Renfrew DL, Franken EA, Berbaum KS et al (1992) Error in radiology: classification and lessons in 182 cases presented at a problem case conference. Radiology 183:145-150
39. Gunderman R, Chan S (2003) Knowledge sharing in radiology. Radiology 229:314-317
40. Adam J (2008) Revalidation of doctors. Clin Radiol 63:853-855

Subject Index

MIX
Papier aus verantwortungsvollen Quellen
Paper from responsible sources
FSC® C105338

If you have any concerns about our products,
you can contact us on
ProductSafety@springernature.com

In case Publisher is established outside the EU,
the EU authorized representative is:
Springer Nature Customer Service Center GmbH
Europaplatz 3, 69115 Heidelberg, Germany

Printed by Libri Plureos GmbH
in Hamburg, Germany